APPLIED MICROBIOLOGY for B.Sc. NURSING

(Including Infection Control and Safety)

(As per the Revised INC Syllabus for B.Sc. Nursing)

Dr C P Baveja
MD (Gold Medalist), MNAMS

Professor of Excellence
Department of Microbiology, Maulana Azad Medical College
New Delhi, India

Formerly:
Director Principal, BSA Medical College, Rohini, Delhi
Director Professor & Head, Department of Microbiology Maulana Azad Medical College, New Delhi
Additional Director General, Ministry of Health and Family Welfare, New Delhi

arya™

ARYA PUBLISHING COMPANY
Village Johron, Trilokpur Road, Kala Amb 173030, Dist. Sirmour (HP)
Delhi Office: 1569/30, Naiwala Street, Karol Bagh, New Delhi-110005 (India)

arya®

Published by:
Dr Vipin Gupta
ARYA PUBLISHING COMPANY
Village Johron, Trilokpur Road
Kala Amb, Dist. Sirmour (HP)

Delhi Office:
1569/30, Naiwala Street
Karol Bagh, New Delhi 110 005 (India)
Ph.: 011-41067632
E-mail: info@aryapublishing.com
Website: www.aryapublishing.com

ISBN–978-93-9479-279-1

First Edition: 2005
Reprint: 2006
Second Edition: 2007
Reprint: 2008, 2009
Third Edition: 2010
Reprint: 2011, 12, 13
Fourth Edition: 2014
Reprint: 2015, 16
Fifth Edition: 2017
Reprint: 2018
Sixth Edition: 2019
Reprint: 2019, 20, 21, 22
Seventh Edition: 2023
Reprint: 2024
Reprint: 2025

Price: ₹ 695.00

Typeset & Designed at:
Laser Tech Prints (D)

Printed at:
Goyal Offset Works (P) Ltd.
Kundli Industrial Area, Haryana

Dedicated to

My parents

(Late) Shrimati Hari Devi

and

(Late) Shri Kishan Chand Baweja

PREFACE

TO THE FIRST EDITION

Nursing is an important profession as far as medical sciences are concerned. They have direct involvement in patient care, therefore, they must acquire a knowledge of microbes and preventive measures against them. There is a paucity of books on the subject of Microbiology for nurses. Hence, the main object of writing the "Textbook of Microbiology for Nurses" is to consolidate the necessary information for nursing profession. Though this book has been designed primarily for the students pursuing undergraduate nursing course, it will also be of immense use to all nursing personnel involved in providing comprehensive health care. Salient features of the book include the following:

1. It is presented in simple and lucid language.
2. To make learning easier, well labelled diagrams and tables have been furnished at appropriate places.
3. The book has been written as per the prescribed course for Microbiology by Nursing Council of India (NCI).
4. The chapter on "Medical Parasitology" has been especially written for nursing students alongwith few diagrams for better understanding.

It was difficult, if not impossible, to write a book for nursing students because of the difficulty in deciding what to include and what not to. Still I have tried my best to include the relevant topics which appeal to nursing students. Suggestions and new ideas for further improvement of this book shall be greatly appreciated and promptly acknowledged.

I could not have come out with this book, had it not been for the help and encouragement put forth by undergraduate nursing students of Microbiology. I am thankful to Dr. V.K. Sharma, Director-Professor and Head, Microbiology Department, Maulana Azad Medical College, New Delhi for invaluable suggestions from time to time.

I extend my thanks to Sh. Amit Gupta of Digigrafics, New Delhi for the preparation of its format and its appropriate presentation.

I am immensely grateful to my family members for their constant encouragement without which I would have never contemplated, let alone complete, this book.

Finally, I acknowledge the pleasure of working with the publishing team—M/s Arya Publishing Company, New Delhi. I extend my heartfelt thanks and sincere regards to all of them, especially Dr. Vipin Gupta for his constant inspiration and magnificent support throughout.

New Delhi

Dr. C P BAVEJA

PREFACE

TO THE SEVENTH EDITION

The seventh edition of **Applied Microbiology for Nursing** has been updated and written as per Indian Nursing Council Syllabus for B.Sc. nursing students. Recent advances have been incorporated in all the chapters. A new unit on **Hospital Infection Control and Safety** has been included, which is of utmost importance to control hospital infection and also for patient safety, New chapters on **Blood Stream Infections, Prophylactic Immunisation, Specimen Collection and Transport** have been incorporated. These will be helpful to nursing students for day to day patient care. A chapter on **Prophylactic Immunisation** will help students to acquire knowledge of immunisation especially for 'Hepatitis B vaccination for health workers'. A chapter 'Essentials of Microbiology at glance' is incorporated to revise the important aspects of Microbiology in no time. This knowledge will be helpful to students during the examination. Constructive suggestions from students and teachers were also included while revising the book. Like the previous editions, I hope the readers will find this edition more informative and up-to-date.

I am thankful to Sh. Rajiv Manchanda and Ms. Shobha of Laser Tech Prints, New Delhi for formatting the book appropriately.

I am extremely grateful to my family members for the support which was very much required to complete the project.

Finally, I am thankful to the entire publishing team – M/s Arya Publishing Company, New Delhi. I express my heartfelt gratitude to Dr. Vipin Gupta and Mr. Arnav Gupta for their deep concern and untiring efforts throughout the project.

New Delhi
January 2023

Dr. C P Baveja

SYLLABUS

FOR B.Sc. (NURSING)

APPLIED MICROBIOLOGY AND INFECTION CONTROL INCLUDING SAFETY

PLACEMENT: III SEMESTER

THEORY: 2 Credits (40 hours)

PRACTICAL: 1 Credit (40 hours) (Lab/Experiential Learning – L/E)

SECTION A: APPLIED MICROBIOLOGY

THEORY: 20 hours

PRACTICAL: 20 hours (Lab/Experiential Learning – L/E)

DESCRIPTION: This course is designed to enable students to acquire understanding of fundamentals of Microbiology, compare and contrast different microbes and comprehend the means of transmission and control of spread by various microorganisms. It also provides opportunities for practicing infection control measures in hospital and community settings.

COMPETENCIES: On completion of the course, the students will be able to:

1. Identify the ubiquity and diversity of microorganisms in the human body and the environment.
2. Classify and explain the morphology and growth of microbes.
3. Identify various types of microorganisms.
4. Explore mechanisms by which microorganisms cause disease.
5. Develop understanding of how the human immune system counteracts infection by specific and non-specific mechanisms.
6. Apply the principles of preparation and use of vaccines in immunization.
7. Identify the contribution of the microbiologist and the microbiology laboratory to the diagnosis of infection.

COURSE OUTLINE

T – Theory, L/E – Lab/Experiential Learning

Unit	Time (Hrs)		Learning Outcomes	Content	Teaching/Learning Activities	Assessment Methods
	T	P				
I	3		Explain concepts and principles of microbiology and its importance in nursing	**Introduction** • Importance and relevance to nursing • Historical perspective • Concepts and terminology • Principles of microbiology	• Lecture cum Discussion	• Short answer • Objective type
II	10	10 (L/E)	• Describe structure, classification morphology and growth of bacteria • Identify Microorganisms	**General Characteristics of Microbes** • Structure and classification of Microbes • Morphological types • Size and form of bacteria • Motility • Colonization • Growth and nutrition of microbes • Temperature • Moisture • Blood and body fluids • Laboratory methods for Identification of Microorganisms	• Lecture cum discussion • Demonstration • Experiential Learning through visual	• Short answer • Objective type

				• Types of Staining – simple, differential (Gram's, AFB), special – capsular staining (negative), spore, LPCB, KOH mount. • Culture and media preparation – solid and liquid. Types of media – semi synthetic, synthetic, enriched, enrichment, selective and differential media. Pure culture techniques – tube dilution, pour, spread, streak plate. Anaerobic cultivation of bacteria		
III	4	6 (L/E)	Describe the different disease producing organisms	**Pathogenic organisms** • Micro-organisms: Cocci – gram positive and gram negative; Bacilli – gram positive and gram negative • Viruses • Fungi: Superficial and Deep mycoses • Parasites • Rodents & Vectors o Characteristics, Source, portal of entry, transmission of infection, Identification of disease producing micro-organisms	• Lecture cum discussion • Demonstration • Experiential learning through visual	• Short answer • Objective type
IV	3	4 (L/E)	Explain the concepts of immunity, hyper sensitivity and immunization	**Immunity** • Immunity: Types, classification • Antigen and antibody reaction • Hypersensitivity reactions • Serological tests • Immunoglobulins: Structure, types & properties • Vaccines: Types & classification, storage and handling, cold chain, Immunization for various diseases • Immunization Schedule	• Lecture • Discussion • Demonstration • Visit to observe vaccine storage • Clinical practice	• Short answer • Objective type • Visit report

SECTION B: INFECTION CONTROL & SAFETY

THEORY: 20 hours

PRACTICAL: 20 hours (Lab/Experiential Learning – L/E)

DESCRIPTION: This course is designed to help students to acquire knowledge and develop competencies required for fundamental patient safety and infection control in delivering patient care. It also focuses on identifying patient safety indicators, preventing and managing hospital acquired infections, and in following universal precautions.

COMPETENCIES: The students will be able to:

1. Develop knowledge and understanding of Hospital acquired Infections (HAI) and effective practices for prevention.
2. Integrate the knowledge of isolation (Barrier and reverse barrier) techniques in implementing various precautions.
3. Demonstrate and practice steps in Hand washing and appropriate use of different types of PPE.
4. Illustrate various disinfection and sterilization methods and techniques.
5. Demonstrate knowledge and skill in specimen collection, handling and transport to optimize the diagnosis for treatment.
6. Incorporate the principles and guidelines of Bio Medical waste management.
7. Apply the principles of Antibiotic stewardship in performing the nurses' role.
8. Identify patient safety indicators and perform the role of nurse in the patient safety audit process.
9. Apply the knowledge of International Patient Safety Goals (IPSG) in the patient care settings.
10. Identify employee safety indicators and risk of occupational hazards.
11. Develop understanding of the various safety protocols and adhere to those protocols.

COURSE OUTLINE

T – Theory, L/E – Lab/Experiential Learning

Unit	Time (Hrs)		Learning Outcomes	Content	Teaching/Learning Activities	Assessment Methods
	T	P				
I	2	2 (E)	Summarize the evidence based and effective patient care practices for the prevention of common healthcare associated infections in the healthcare setting	**HAI (Hospital acquired Infection)** • Hospital acquired infection • Bundle approach - Prevention of Urinary Tract Infection (UTI) - Prevention of Surgical Site Infection (SSI) - Prevention of Ventilator Associated events (VAE) - Prevention of Central Line Associated Blood Stream Infection (CLABSI) • Surveillance of HAI – Infection control team & Infection control committee	• Lecture & Discussion • Experiential learning	• Knowledge assessment • MCQ • Short answer
II	3	4 (L/E)	Demonstrate appropriate use of different types of PPEs and the critical use of risk assessment	**Isolation Precautions and use of Personal Protective Equipment (PPE)** • Types of isolation system, standard precaution and transmission-based precautions (Direct Contact, Droplet, Indirect) • Epidemiology & Infection prevention – CDC guidelines • Effective use of PPE	• Lecture • Demonstration & Re-demonstration	• Performance assessment • OSCE
III	1	2 (L)	Demonstrate the hand hygiene practice and its effectiveness on infection control	**Hand Hygiene** • Types of Hand hygiene. • Hand washing and use of alcohol hand rub • Moments of Hand Hygiene • WHO hand hygiene promotion	• Lecture • Demonstration & Re-demonstration	• Performance assessment
IV	1	2 (E)	Illustrates disinfection and sterilization in the healthcare setting	**Disinfection and sterilization** • Definitions • Types of disinfection and sterilization • Environment cleaning • Equipment Cleaning • Guides on use of disinfectants • Spaulding's principle	• Lecture • Discussion • Experiential learning through visit	• Short answers • Objective type
V	1		Illustrate on what, when, how, why specimens are collected to optimize the diagnosis for treatment and management.	**Specimen Collection (Review)** • Principle of specimen collection • Types of specimens • Collection techniques and special considerations • Appropriate containers • Transportation of the sample • Staff precautions in handling specimens	• Discussion	• Knowledge evaluation • Quiz • Performance assessment • Checklist
VI	2	2(E)	Explain on Bio Medical waste management & laundry management	**BMW (Bio Medical Waste Management)** *Laundry management process and infection control and prevention* • Waste management process and infection prevention • Staff precautions • Laundry management • Country ordinance and BMW National guidelines 2017: Segregation of wastes, Colour coded waste containers, waste collection & storage, Packaging & labeling, Transportation	• Discussion • Demonstration • Experiential learning through visit	• Knowledge assessment by short answers, objective type • Performance assessment

Unit	Time (T)	Time (L/E)	Learning Outcomes	Content	Teaching/Learning Activities	Assessment Methods
VII	2		Explain in detail about Antibiotic stewardship, AMR Describe MRSA/ MDRO and its prevention	**Antibiotic stewardship** • Importance of Antibiotic Stewardship • Anti-Microbial Resistance • Prevention of MRSA, MDRO in healthcare setting	• Lecture • Discussion • Written assignment – Recent AMR (Antimicrobial resistance) guidelines	• Short answer • Objective type • Assessment of assignment
VIII	3	5 (L/E)	Enlist the patient safety indicators followed in a health care organization and the role of nurse in the patient safety audit process	**Patient Safety Indicators** • Care of Vulnerable patients • Prevention of Iatrogenic injury • Care of lines, drains and tubing's • Restrain policy and care – Physical and Chemical • Blood & blood transfusion policy • Prevention of IV Complication • Prevention of Fall • Prevention of DVT • Shifting and transporting of patients • Surgical safety • Care coordination event related to medication reconciliation and administration • Prevention of communication errors • Prevention of HAI • Documentation	• Lecture • Demonstration • Experiential learning	• Knowledge assessment • Performance assessment • Checklist/ OSCE
			Captures and analyzes incidents and events for quality improvement	**Incidents and adverse Events** • Capturing of incidents • RCA (Root Cause Analysis) • CAPA (Corrective and Preventive Action) • Report writing	• Lecture • Role play • Inquiry Based Learning	• Knowledge assessment • Short answer • Objective type
IX	1		Enumerate IPSG and application of the goals in the patient care settings.	**IPSG (International Patient safety Goals)** • Identify patient correctly • Improve effective communication • Improve safety of High Alert medication • Ensure safe surgery • Reduce the risk of health care associated infection • Reduce the risk of patient harm resulting from falls • Reduce the harm associated with clinical alarm system	• Lecture • Role play	• Objective type
X	2	3 (L/E)	Enumerate the various safety protocols and its applications	**Safety protocol** • 5S (Sort, Set in order, Shine, Standardize, Sustain) • Radiation safety • Laser safety • Fire safety - Types and classification of fire - Fire alarms - Firefighting equipment • HAZMAT (Hazardous Materials) safety - Types of spill - Spillage management - MSDS (Material Safety Data Sheets)	• Lecture • Demonstration/ Experiential learning	• Mock drills • Post tests • Checklist

			• Environmental safety - Risk assessment - Aspect impact analysis - Maintenance of Temp and Humidity (Department wise) - Audits • Emergency Codes • Role of Nurse in times of disaster		
XI	2	Explain importance of employee safety indicators	**Employee Safety Indicators** • Vaccination • Needle stick injuries (NSI) prevention • Fall prevention • Radiation safety • Annual health check	• Lecture • Discussion • Lecture method • Journal review	• Knowledge assessment by short answers, objective type • Short answer
		Identify risk of occupational hazards, prevention and post exposure prophylaxis.	**Healthcare Worker Immunization Program and management of occupational exposure** • Occupational health ordinance • Vaccination program for healthcare staff • Needle stick injuries and prevention and post exposure prophylaxis		

Experiential Learning:

Experiential learning is the process by which knowledge is created through the process of experience in the clinical field. Knowledge results from the combination of grasping and transforming experience. (Kolb, 1984). The experiential learning cycle begins with an experience that the student has had, followed by an opportunity to reflect on that experience. Then students may conceptualize and draw conclusions about what they experienced and observed, leading to future actions in which the students experiment with different behaviors. This begins the new cycle as the students have new experiences based on their experimentation. These steps may occur in nearly and order as the learning progresses. As per the need of the learner, the concrete components and conceptual components can be in different order as they may require a variety of cognitive and affective behaviors.

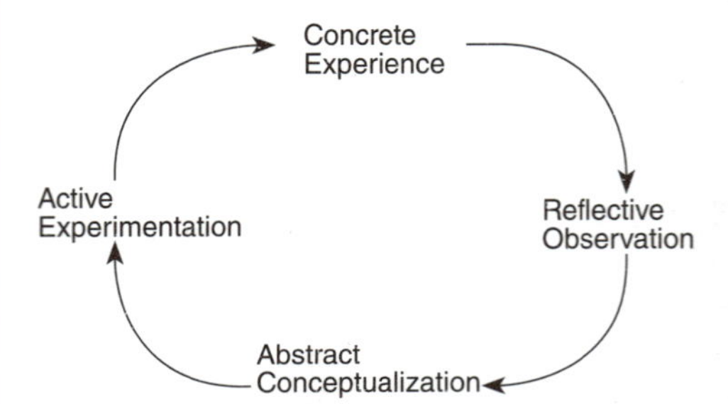

Kolb's Cycle of Experiential Learning

CONTENTS

Unit I: General Microbiology

Unit II: Immunology

Unit III: Systemic Bacteriology

Unit IV: Virology

Unit V: Mycology

Unit VI: Parasitology

Unit VII: Hospital Infection Control and Safety

Unit VIII: Applied Microbiology

Unit IX: Microbiology at a Glance

Unit X: Practical Microbiology

Unit I

GENERAL MICROBIOLOGY

Historical Introduction

1

I. INTRODUCTION

Microbiology is the science of living organisms that are only visible under the microscope. *Medical microbiology* deals with the causative agents of infectious diseases of man, his reaction to *such* infections, the ways in which they produce disease and the methods for their diagnosis.

The fact that the disease is transmitted by contact, from man to man, was known since biblical times. *Varo* and *Columella* (first century B.C.) postulated that diseases were caused by invisible organisms which they called '*Animalia minuta*'. As microbes are invisible to the unaided eye, definitive knowledge about them had to await till microscopes were developed. The credit for observation and description of bacteria goes to ***Antony van Leeuwenhoek*** (1632-1723), a draper from Delft, Holland, whose hobby was grinding lenses. He described three major morphological forms of bacteria. The significance of these observations was not then realised. In 1678, ***Robert Hook*** developed compound microscope and confirmed Leeuwenhoek's observations.

II. SCIENTIFIC DEVELOPMENT OF MICROBIOLOGY

Scientific development of microbiology was ushered by *Louis Pasteur*, perfection on microbiological studies by *Robert Koch*, the introduction of antiseptic surgery by *Lord Lister* and the contributions of *Paul Ehrlich* in chemotherapy.

A. Louis Pasteur (1822-1895) (Fig. 1.1)

He was a trained chemist of France. He established that fermentation was caused by microbial agents. He is also known as ***father of microbiology.***

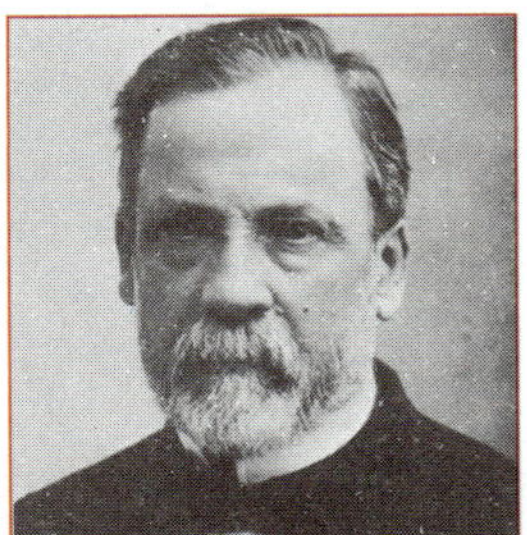

Fig. 1.1 Louis Pasteur

Important Contributions of Louis Pasteur in Microbiology

1. Development of methods and techniques of bacteriology.
2. Proved conclusively that all forms of life, even microbes, arose only from their like and not *de novo*.
3. Introduction of sterilisation techniques and development of steam steriliser, autoclave and hot-air oven.
4. Studies on anthrax, chicken cholera and hydrophobia. During studies on rabies, though Pasteur could not isolate any microorganism from man and dog but he suggested that the causative agent of rabies was too small to be seen by microscope.
5. Live vaccine: He introduced attenuated live vaccine for prophylactic use. He attenuated the anthrax bacillus by incubation at high temperature (42°–43°C) and proved that inoculation of such bacilli in animals induced specific protection against anthrax. Pasteur coined the term vaccine for such prophylactic preparations to commemorate the first of such preparations, namely, cowpox, employed by Jenner for protection against smallpox.

Pasteur's development of a vaccine for hydrophobia marked a milestone in development of immunisation in medicine. This work was acclaimed throughout the world. The Pasteur Institute, Paris, was built by public contribution for the preparation of vaccines and for the investigation of infectious diseases.

B. Joseph Lister (1827-1912)

He was a Professor of Surgery in Glasgow Royal Infirmary. He applied Pasteur's work and introduced antiseptic techniques in surgery (1867) effecting a pronounced drop in mortality and morbidity due to surgical sepsis. It was a milestone in the evolution of surgical practice from the era of 'laudable pus' to modern aseptic techniques. His antiseptic surgery involved the use of carbolic acid. He is known as ***father of antiseptic surgery.***

C. Robert Koch (1843-1910) (Fig. 1.2)

Robert Koch was a German general practitioner. He is also known as the *father of bacteriology*. His contributions are as follows:

1. Perfected bacteriological techniques and introduced methods for isolation of pure strains of bacteria.
2. Introduced methods of obtaining bacteria in pure cultures using solid media.

3. Introduced staining techniques.
4. Discovered the anthrax bacillus (1876), tubercle bacillus (1882) and the cholera vibrios (1883).

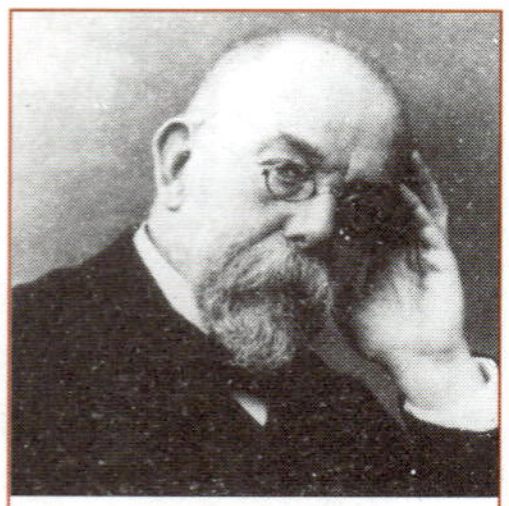

Fig. 1.2 Robert Koch

5. ***Koch's postulates:*** According to Koch's postulates, a microorganism can be accepted as the causative agent of an infectious disease only if the following conditions are fulfilled.
   (i) The organism should be constantly associated with the lesions of the disease.
   (ii) It should be possible to isolate the organism in pure culture from the lesions of the disease.
   (iii) The isolated organism (in pure culture) when inoculated in suitable laboratory animals should produce a similar disease.
   (iv) It should be possible to re-isolate the organism in pure culture from the lesions produced in the experimental animals.

   An additional criterion introduced subsequently requires that specific antibodies to the organisms should be demonstrable in the serum of patients. These postulates have proved to be useful in confirming doubtful claims made regarding the causative agents of infectious diseases. However, it may not always be possible to satisfy all the postulates in every case. An important example of not fulfilling the Koch's postulates is lepra bacillus.
6. ***Koch's phenomenon:*** Robert Koch observed that guineapigs already infected with tubercle bacillus responded with an exaggerated inflammatory response when injected with the tubercle bacillus or its protein. This hypersensitivity reaction is called ***Koch's phenomenon***.

D. Paul Ehrlich (1854-1915)

Paul Ehrlich was a German scientist and is also known as ***father of chemotherapy***. His contributions are as follows:

1. Applied stains to cells and tissues for study of their functions.
2. Reported the acid-fast nature of tubercle bacillus.
3. Proposed '***side chain theory***' of antibody production.
4. Discovered *salvarsan*, an arsenical compound, sometimes called the '***magic bullet***'. It was capable of destroying the spirochaete of syphilis. Later on he discovered '***neosalvarsan***' and thus created a new branch of medicine known as ***chemotherapy***.
5. Introduced methods of standardising toxin and antitoxin.

A number of scientists in medicine and physiology have been awarded Nobel Prizes for their contributions in microbiology (Table 1.1).

III. IMPORTANCE OF MICROBIOLOGY

Nurses play an important role in collection, labelling and transportation of specimens to the laboratory. If proper precautions are taken in collection and transport of clinical specimens, it results in quality examination and appropriate reporting and thus contributes in proper patient care. Health care associated infections or nosocomial infection are of great concern in hospitals. Nurses can help in prevention of nosocomial infections by providing sterile instruments, dressings, surgical gloves, face masks and implementing hand hygiene after any procedure involving nursing care for the patient. Microbiology helps nurses in basic understanding of sterilisation and disinfection procedures. Maintenance of cold chain for vaccines is another aspect which nurses may contribute with the help of microbiology.

Table 1.1: Nobel Laureates

	Nobel Laureate	Research work
1901	Emil A. Von Behring	Developed diphtheria antitoxin
1902	Sir Ronald Ross	Life cycle of malarial parasite
1905	Robert Koch	Tuberculosis—discovery of causative agent
1907	C. L. A. Laveran	Discovery of malarial parasite in unstained preparation of blood.
1908	Paul Ehrlich and Elie Metchnikoff	Role of phagocytes in immunity, the first selective theory of antibody formation
1913	Charles Richet	Anaphylaxis
1919	Jules Bordet	Developed complement fixation test
1928	Charles Nicolle	Typhus fever
1930	Karl Landsteiner	Described ABO blood groups
1939	Gerhardt Domagk	Antibacterial effect of prontosil
1945	Sir Alexander Fleming, Sir Howard Florey and E. B. Chain	Discovery of drug 'penicillin'
1951	Max Theiler	Yellow fever vaccine
1952	Selman A. Waksman	Discovery of streptomycin
1954	J.F. Enders, F. C. Robbins and T. H. Weller	Cultivation of poliovirus in tissue culture
1958	G.W. Beadle, Joshua Lederberg and E. L. Tatum	Genetic mechanisms, transmission of hereditary characteristics
1960	Sir Macfarlane Burnet and Sir Peter Brian Medawar	Immunological tolerance, clonal selection theory
1962	Watson and Crick	Double helix structure of deoxyribonucleic acid (DNA)
1965	Francois Jacob, Andre Lwoff and Jacques Monod	Operon hypothesis and protein synthesis
1966	Peyton Rous	Viral oncogenesis (avian sarcoma)
1968	Holley, Khurana and Nirenberg	Genetic code
1969	Max Delbruck, A. D. Hershey and Salvador Luria	Mechanisms of virus infection in living cells
1972	Gerald Edelman and Rodney Porter	Chemical structure of antibody
1975	David Baltimore, Renato Dulbecco and Howard M. Temin	Interaction between tumour viruses and genetic material of cells, discovered reverse transcriptase
1976	Baruch S. Blumberg and Carleton Gajdusek	Australia antigen—Blumberg Kuru virus—Gajdusek
1977	Rosalyn Yallow	Developed radioimmunoassay
1980	Baruj Benacerraf, Jean Dausset and George Snell	HLA antigens
1983	Barbara McClintoch	Mobile genetic elements
1984	Cesar Milstein and Georges Kohler Niels Jerne	Monoclonal antibodies and hybridoma technology Idiotype network hypothesis—Jerne, N
1987	Susumu Tonegawa	Elucidated nature of antibody diversity
1989	J. Michael Bishop and Hanold E. Varmus	Identified first cellular oncogenes
1990	J. Murray and E. D. Thomas	Organ and cell transplantation
1993	Kary Mullis	Polymerase chain reaction (PCR)
1996	Peter C. Doherty and Rolf M. Zinkernagel	Cell mediated immune defences
1997	Stanley B. Prusiner	Discovery of prions
2005	Marshell and Warren	Helicobacter pylori and its role in peptic ulcer.

Contd.

Table 1.1: Nobel Laureates

	Nobel Laureate	Research work
2008	Luc Montagnier and Francoise Barre-Sinoussi	Discovery of human immunodeficiency virus
	Herald zur Hausen	Human papilloma viruses causing cervical cancer—Hausen H.Z.
2011	Bruce A. Beutler and Jules A. Haffmann	Discoveries concerning the cultivation of innate immunity
	Ralph M. Steinman	Discovery of the dendritic cell and its role in active immunity—Steinman
2015	William C Campbell and Satoshi Omura	Discoveries concerning a novel therapy against infections caused by roundworm parasites.
	Youyou Tu.	Discoveries concerning a novel therapy against Malaria - Youyou Tu.
2020	Harey J. Alter, Michael Houghton and Charles M. Rice	Discovery of hepatitis C virus

KEY POINTS

1. *Microbiology* is the science of living organisms that are only visible under microscope.
2. Scientific development of microbiology is contributed by several scientists.
3. A microorganism can be accepted as the causative agent of infectious disease only if it fulfills the *Koch's postulates*.
4. Nobel prize has been awarded to various scientists for their discoveries.

STUDY QUESTION

1. Write short notes on:
   (i) Robert Koch
   (ii) Louis Pasteur
   (iii) Koch's postulates
   (iv) Koch's phenomenon
   (v) Paul Ehrlich

MULTIPLE CHOICE QUESTIONS (MCQs)

1. Who is known as the Father of Microbiology?
   (a) Paul Ehrlich
   (b) Joseph Lister
   (c) Louis Pasteur
   (d) Kitasato
2. Who introduced the techniques of sterilisation?
   (a) Robert Koch
   (b) Louis Pasteur
   (c) John Needham
   (d) Joseph Lister
3. The term vaccine was coined by:
   (a) Louis Pasteur
   (b) Robert Koch
   (c) Joseph Lister
   (d) Edward Jenner
4. Who introduced methods of obtaining bacteria in pure cultures using solid media?
   (a) Robert Koch
   (b) Louis Pasteur
   (c) Joseph Lister
   (d) Paul Ehrlich
5. Who discovered *Mycobacterium tuberculosis*?
   (a) Louis Pasteur
   (b) Robert Koch
   (c) Loeffler
   (d) Yersin
6. Who is known as the '*Father of Chemotherapy*'?
   (a) Robert Koch
   (b) Louis Pasteur
   (c) Paul Ehrlich
   (d) Joseph Lister

ANSWERS (MCQs)

1. (c) 2. (b) 3. (a) 4. (a) 5. (b) 6. (c)

Microscopy and Morphology of Bacteria

2

I. INTRODUCTION

Microorganisms are living structures of microscopical size. These were originally classified under plant and animal kingdoms. This classification proved unsatisfactory, therefore, a third kingdom *Protista* was formed.

Protista

It is divided into two groups—*prokaryotes* and *eukaryotes* (Table 2.1).

Table 2.1: Differences between Prokaryotic and Eukaryotic Cells

Structure	Prokaryotes	Eukaryotes
Nucleus		
Nuclear membrane	Absent	Present
Nucleolus	Absent	Present
Chromosome	One	More than one
Deoxyribonucleoprotein	Absent	Present
Division	By binary fission	By mitosis
Cytoplasm		
Mitochondria, Golgi apparatus, Lysosomes, Pinocytosis, Endoplasmic reticulum	All are absent	All are present
Chemical Composition		
Sterols	Absent	Present
Muramic acid	Present	Absent

1. Eukaryotes

Fungi, algae, protozoa and slime moulds are included in this group.

2. Prokaryotes

Bacteria belong to this group.

Bacteria

The size of bacteria is measured in unit of a micron (micrometre).

1 micron (μ) or micrometre (μm) = 1/1000 millimetre

1 millimicron (mμ) or nanometre (nm) = 1/1000 μm (micron) or one millionth of a millimetre

1 Angstrom unit (Å) = 1/10 nm (nanometre)

Bacteria of medical importance measure 2-5 μm (L) × 0.2–1.5 μm (W). The resolution power of an unaided eye is about 200 microns. Bacteria, being much smaller than the resolution limit, can be visualised only under magnification. Hence, the study of bacteria requires the use of microscopes.

II. MICROSCOPY

Microscopy is done for following purposes:

1. Magnification of an object
2. Maximisation of resolution
3. Optimisation of the contrast between structures, organisms and background.

A. Parts of Microscope

An ordinary light microscope consists of different parts such as the stand, the optical system, the body, the stage, the substage and the mirror (Fig. 2.1).

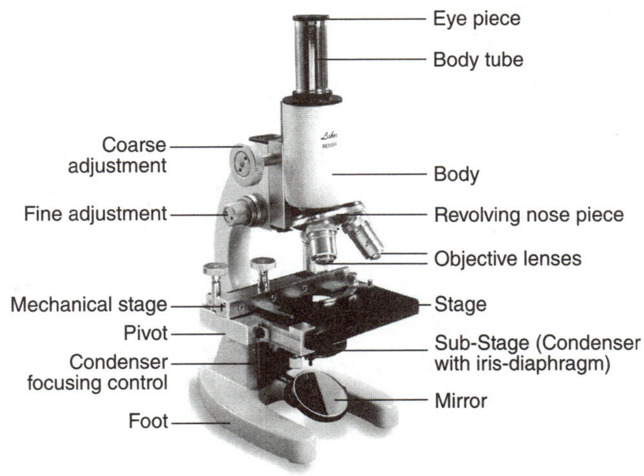

Fig. 2.1 Light Microscope

1. The Stand

The stand comprises a heavy *foot*, often horseshoe shaped and the *limb* which bears the optical system. The limb is attached to the foot by a *hinged joint*.

2. The Optical System

The optical system is mounted in a tube which is usually in two parts: (i) an *external tube* which bears at its lower end a revolving *nose piece* in which interchangeable three *objective lenses* of various magnifications such as low power (X10), high power (X40) and oil immersion (X100); (ii) an *inner draw tube* that carries the eye piece (magnification X5, X6 or X10) at its upper end.

3. The Body

The whole assembly is held in position by the body which consists of two mechanisms: the *coarse* and *fine adjustments*. With the help of these adjustments, the height of the tube can be adjusted for optimal viewing.

4. The Stage

The stage is a platform that accommodates a glass microslide on which the object to be examined is mounted. A *mechanical* stage is fitted to the fixed stage so that object can be moved from side to side and before backwards.

5. The Substage

Beneath the stage is the substage that carries a *condenser* whose lenses serve to condense the rays of light and to focus them on the object. The height as well as horizontal position of the condenser are adjustable. Immediately below the condenser is the *iris diaphragm* which can control the amount of light reaching the object. Beneath it is a ring-shaped filter holder.

6. The Mirror

Fitted to the tail piece below the condenser is a hinged mirror to focus light from the source of illumination onto the object. This mirror is *plane* on one side and *concave* on the other. The mirror can be tilted and rotated in all directions. In modern microscopes, however, the mirror has been replaced with a compact source of illumination. To avoid excessive strains on eyes in case of prolonged work, binocular microscopes are useful.

B. Focussing of an Object

1. Under Low Power

(i) Place the slide to be focussed on the stage and fit it into the mechanical stage. Bring the object to be examined on the central aperture in the stage by using the screw of the mechanical stage.

(ii) By adjusting the plane mirror, focus the light on the object. Partially close the iris diaphragm and lower the objective (X 10) lens near the slide by use of coarse adjustment.

(iii) Now look into the eye-piece and focus the object by using coarse adjustment. The object can be brought to a sharp focus with the fine adjustment. *The condenser usually occupies a low position* while examining the object under low-power.

2. Under High Power

(i) Simply rotate the nose-piece so that the high power objective (X40) lens comes to lie above the slide to a sharp focus.

(ii) The iris diaphragm is fully opened and concave mirror is used to condense the light on the object.

(iii) *The condenser usually occupies a higher position* than for focussing under the low power.

(iv) For a sharp focus, the fine adjustment can be used.

3. Under Oil Immersion Lens

(i) A drop of oil is placed on the slide and then turn the nose piece further so that the oil immersion (X100) lens is in use. It will automatically dip into the drop of the oil.

(ii) The iris diaphragm is kept fully opened and *the condenser is kept in the top position*. The fine adjustment only is used to focus the necessary area.

C. Precautions

(i) Before using a microscope, make sure that the eye piece as well as all the objectives are clean.

(ii) The plane side of mirror is in position.

(iii) Make minimal and careful use of only the fine adjustment while examining the object under high power and oil immersion lenses.

(iv) Never clean the objective with alcohol, as it may dissolve the cement which unites the component lenses.

(v) Higher the magnification, smaller the area that can be examined at a time. *It is always advisable to focus the object under low power (X10) first and then switch over to next high power.*

III. STUDY OF BACTERIA

A. Unstained (Wet) Preparations

Unstained preparations are examined mainly for bacterial motility (e.g. hanging drop preparation) and for demonstration of spirochaetes (e.g. dark ground microscopy).

B. Stained Preparations

Smear made from bacterial culture or specimen is first dried and then fixed with heat by flaming the slide from underneath. Heat kills and fixes the bacteria on slide due to coagulation of bacterial proteins. The fixed smear is stained by appropriate staining technique.

Common Staining Techniques

1. Simple Stains

Basic dyes such as methylene blue or basic fuchsin are used as simple stains. They provide the colour contrast, but impart the same colour to all the bacteria in a smear.

2. Negative staining

Bacteria are mixed with dyes such as India ink or nigrosin. The background gets stained and unstained bacteria stand out in contrast. This is very useful in the demonstration of bacterial capsules which do not take simple stains.

3. Differential stains

They impart different colours to different bacteria or bacterial structures. The two most commonly employed differential stains are the *Gram stain* and the *acid-fast stain*.

Gram's Stain (Fig. 2.2)

It is the most widely used stain in bacteriology.

Method

1. Heat fixed smear, of specimen or the bacterial culture, is stained with crystal violet (primary stain) for one minute. Other pararosaniline dyes such as gentian violet or methyl violet may also be used as primary stain.
2. Pour Gram's iodine (dilute solution of iodine) over the slide for one minute. Gram's iodine acts a mordant.
3. Wash the smear with water.
4. Decolourise with acetone for 10-30 seconds. Alcohol can be substituted for acetone.
5. Wash the smear with water
6. Counterstain with a dye safranin for 30 seconds. Dilute carbol fuchsin or neutral red may also be used as counterstain.
7. Wash the smear with water.
8. The smear is then blot dried.
9. Examine under oil immersion (×100) objective.

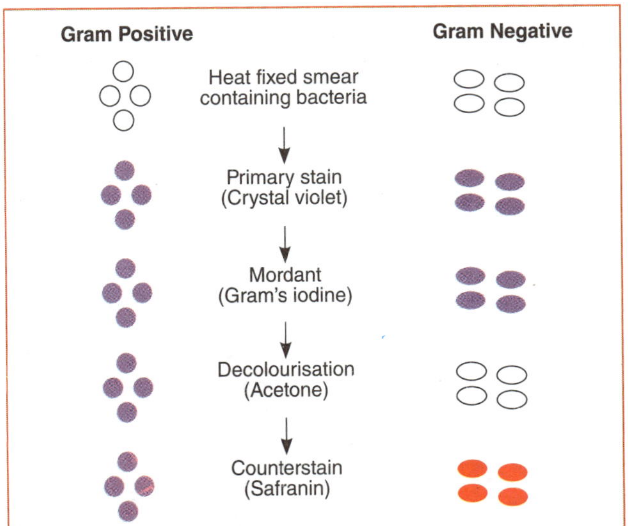

Fig. 2.2 Principle and method of Gram staining

Differentiation on Gram Staining

Two broad groups – Gram positive
– Gram negative

Gram positive – resist decolourisation and retain the colour of primary stain i.e. violet.

Gram negative – are decolourised by acetone/alcohol and, therefore, take counter-stain and appear red.

Mechanism of Gram Staining

The exact mechanism is not understood. It may, however, be attributed to the following.

1. Permeability of bacterial cell wall and cytoplasmic membrane

The Gram positive cells have a more acidic protoplasm, which accounts for retaining the basic dye more strongly than the Gram negative bacteria. Iodine makes the protoplasm more acidic and serves as mordant, i.e. iodine combines with dye to form a dye-iodine complex and fixes the dye in bacterial cell. The Gram positive cell wall or cytoplasmic membrane being less permeable, the dye-iodine complex gets trapped within the cell. The Gram negative cell wall has increased permeability to acetone or alcohol, permitting the outflow of complex during decolourisaton.

2. Integrity of cell wall

The integrity of the cell wall is essential for a positive stain. The Gram positive bacteria become Gram negative when cell wall is damaged.

Acid-Fast Stain (Ziehl-Neelsen stain)

The acid-fast stain was discovered by Ehrlich and subsequently modified by Ziehl and Neelsen. Staining of Mycobacteria (usually tubercle and lepra bacilli) is done by this technique.

Method

1. The carbol fuchsin stain is poured on a slide containing fixed smear. Gentle heat is applied to the underside of the slide, by means of a spirit flame, until the stain just commences to steam. The carbol fuchsin is left on the slide for 5-10 minutes with intermittent heating during that period. Care must be taken to ensure that the stain does not dry out, to counteract drying more solution of stain is added to the slide and the slide reheated. Heating of the stain is required for penetration of the dye into the cell wall.
2. Wash in tap water.
3. The stained smear is decolourised with 20% sulphuric acid and washed with water. This step should be repeated till the pink/red colour stops coming out. In case of lepra bacilli 5% sulphuric acid is used as *M. leprae* is less acid-fast. Another alternative for decolourisation is acid-alcohol (3 ml HCl and 97 ml ethanol).

4. The smear is counterstained with 2% methylene blue for 1-2 minute. Malachite green can also be used as counterstain instead of methylene blue.
5. Wash with water and air dry.

Microscopic Examination of the Smear

Acid-fast bacilli appear red (colour of carbol fuchsin) in blue (colour of methylene blue) background of pus cells and epithelial cells.

Principle

Acid-fastness is due to the high content of lipids, fatty acids and higher alcohols found in the cell wall of mycobacterium. Mycolic acid (a wax), acid-fast in the free state, is found in all acid-fast bacteria. Besides lipid contents, acid-fastness depends also on the integrity of the cell wall.

C. Morphology of Bacteria

Depending on their shape, bacteria are classified into several types (Fig. 2.3):

1. Cocci (from kokkos, meaning berry): These are oval or spherical cells. These cocci may be arranged in pairs (diplococci), chains (streptococci), and clusters (staphylococci).
2. Bacilli (bacillus, meaning rod): These are rod shaped cells. Some of these bacilli may be having peculiar arrangement or shape as follows:
   (i) Coccobacilli—length of bacteria is approximately same as its width e.g. Brucella.
   (ii) Streptobacilli—These bacilli are arranged in chains e.g. Streptobacillus.
   (iii) Chinese letter or cuneiform pattern—arranged at angles to each other e.g. Corynebacterium.
   (iv) Comma-shaped—curved appearance e.g. Vibrio.
   (v) Spirilla—rigid spiral forms e.g. Spirillum.
3. Spirochaetes (from spiera meaning coil; chaite meaning hair): These are slender, flexous spiral forms e.g. Treponema.
4. Actinomycetes (from actis, meaning ray, mykes meaning fungus): These are branching filamentous bacteria resembling fungi.
5. Mycoplasmas: These bacteria are cell wall deficient and hence do not possess a stable shape.

D. Bacterial Anatomy

The outer layer or cell envelope of a bacterial cell consists of two components—

(a) a rigid cell wall;
(b) underlying cytoplasmic or plasma membrane.

The cell envelope encloses the protoplasm which comprises cytoplasm, cytoplasmic inclusions (mesosomes, ribosomes, inclusion granules, vacuoles) and a single circular chromosome of deoxyribonucleic acid (DNA) (Fig. 2.4). Besides these essential components, some bacteria may possess additional structures, such as, capsule, flagella and fimbriae.

1. The Cell Wall (Table 2.2)

The cell wall is a tough and rigid structure, surrounding the bacterium like a shell. The rigid part of the cell wall is a peptidoglycan.

Table 2.2: Differences between Cell Wall of Gram positive and Gram negative Bacteria

Character	Gram positive	Gram negative
Thickness	Thicker	Thinner
Periplasmic space	Absent	Present
Lipids	Absent or small	Present
Teichoic acid	Present	Absent
Peptidoglycan	16-80 nm	2 nm

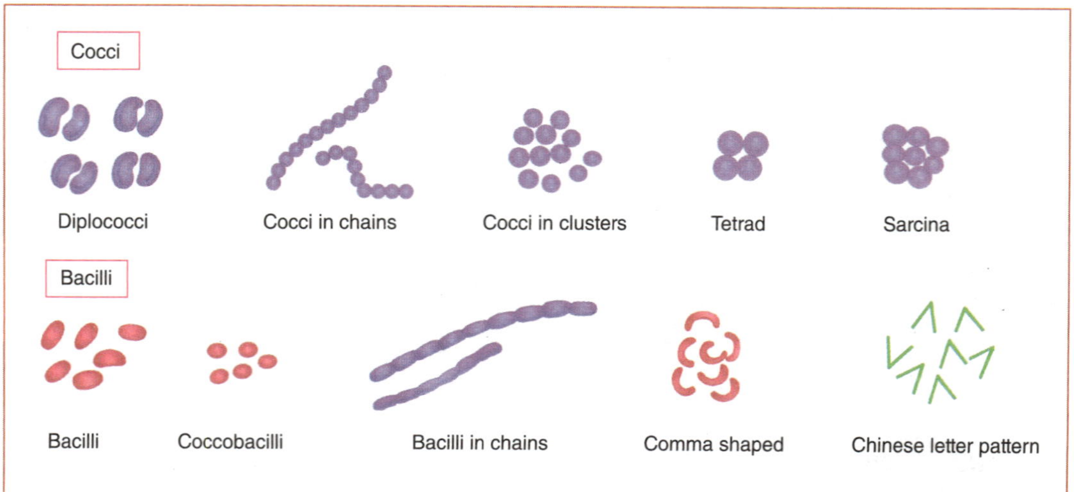

Fig. 2.3 Shapes and different arrangements of bacteria

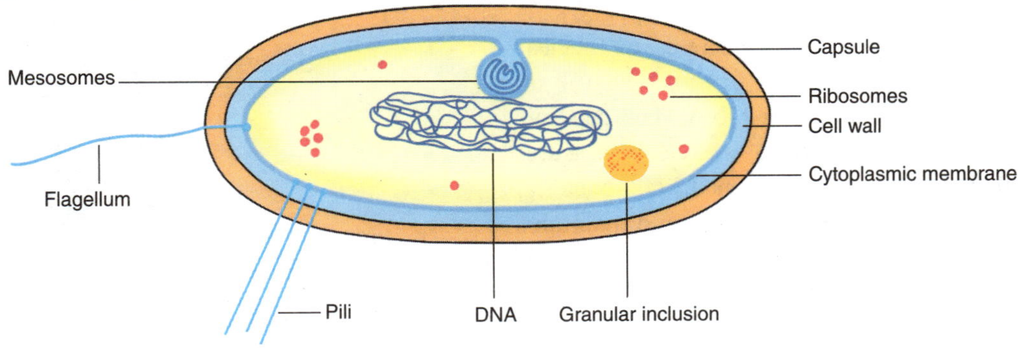

Fig. 2.4 Bacterial cell

(I) Gram-negative Cell Wall

The Gram negative cell wall is a complex structure with the following components (Fig. 2.5).

(a) **Lipoprotein layer:** It connects the peptidoglycan to outer membrane.

(b) **Outer membrane:** This contains certain proteins named outer membrane proteins. These are target sites for phages, antibiotics and bacteriocins.

(c) **Lipopolysaccharide (LPS):** This layer consists of lipid A, to which is attached a polysaccharide. LPS constitutes the endotoxin of gram-negative bacteria. The polysaccharide determines a major surface antigen, the O antigen. The toxicity (pyrogenicity, lethal effect, tissue necrosis) of bacteria is associated with lipid A.

(d) **The periplasmic space:** It is the space in between the inner and outer membranes.

(e) **Peptidoglycan**.

(II) Gram-positive Cell Wall

(a) **Peptidoglycan:** This layer in Gram positive bacteria is thicker (16-80 nm) than that in Gram negative bacteria (2 nm) (Fig. 2.5).

(b) **Teichoic acid:** Gram positive cell wall contains significant amount of teichoic acid which is absent in Gram negative bacteria. The teichoic acids constitute major surface antigens of Gram positive bacteria.

2. Cytoplasmic Membrane

It is 5-10 nm thick elastic semipermeable layer which lies beneath the cell wall separating it from the cell cytoplasm (Fig. 2.3).

Cytoplasmic membrane acts as an osmotic barrier. It acts as a semipermeable membrane controlling the inflow and outflow of metabolites to and from the protoplasm.

3. Cytoplasm

It contains ribosomes, mesosomes, vacuoles and inclusions.

(I) Ribosomes

These are the centres of protein synthesis. These are composed of ribosomal RNA (rRNA) and ribosomal proteins.

(II) Intracytoplasmic Inclusions

These are sources of stored energy and present in some species of bacteria. Their function and significance are uncertain.

(III) Mesosomes (Chondroids)

Mesosomes are vesicular, multilaminated or convoluted structures formed as invaginations of the plasma membrane into the cytoplasm (Fig. 2.3). They are the principal centres of respiratory enzyme and are analogous to mitochondria of eukaryotes.

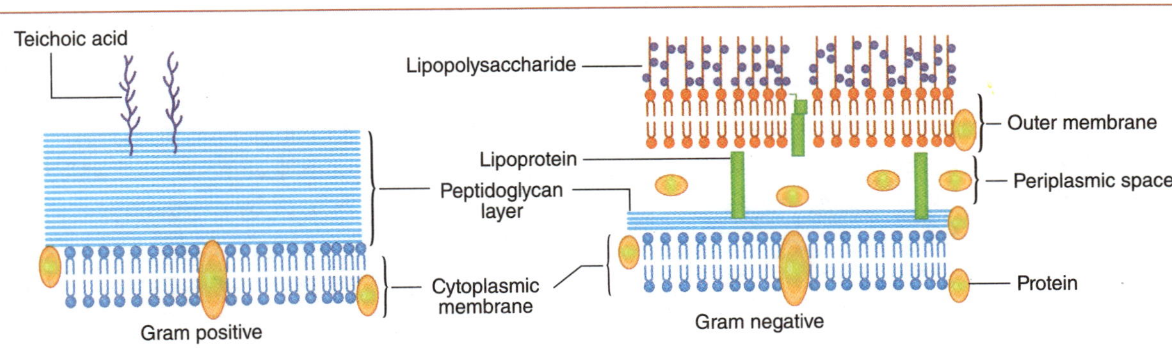

Fig. 2.5 Structure of Gram positive and Gram negative bacterial cell wall

4. Nucleoid

Bacteria do not have true nucleus. There is no nuclear membrane or nucleolus. Nucleoid is present which is an irregularly shaped region containing DNA. The genomic DNA is double stranded in the form of a circle. It measures about 1 mm (1000 μm) when straightened. The bacterial DNA is haploid, replicates by simple fission and maintains bacterial genetic characteristics.

Some bacteria may possess extranuclear genetic material in the cytoplasm consisting of DNA named as plasmids or episomes. The plasmid replicates autonomously. They are not essential for the life of the cell, but may confer on the bacteria certain properties, such as drug resistance and toxigenicity which constitute a survival advantage to the bacteria.

5. Bacterial Capsule and Slime Layer

It is the amorphous viscid bacterial secretion which surrounds some bacteria as their outermost layer (Fig. 2.4). When it diffuses into the surrounding medium and remains as a loose undemarcated secretion it is known as slime layer. When this secretion is organised into a sharply defined structure, as in *Streptococcus pneumoniae* (pneumococcus), it is known as the capsule. The slime layer or capsule is generally polysaccharide in nature but it is polypeptide in anthrax bacillus.

Functions

(i) Capsule enhances bacterial virulence by inhibiting phagocytosis.
(ii) It acts as protective covering against antibacterial substances such as, bacteriophages, phagocytes, enzymes.
(iii) Capsular antigen is specific for bacteria and can be used for identification and typing of bacteria.

Capsulated Organisms

Streptococcus pneumoniae, Klebsiella sp. Bacillus anthracis, Cryptococcus neoformans (a fungus).

Demonstration of Capsule

Capsule has little affinity for basic dyes, therefore, it can't be stained by Gram staining. The following methods have been used for demonstration of capsule.

(I) India ink staining (negative staining)

Capsule appears as a clear halo around bacterium as the ink can't penetrate the capsule (Fig. 2.6).

(II) Serological methods

When a suspension of capsulated bacterium is mixed with its specific anticapsular serum and examined under the

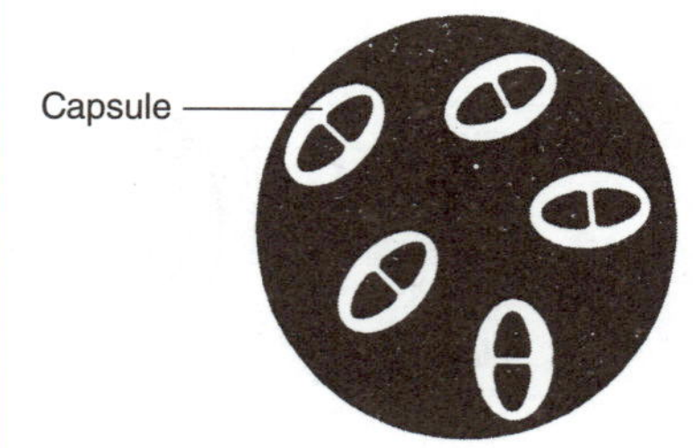

Fig. 2.6 Pneumococci stained with India ink to show capsule

microscope, the capsule appears 'swollen' due to increase in its refractivity. This phenomenon is called capsule swelling reaction or Quellung phenomenon. This is also named as Neufeld reaction after the person who described it.

6. Flagella

Flagella are cytoplasmic appendages protruding through cell wall. These are thread like structures composed of a protein (flagellin), 5-20 μm in length and 0.01-0.02 μm in diameter. They are organ of locomotion.

Parts and Composition

Each flagellum consists of three parts.
(i) filament
(ii) hook
(iii) basal body

The basal body contains outer and inner rings by which the basal body is attached to the cytoplasmic membrane. Outer rings are absent in Gram positive bacteria.

Arrangement/Types (Fig. 2.7)

(i) Monotrichous—Single polar flagellum (at one end) e.g. *Vibrio cholerae*.
(ii) Amphitrichous—Single flagellum at both the ends e.g. *Alcaligenes faecalis*.
(iii) Lophotrichous—Tuft of flagella at one or both ends e.g. *Spirilla*.
(iv) Peritrichous—Flagella arranged all round the cell e.g. *Salmonella typhi*.

Demonstration

Flagella are about 0.02 μm in thickness and hence beyond the resolution limit of the light microscope. The following methods are used for its demonstration:
(i) Dark ground illumination.
(ii) Special staining techniques in which thickness of flagella is increased by mordanting.
(iii) Electron microscopy.
(iv) Indirect methods by which motility of bacteria can be seen or demonstrated.
   (a) Spreading type of growth on a medium e.g. swarming growth of Proteus sp.

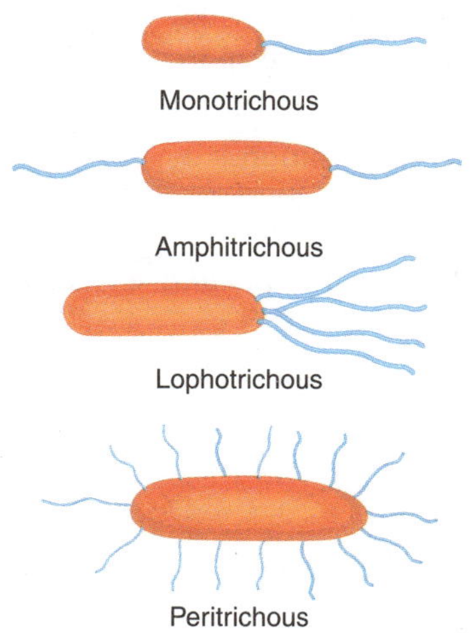

Fig. 2.7 Arrangement of flagella

(b) Motility under the microscope e.g. hanging drop preparation.
(c) Spreading of a bacteria in semisolid agar e.g. Craigie's tube method.

7. *Fimbriae*

These are hair-like appendages projecting from the cell surface as straight filaments. They are also called pili. They are 0.1 to1.0 µm in length and less than 10 nm thick (shorter and thinner than flagella). Fimbria is composed of protein called pilin.

Functions

(i) Adhesion—Fimbriae are organs of adhesion. This property enhances the virulence of bacteria.
(ii) Transfer of genetic material.

Detection of Fimbriae

(i) Electron microscopy.
(ii) Haemagglutination.

8. *Bacterial Spore*

Spores are highly resistant resting stage formed in unfavourable environmental conditions presumed to be related to the depletion of exogenous nutrients. As bacterial spores are formed within the parent cell, these are called endospores. Sporulation is not a method of reproduction.

Morphology of Spore

The cell membrane grows inward and forms spore wall around the core (forespore). The inner-most layer of the spore wall forms the spore membrane from which the cell wall of future vegetative bacterium develops. Outside this membrane is thick layer, the cortex and a multilayered tough spore coat. Some spores have an additional apparently rather loose, outercovering called exosporium (Fig. 2.8).

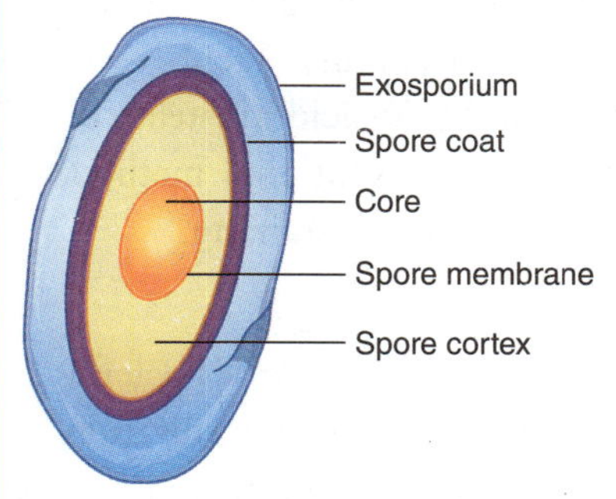

Fig. 2.8 Structure of bacterial spore

Shape and Position of Spores

Spores may be central, subterminal or terminal (Fig. 2.9). They may be oval or spherical in shape. The diameter of spore may be same or less than the width of bacteria (*Bacillus*), or may be wider than the bacillary body producing a distension or bulge in the cell (*Clostridium*).

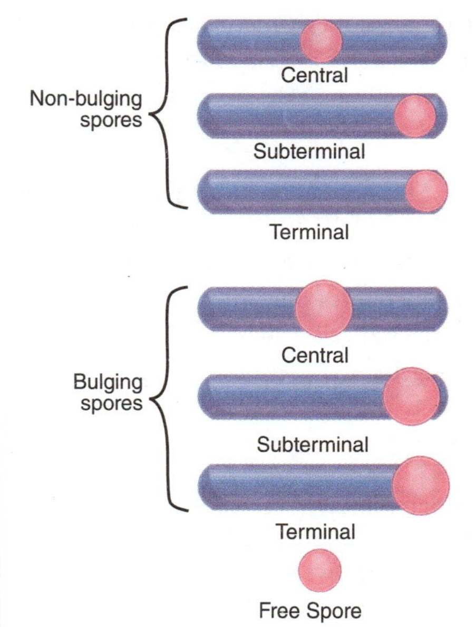

Fig. 2.9 Types of bacterial spores

Resistance

Bacterial spores are extremely resistant to ordinary boiling, disinfectants and heating. However, spores of all medically important bacteria are destroyed by autoclaving at 121°C for 15 minutes. Methods of disinfection and sterilization should ensure destruction of spores also.

Germination

The process of conversion of a spore into vegetative cell under suitable conditions is known as germination.

Demonstration

(i) Gram staining—Spores appear as an unstained refractile body within the cell.

(ii) Modified Ziehl-Neelsen (ZN) staining—Spores appear as acid-fast (red colour). Ziehl-Neelsen staining with 0.25-0.5% sulphuric acid (instead of 20% sulphuric acid as used in conventional method) as decolouring agent is used for spore staining.

Uses of Spores

Spores of certain species of bacteria are employed as indicator for proper sterilisation e.g. *Bacillus stearothermophilus* which is destroyed at a temperature of 121°C for 10–20 minutes (same temperature and time as used in autoclaving). These spores may be kept in autoclave prior to its use. Absence of the spores after autoclaving indicates proper sterilisation.

Spore Forming Bacteria

Obligate aerobes—genus *Bacillus* e.g. *B. anthracis* and *B. subtilis*

Obligate anaerobes—genus *Clostridia e.g. Cl. tetani, Cl. welchii, Cl. botulinum.*

KEY POINTS

1. Microorganisms are living structures of microscopical size. They belong to *prokaryotes*.
2. Microscopy can be done to observe these microorganisms.
3. Bacteria are either *Gram positive* or *Gram negative* on Gram staining.
4. Broadly bacteria are classified into *cocci* or *bacilli*.
5. Bacterial cell possesses several components such as *the cell wall, the cytoplasmic membrane, the cytoplasm, the nucleus, the bacterial capsule, the flagella, the fimbriae and the bacterial spore*.

STUDY QUESTIONS

1. Draw a labelled diagram of bacterial cell.
2. Write short notes on:
   (i) Bacterial cell wall
   (ii) Bacterial capsule
   (iii) Flagella
   (iv) Bacterial spore

MULTIPLE CHOICE QUESTIONS (MCQs)

1. Peptidoglycan layer of cell wall is thicker in:
   (a) Gram positive bacteria
   (b) Gram negative bacteria
   (c) Fungi
   (d) Parasites
2. Lipopolysaccharide is a major component of cell wall in:
   (a) Gram positive bacteria
   (b) Gram negative bacteria
   (c) Fungi
   (d) Parasites
3. A tuft of flagella present at one or both ends of bacterial cell, is known as:
   (a) Monotrichous
   (b) Amphitrichous
   (c) Lophotrichous
   (d) Peritrichous
4. Which one of the following bacteria is cell wall deficient?
   (a) *Escherichia coli*
   (b) *Salmonella typhi*
   (c) *Mycoplasma*
   (d) *Treponema pallidum*
5. All of the following are spore forming bacteria except:
   (a) *Clostridium botulinum*
   (b) *Bacillus subtilis*
   (c) *Bacillus anthracis*
   (d) *Pseudomonas aeruginosa*
6. Indian ink staining is used to demonstrate:
   (a) Cell wall
   (b) Bacterial capsule
   (c) Bacterial flagella
   (d) Bacterial spore

ANSWERS (MCQs)

1. (a) 2. (b) 3. (c) 4. (c) 5. (d) 6. (b)

3 Growth and Nutrition of Bacteria

The minimum nutritional requirement for growth and multiplication of bacteria include sources of carbon, nitrogen, hydrogen, oxygen and some inorganic salts.

I. BACTERIAL GROWTH

A. Bacterial Cell Division

Bacteria divide by binary fission. When a bacterial cell reaches a critical mass in its cellular constituents, the cell division starts. Bacterial nucleus or chromosome is a circular double stranded DNA molecule. The nuclear division precedes bacterial cell division. During replication, the two strands of DNA are separated and new complementary strands are formed. Thus two identical double stranded DNA molecules are formed.

The replicated DNA molecules are distributed to the two daughter cells. A transverse septum grows across the cell from the cell membrane. This is followed by the deposition of cell wall material and the two daughter cells separate.

B. Generation Time

The time required for a bacterium to give rise to two daughter cells under optimum conditions, is known as the **generation time**. The generation time in most of the medically important bacteria is about 20 minutes. In *Mycobacterium tuberculosis* it is about 20 hours and in lepra bacilli it is 20 days.

Clinical Significance

When generation time is about 20 minutes (most of the medically important bacteria), bacteria take 18-24 hrs to grow on culture media. In contrast *M.tuberculosis* take longer duration (in weeks) to grow as its generation time is longer, i.e., 20 hrs. *M.leprae* takes months to grow in animal models as its generation time is 20 days.

C. Bacterial Count

1. *Total count*: This indicates total number of bacteria in the specimen, irrespective of whether they are living or dead.
2. *Viable count*: It measures the number of living (viable) cells.

D. Bacterial Growth Curve

When a bacterium is inoculated into a suitable culture medium and incubated, its growth follows a definite course. When bacterial count of such culture is determined at different intervals and plotted in relation to time, a growth curve is obtained (Fig. 3.1). The growth curve has four phases.

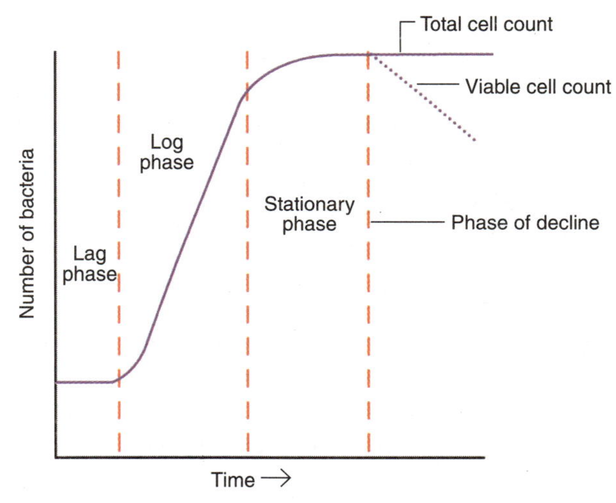

Fig. 3.1 Bacterial growth curve

1. Lag Phase

After inoculation of the culture medium, multiplication usually does not begin immediately. The period between inoculation and beginning of multiplication is known as lag phase. During this period the organisms adapt to the new environment, during which necessary enzymes and intermediate metabolites are built up in adequate quantities for multiplication to proceed. There is increase in the size of the cells but there is no appreciable increase in numbers.

2. Log (Logarithmic) or Exponential Phase

The cell division starts and their numbers increase exponentially or by geometric progression with time. If the logarithm of the v iable count is plotted against time, a straight line is obtained.

3. Stationary Phase

After log phase, the bacterial growth ceases almost completely due to exhaustion of nutrients and accumulation of toxic products. The number of progeny cells formed is just enough to replace the number of cells that die. The number of viable cells remain stationary as there is almost a balance between the dying cells and the new-formed cells.

4. Phase of Decline

After a period of stationary phase, the bacterial population decreases due to the death of cells. The decline phase starts due to exhaustion of nutrients, accumulation of toxic products and autolytic enzymes. There is decline in viable count and not in total count.

II. BACTERIAL NUTRITION

The principal constituent of bacterial cell is water, which is about 80% of the total weight. For growth of bacteria, the minimum nutritional requirement is water, a source of carbon, a source of nitrogen and some inorganic salts. These nutritional elements may be supplied in suitable artificial culture media. In addition to these, bacteria require sulphur, phosphorus and other elements such as sodium, potassium, magnesium, iron and manganese in small amounts.

Clinical Significance

The knowledge of compounds required by different bacteria is helpful in preparation of culture media for growing that particular bacterium. Some bacteria may require some special nutrients to be incorporated in the culture media.

ENVIRONMENTAL FACTORS AFFECTING GROWTH

1. Moisture

Moisture is an essential requirement for the growth of bacteria because 80% of the bacterial cell consists of water.

2. Oxygen

On the basis of requirement of oxygen, bacteria are divided into *aerobes* and *anaerobes*.

(a) **Aerobes:** They require oxygen for their growth. They may be *obligate aerobes*, which grow only in the presence of oxygen, or *facultative anaerobes* that are ordinarily aerobes but can also grow without oxygen. Most of the pathogenic bacteria are facultative anaerobes. Example of obligate aerobe is *Pseudomonas aeruginasa*. Microaerophilic bacteria **(microaerophiles)** can grow in the presence of traces of oxygen. *Campylobacter* and *Helicobacter pylori* are examples of microaerophilic bacteria.

(b) **Anaerobes:** The *obligate* or *strict* anaerobes can grow only in the absence of oxygen. *Clostridium tetani* is one such example. Obligate anaerobes cannot grow even in the presence of traces of oxygen.

3. Carbon Dioxide

Small amount of carbon dioxide is required by all bacteria. Some organisms such as *Brucella abortus* require much higher level of carbon dioxide (5-10 per cent) for their growth especially for primary isolation. These bacteria are called *capnophilic bacteria*.

4. Temperature

The temperature at which growth occurs best is known as *Optimum temperature*.

The optimal temperature range varies with different bacterial species. Most of the pathogenic bacteria grow optimally at 37 °C (our body temperature).

5. pH

Most of the medically important bacteria can grow at pH 7.2-7.6. However, some bacteria such as lactobacilli and cholera vibrio grow at acidic and alkaline pH respectively.

Clinical Significance

Culture media having alkaline pH are used for growing *Vibrio cholerae*.

KEY POINTS

1. Bacterial cell division occurs by binary fission.
2. The time required for the bacterium to give rise to two daughter cells under optimum conditions is known as the *generation time*.
3. Bacterial growth curve has four phases namely *lag phase*, *log phase*, *stationary phase* and *phase of decline*.
4. Majority of the pathogenic bacteria grow optimally at *37°C*.

STUDY QUESTION

1. Write briefly about Bacterial growth curve.

MULTIPLE CHOICE QUESTIONS (MCQs)

1. Generation time of *Mycobacterium tuberculosis* is about:
   (a) 20 seconds
   (b) 20 minutes
   (c) 20 hours
   (d) 20 days
2. Bacteria which can grow at temperature between 25°C and 40°C are known as:
   (a) Mesophiles
   (b) Psychrophiles
   (c) Thermophiles
   (d) None of the above
3. Which one of the following bacteria can grow in acidic pH?
   (a) Klebsiella sp.
   (b) Lactobacilli
   (c) *Pseudomonas aeruginosa*
   (d) *Vibrio cholerae*
4. The bacteria which require higher level of carbon dioxide for their growth are known as:
   (a) Microaerophilic bacteria
   (b) Capnophilic bacteria
   (c) Aerobic bacteria
   (d) None of the above

ANSWERS (MCQs) ...✓

1. (c) 2. (a) 3. (b) 4. (b)

Culture Media and Culture Methods

4

I. CULTURE MEDIA

Culture media are required to grow the organisms from infected material to identify the causative agent. After identification of organism, culture media are also used for antibiotic sensitivity testing.

Types of Media

Simple Media

Nutrient broth is an example of simple medium (basal medium). It contains peptone water and meat extract 1%. When glucose (0.5%) is added to nutrient broth, it becomes glucose broth. **Peptone water** and **glucose broth** are shown in Fig. 4.1 and Fig. 4.2 respectively. Brain-heart infestion (BHI) broth is a commonly used liquid medium for the culture of non-fastidious and moderately fastidious organisms.

When 2-3% agar is added to nutrient broth, it becomes **nutrient agar** (Fig. 4.3). This is the simplest and routinely employed medium in laboratory for diagnostic purposes.

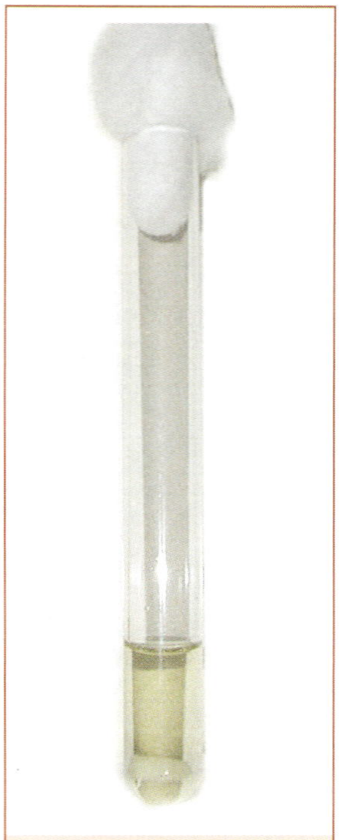

Fig. 4.1 Peptone water

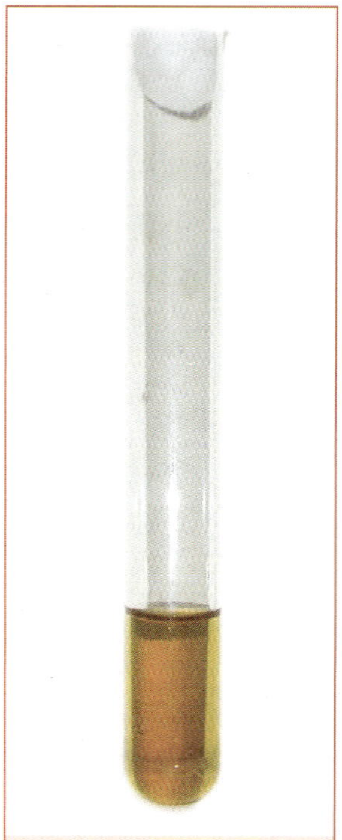

Fig. 4.2 Glucose broth

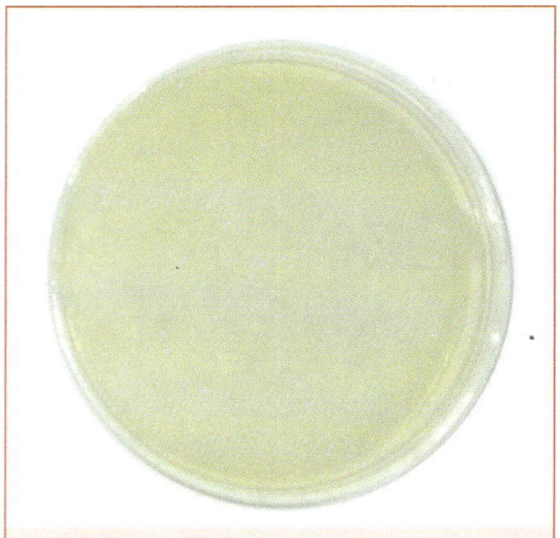

Fig. 4.3 Nutrient agar

Complex Media

All media other than simple media are complex. Complex media have added ingredients for bringing out certain properties or providing special nutrients required for the growth of the bacterium in question.

Special Media

(a) Enriched Media

When basal medium is added with some nutrients such as blood, serum or egg, it is called enriched medium.

Example:

Blood agar (Fig. 4.4) – Blood is added to nutrient agar.

Fig. 4.4 Blood agar

(b) Enrichment Media

Some substances are incorporated in the liquid medium which have a stimulating effect on the bacteria to be grown or inhibits its competitors. This results in an absolute increase in the number of wanted bacteria related to other bacteria. Such media are called enrichment media. These are very useful for culture of faeces where the non-pathogenic or commensal bacteria tend to overgrow the pathogenic ones, e.g., Salmonella being overgrown by *Esch. coli.*

Tetrathionate broth – Tetrathionate is added which inhibits coliforms while allowing typhoid-paratyphoid bacilli to grow.

(c) Selective Media

Selective media contain substances that inhibit all but a few types of bacteria and facilitate the isolation of a particular species. These media are used to isolate a particular bacteria from specimens where mixed bacterial flora are expected. Selective media are solid in contrast to enrichment media which are liquid.

Deoxycholate citrate agar (DCA) – Addition of deoxycholate acts as a selective agent for enteric bacilli (Salmonella, Shigella).

(d) Differential Media

When a medium contains substances which help to distinguish differing characteristics of bacteria, it is called "differential medium" e.g. MacConkey's medium, which contains peptone, lactose, agar, sodium taurocholate and neutral red. The lactose fermenters (LF) form pink coloured colonies whereas non-lactose fermenters (NLF) produce colourless or pale colonies.

(e) Indicator Media

These media contain an indicator which changes colour when a bacterium grows in them. *Salmonella typhi* grow as black colonies on **Wilson and Blair medium** containing sulphite. **MacConkey's medium** is differential as well as indicator medium.

(f) Transport Media

These are used in the case of delicate organisms (e.g. gonococci) which may not survive the time taken for transit or may be overgrown by non-pathogenic bacteria (e.g. cholera organisms). For transport of specimens to the laboratory, special media are devised and these are termed transport media.

Example:

Stuart's transport medium – It may be used for organisms such as gonococci.

Dehydrated media

Dehydrated media are commercially available. These are simply reconstituted in distilled water and sterilised before use. With dehydrated media, the process of media making has become simpler and its quality more uniform.

Table 4.1 and Table 4.2 show some of the liquid media and solid media respectively.

II. CULTURE METHODS

A. Streak Culture (Surface Plating)

It is the routine method employed for bacterial isolation in pure culture. A platinum or nichrome wire loop of 2-4 mm in diameter is used. Due to high cost of platinum, loops for routine laboratory work are made of nichrome

Table 4.1: Composition and Uses of Liquid Media

	Medium	Composition	Uses
1.	Peptone water	Peptone – 1% NaCl – 0.5% Water – 100 ml (pH 7.4)	Routine culture, Sugar fermentation tests
2.	Nutrient broth	Peptone water + Meat extract—1%	Routine culture
3.	Glucose broth	Nutrient broth + Glucose – 0.5%	Blood culture, Culture of certain organisms e.g. Streptococci
4.	Brain-Heart Infusion (BHI) broth	Brain and beef heart, peptones, glucose, sodium chloride and buffers	Blood culture, culture of certain organisms, antibiotic sensitivity testing
5.	Enrichment media		
	(i) Alkaline peptone water	Peptone water (pH 9.0)	Culture of Vibrio
	(ii) Selenite F broth	Peptone water, Sodium selenite	Culture of faeces for salmonellae and shigellae
	(iii) Tetrathionate broth	Nutrient broth, Sodium thiosulphate, Calcium carbonate, Iodine solution	Culture of faeces especially for salmonellae
	(iv) Robertson's cooked meat broth (RCM)	Nutrient broth, Predigested cooked meat of ox heart	Culture of anaerobic bacteria

Table 4.2: Composition and Uses of Solid Media		
Medium	**Composition**	**Uses**
1. Simple medium		
(i) Nutrient agar	Nutrient broth, Agar (2-3%)	Routine culture
2. Enriched media		
(i) Blood agar	Nutrient agar, Sheep blood (5-10%)	Routine culture
(ii) Chocolate agar	Heated blood agar (55°C × 2hr)	Culture of Neisseria, *H. influenzae*
(iii) Loeffler's serum slope (LSS)	Nutrient broth, Glucose, Horse serum	Culture of *C. diphtheriae*
3. Indicator medium		
(i) MacConkey's medium	Peptone Lactose Sodium taurocholate Agar Neutral red	Culture of Gram negative bacilli
4. Selective media		
(i) Deoxycholate citrate agar (DCA)	Nutrient agar, Sodium deoxycholate, Sodium citrate, Lactose, Neutral red	Culture of *Salmonellae* and *Shigellae*
(ii) Bile salt agar (BSA)	Nutrient agar, Sodium taurocholate (0.5%) pH 8.2	Culture of *Vibrio cholerae*

wire (24 S.W.G. size). This loop is first sterilised in the bunsen flame by making it red hot and cooled by touching an uninoculated part of the medium. Then a loopful of specimen is smeared onto the surface of a dried plate near the peripheral area. This is named as primary inoculum. From the primary inoculum, it is spread thinly over the plate by streaking with the loop in parallel lines (Fig. 4.5). The loop is flamed and cooled in between the different sets of streaks. It is done to obtain isolated colonies over the final series of streaks. The culture plate is incubated at 37°C for overnight. Confluent growth occurs at the primary inoculum and well separated colonies are obtained on the final streaks. Single isolated colony is the best to study the various properties of bacteria.

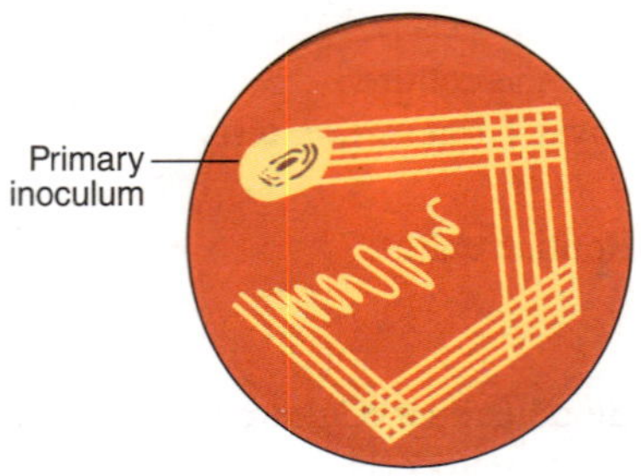

Fig. 4.5 Streak culture (surface plating) on solid medium

B. Lawn Culture

This type of culture method is employed in antibiotic sensitivity testing (disc diffusion method) and in bacteriophage typing. Lawn cultures are obtained by flooding the surface of the plate with a liquid culture or suspension of the bacterium. Culture plate is kept for a minute and then excess material is poured off. Alternatively, the culture plate may be inoculated by a sterile swab soaked in liquid bacterial culture or suspension **(swabbing)**. Plate is then incubated at 37°C overnight to obtain bacterial colonies.

ANAEROBIC CULTURE METHODS

Anaerobic bacteria grow only in the absence of oxygen (anaerobic conditions). These anaerobic conditions or anaerobiosis can be established by various methods.

Anaerobiosis obtained by "McIntosh and Filde's" anaerobic jar (Fig. 4.6) is the most reliable and widely used method.

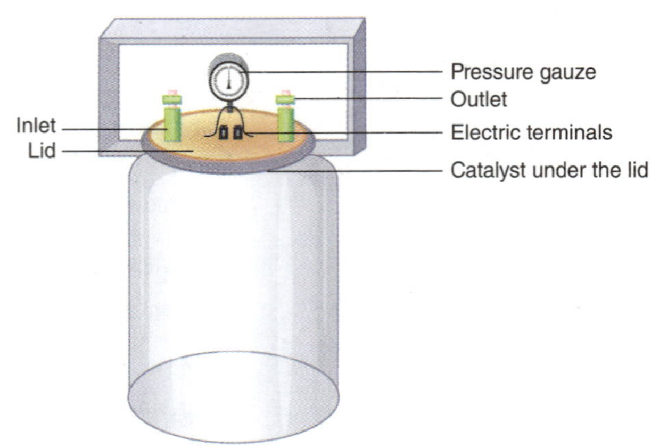

Fig. 4.6 McIntosh and Filde's anaerobic jar

Procedure

McIntosh and Filde's anaerobic jar consists of a stout glass or metal jar with a metal lid which can be clamped air-tight with a screw. The lid is fitted with two tubes with taps, one acting as inlet for introduction of gas and the other as the outlet. The lid also contains two terminals which can be connected to an electrical supply. A catalyst (alumina pellets coated with palladium) is suspended under the lid by stout wires which are connected with the terminals to heat the catalyst for its activity. Nowadays catalyst (without heating) at room temperature is used.

Culture plates inoculated with specimens are placed inside the anaerobic jar with an indicator. The lid is clamped tight. The outlet tube is connected to a vacuum pump while inlet tube is closed. The air inside is evacuated. The outlet tube is then closed and hydrogen gas is passed through inlet tube till reduced atmospheric pressure is brought to normal atmospheric pressure (i.e., 760 mm Hg) which is monitored on the vacuum gauze as zero. Electric terminals are switched on to heat the catalyst and if 'room temperature catalyst' is used, heating is not required. The catalyst helps to combine hydrogen and residual oxygen to form water.

Reduced methylene blue is generally used as indicator of anaerobiosis in the jar. It remains colourless in anaerobic conditions, but turns blue on exposure to oxygen.

KEY POINTS

1. *Culture media* are required to grow the organisms from infected material to identify the causative agent.
2. *Anaerobic media* are used for cultivation of anaerobic bacteria, e.g., *cooked meat broth* (*CMB*).
3. Streak culture (surface plating) is the routine culture method employed for bacterial isolation in pure culture.
4. Anaerobic bacteria grow only in the absence of oxygen (anaerobic conditions). "McIntosh and Filde's" anaerobic jar is the most reliable and widely used method to obtain anaerobic conditions.

STUDY QUESTIONS

1. Write short notes on:
   (i) Enriched media (ii) Enrichment media (iii) Selective media.
2. Write short notes on:
   (i) Streak culture (ii) Lawn culture.

MULTIPLE CHOICE QUESTIONS (MCQs)

1. All of the following are examples of enriched media except:
   (a) Blood agar
   (b) Chocolate agar
   (c) Loeffler's serum slope
   (d) Bile salt agar
2. When a solid medium contains a substance that inhibits all unwanted bacteria but facilitates the isolation of particular bacteria, it is known as:
   (a) Selective medium
   (b) Enriched medium
   (c) Indicator medium
   (d) None of the above
3. When a liquid medium contains a substance that inhibits all unwanted bacteria but stimulates the growth of particular bacteria, it is known as:
   (a) Selective medium
   (b) Enriched medium
   (c) Enrichment medium
   (d) None of the above
4. Anaerobic jar is commonly used to grow:
   (a) *Clostridium tetani*
   (b) *Klebsiella sp.*
   (c) *Pseudomonas aeruginosa*
   (d) None of the above

ANSWERS (MCQs) ...✓

1. (d) 2. (a) 3. (c) 4. (a)

Processing of Specimens

5

I. COLLECTION AND TRANSPORT OF SPECIMENS

There are certain specimens such as blood and cerebrospinal fluid which are normally sterile. Other specimens such as sputum and faeces contain a large number of commensals. For collection of such normally nonsterile specimens the container may not be absolutely sterile; but must be chemically clean.

The following general points, although glaringly obvious are ignored from time to time.

1. No antiseptic or antimicrobial agents should come into contact with the specimen; all specimen containers should be sterile before use.
2. In collection of specimen, care must be taken to avoid contamination of the outside of the container otherwise the person delivering the specimen to the laboratory and the laboratory staff may be infected.
3. Specimen should be transported to the laboratory immediately. In case of unavoidable delay suitable transport medium has to be used.
4. Proper disposal of the specimen, after use, must be ensured.

II. PROCESSING OF SPECIMENS

A. Microscopy

Microscopic examination of unstained wet preparation of urine and cerebrospinal fluid reveals pus cells and red blood cells but for the demonstration of the bacteria, stained preparations are necessary. For the demonstration of *Treponema pallidum* (agent of syphillis)—unstained wet preparations are examined by *dark ground illumination.*

Microscopy of Gram stained preparations is useful in infections caused by organisms with characteristic morphology *e.g.* in gonorrhoea, and Vincent's angina. For the demonstration of tubercle bacilli, films are stained by Ziehl-Neelsen method.

In recent years, the fluorescent antibody technique is being used for the direct demonstration of *organism* or the *antigen* in the clinical material and this method has permitted a rapid diagnosis than culture examination.

B. Culture

Isolation by culture not only permits precise identification based on the characteristics of the organism, but is also a *more sensitive method* than microscopy for the detection of the organism. Furthermore, it is also used to determine the sensitivity of the etiological agent to chemotherapeutic agents.

Blood agar is used as the routine culture medium for inoculation of specimens; however, special media are required for certain pathogens. Selective media are used for the specimens which are normally non-sterile.

For identification of the bacteria isolated in the laboratory a number of characteristics are to be taken into account.

C. Identification

1. Colony Appearance

Colour, size, shape and surface of colony are important. If bacterial colony is on blood agar, haemolysis is noted; the type of haemolysis is significant.

2. Morphology of the Bacteria

Size, shape, arrangement and staining character are determined by Gram's method. The presence of matachromatic granules in *Corynebacterium diphtheriae* is ascertained by Albert's method of staining. Motility is tested by hanging drop preparation. Besides motility, morphology of the bacteria may also be appreciated on hanging drop preparation.

3. Biochemical Reactions

The biochemical properties which are of value in identification include (i) presence of a particular enzyme and (ii) presence of certain metabolic end products in the culture of unknown bacteria.

The enzymes commonly tested include coagulase, catalase, phosphatase, oxidase, urease, gelatinase etc. These tests are used in the preliminary identification of bacteria.

4. Antigenic Composition

Identity of an isolate is best confirmed by testing it with

known specific antiserum. The best way to identify a Gram negative bacillus is by *slide agglutination test* using known antisera. Such tests are ordinarily required for the identification of shigella and salmonella.

5. Pathogenicity Tests

In-vivo tests for virulence of a particular strain of bacteria are done in animals such as guineapig, rabbit or mouse. These tests have been used for the identification of tubercle bacilli, diphtheria bacilli, clostridia etc.

D. Antibiotic Susceptibility Testing

One of the most important functions of the diagnostic laboratory is to test the susceptibility of microbial pathogens to commonly used antibiotics. Susceptibility testing is particularly important when sensitivity to a given antibiotic agent cannot be reliably predicted.

KEY POINTS

1. During collection and transport, care must be taken to avoid contamination of the specimens.
2. After isolation of bacteria in pure culture from a specimen, it can be identified by *morphology* of bacterial colony, *staining*, *hanging drop* preparation and various *biochemical tests*.

STUDY QUESTION

1. Write short notes on:
   (i) Collection and transport of specimens (ii) Identification of bacteria.

MULTIPLE CHOICE QUESTIONS (MCQs)

1. Dark ground illuminaiton is generally used for examinaiton of
   (a) *Treponema pallidum*
   (b) *Escherichia coli*
   (c) *Proteus sp.*
   (d) None of the above

ANSWERS (MCQs)

1. (a)

Microbial Pathogenicity

6

The host-parasite relationship is determined by the interaction between host factors and the infecting microorganism. Health or disease depends on the equilibrium between the two.

I. MICROBES AND RELATED TERMS

A. Microbes

Microbes can be divided into saprophytes and parasites, based on their relationship to their hosts.

1. ***Saprophytes:*** These are free-living microbes that live on dead or decaying organic matter. They are generally unable to invade the living body. However, when host resistance is lowered, may cause infection.
2. ***Parasite:*** A parasite is a microorganism which lives on a living host and derives nutrition from the host, without any benefit to the host.

B. Related Terms

1. ***Commensals:*** Commensals live in complete harmony with the host without causing any harm to it.
2. ***Pathogen:*** Microorganism capable of producing disease in the host is called pathogen.
3. ***Opportunistic pathogens:*** Some commensals or saprophytes can produce disease when host resistance is lowered.
4. ***Pathogenicity:*** It refers to the ability of a class of microbes to produce disease.
5. ***Virulence:*** It is the degree of pathogenicity of a microbe.

II. INFECTION

Infection: The lodgement and multiplication of a parasite in the body is known as infection. All infections do not invariably result in disease.

A. Transmission of Infection

There are three links in the chain of transmission of communicable diseases. These links include the *reservoir*, *mode of transmission* and the *susceptible host*.

1. Reservoir

It refers to any human being, animal, plant, soil or inanimate matter in which parasite normally lives, multiplies and depends primarily for its survival.

Sources of infection

These may be endogenous sources or exogenous sources.

(i) Endogenous sources

Organisms of normal flora are usually non-pathogenic but occasionally they behave as pathogens outside their habitat. Viridans streptococci which are the normal flora of the mouth may cause infective endocarditis.

(ii) Exogenous sources

Most of the infections are exogenous in origin. Exogenous sources include:

(a) Human cases and carriers
(b) Animals
(c) Insects
(d) Soil and water
(e) Food

2. Modes of Transmission

Pathogenic organisms can spread from one host to another by a variety of mechanisms as follows:

(i) *Contact*
(ii) *Inhalation*
(iii) *Ingestion*
(iv) *Inoculation*
(v) *Vectors*
(vi) *Transplacental*
(vii) *Iatrogenic and laboratory infections*

3. Susceptible Host

The infectious agent enters the body by one of the following routes: *oral, respiratory, genitourinary, conjunctival or cutaneous.* This is known as *portal of entry*.

The outcome of an infection depends on interaction between microbial factors which predispose to pathogenicity and various host factors which contribute to resistance.

B. Factors Predisposing to Microbial Pathogenicity

Determinants of Virulence

(i) Adhesion

The initial event in the pathogenesis is the attachment of the bacteria to body surfaces.

(ii) Invasiveness

This refers to the ability of an organism to spread within the host tissues after establishing infection. Highly invasive pathogens produce, spreading or generalised lesions (e.g. streptococcal infections), while less invasive pathogens cause localised lesions (e.g. staphylococcal abscess).

(iii) Antiphagocytic factors

Macrophages and polymorphs play role in phagocytosis of microbes. There are certain factors which oppose phagocytosis for survival of bacteria. One such factor is bacterial capsule.

(iv) Bacterial toxins

Bacteria produce two types of toxins, endotoxins and exotoxins (Table 6.1).

(a) *Endotoxins*—They are lipopolysaccharide (LPS) in nature and form an integral part of the cell wall of Gram negative bacteria. They are released from the bacterial surface by natural lysis of the bacteria or by the disintegration of the cell wall. Massive Gram negative septicaemias may cause the syndrome of endotoxic shock.

(b) *Exotoxins*—They are proteins which are secreted by certain species of bacteria. They diffuse readily into the surrounding medium.

(v) Enzymes

Some bacteria produce enzymes which directly damage host tissue.

(a) *Hyaluronidase*—It breaks down hyaluronic acid and helps in spread of infection e.g. streptococcus.

(b) *Coagulase*—It causes deposition of fibrin around the bacteria and thus prevents phagocytosis e.g. staphylococcus.

III. TYPES OF INFECTIOUS DISEASES

Infectious diseases may be *localised* or *generalised.*

A. Localised

There is an acute inflammatory reaction at the site of invasion to arrest infection. When this process fails, the organisms spread to regional lymph nodes and then to blood stream which leads to dissemination of organisms.

B. Generalised

1. *Bacteraemia*: It is the circulation of bacteria in blood.
2. *Septicaemia*: It is the condition where bacteria circulate and multiply in the blood, form toxic products and cause high fever.
3. *Pyaemia*: It is condition where pyogenic bacteria produce septicaemia with multiple abscesses in internal organs e.g. liver, spleen, kidney.

Table 6.1: Differences between Exotoxins and Endotoxins

S. No.	Exotoxins	Endotoxins
1.	Protein (polypeptides)	Lipopolysaccharide in nature.
2.	Heat labile (> 60°C).	Heat stable.
3.	Actively secreted by living cells into medium	Form integral part of the cell wall; released only on disruption of bacterial cell.
4.	Highly antigenic; stimulates formation of antitoxin which neutralises toxin.	Weakly antigenic; antitoxin is not formed but antibodies against polysaccharide are raised.
5.	Converted into toxoid by formaldehyde.	Cannot be toxoided.
6.	Enzymic in action.	No enzymic action.
7.	Specific pharmacological effect for each exotoxin.	Non-specific action of all endotoxins.
8.	Very high potency.	Low potency.
9.	Highly specific for particular tissue e.g. tetanus toxin for CNS.	Non-specific in action.
10.	Don't produce fever in host.	Usually produce fever.
11.	Produced mainly by Gram-positive bacteria and also by some Gram-negative bacteria.	Produced by Gram-negative bacteria.

KEY POINTS

1. A *parasite* is a microorganism which lives on a living host and derives nutrition from the host, without any benefit to the host.
2. *Bacterial toxins* contribute in virulence of bacteria.
3. *Endotoxins* are lipopolysaccharide (LPS) in nature while *exotoxins* are heat labile proteins.
4. Exotoxins can be converted into *toxoids* e.g. tetanus toxoid.

STUDY QUESTION

1. Tabulate the differences between exotoxins and endotoxins.

MULTIPLE CHOICE QUESTIONS (MCQs)

1. Which toxin can be converted into toxoid by formaldehyde?
   (a) Exotoxin
   (b) Endotoxin
   (c) Both of the above
   (d) None of the above
2. Chemical nature of endotoxin is:
   (a) Lipopolysaccharide
   (b) Protein
   (c) Carbohydrate
   (d) None of the above
3. Chemical nature of exotoxin is:
   (a) Lipopolysaccharide
   (b) Protein
   (c) Carbohydrate
   (d) None of the above

ANSWERS (MCQs) ...✓

1. (a) 2. (a) 3. (b)

Unit II

IMMUNOLOGY

Immunity

7

The term 'immunity' is defined as resistance exhibited by the host against any foreign antigen including microorganisms. This resistance plays a major role in prevention of infectious diseases. Immunity may be *innate or acquired.*

I. INNATE IMMUNITY

It is the resistance which individual possesses by birth. It is by virtue of his genetic and constitutional make-up. It does not depend on prior contact with foreign antigen.

Mechanisms of Innate Immunity

1. Epithelial Surfaces

(i) Skin

It not only acts as a mechanical barrier to microorganisms but also provides bactericidal secretions. The high concentration of salt in drying sweat, the sebaceous secretions and long chain fatty acids contribute to bactericidal activity.

(ii) Respiratory tract

The inhaled particles are arrested in the nasal passages on the moist mucous membrane surfaces. The mucous secretions of respiratory tract act as a trapping mechanism and hair like cilia propels the particles towards the pharynx where it is swallowed or coughed out. The cough reflex acts as an important defence mechanism.

(iii) Intestinal tract

The mouth possesses saliva which has an inhibitory effect on many micro-organisms. Some bacteria may be swallowed and are destroyed by acidic pH of gastric juices.

(iv) Conjunctiva

Tears have a major role by flushing away bacteria and other dust particles. In addition, lysozyme present in tears has a bactericidal action.

(v) The Genitourinary tract

The flushing action of urine eliminates bacteria from the urethra. The acidic pH of vaginal secretions in female, due to the fermentation of glycogen by lactobacillus (normal flora), renders vagina free of many pathogens.

2. Antibacterial Substances

Besides specific antibody formation, there are number of nonspecific antibacterial substances present in blood and tissues. These substances are properdin, complement, lysozyme etc.

3. Cellular Factors

Once the infective agent has crossed the barrier of epithelial surfaces, the tissue factors come into play for defence.

When an infective agent invades tissue, an exudative inflammatory reaction occurs by accumulation of phagocytes at the site of infection. Phagocytic cells ingest these organisms and destroy them. However, some bacteria (*M. tuberculosis, M. leprae*) resist this type of killing and can multiply within phagocytes and thus produce disease.

II. ACQUIRED IMMUNITY

The resistance acquired by an individual during life is known as acquired immunity. It is of two types, *active* and *passive*.

A. Active Immunity

Active Immunity is subdivided into two types: Natural and Artificial.

Natural—Through clinical or subclinical infection
Artificial—Induced by vaccinatio

Mechanism

Active immune response stimulates both humoral and cell mediated immunity usually in parallel.

(i) Humoral immunity

It is antibody mediated immunity. It depends on the synthesis of antibodies by plasma cells. These cells produce specific circulating antibody which combines specifically with the antigens and modify their activity.

(ii) Cell mediated immunity (CMI)

It depends on T-lymphocytes developed against certain antigens. The cell mediated immunity by sensitised T-lymphocytes is important in resistance to chronic bacterial infections.

Types

(i) Natural active immunity

It is acquired by natural subclinical or clinical infections. Such immunity is **long lasting**. Persons recovering from smallpox infection develop natural active immunity.

(ii) Artificial active immunity

It is produced by **vaccination**. The vaccines are prepared from live, attenuated or killed microorganisms, or their antigens or toxoids. In killed vaccines the organisms are killed by heat, formalin, phenol and alcohol. Toxoids are prepared from bacterial exotoxins inactivated by formalin (formol toxoid) or by alum (alum precipitated toxoid–APT). Toxoids are immunogenic but not toxigenic.

VACCINES

(a) ***Live vaccines***
BCG for tuberculosis
Sabin vaccine for poliomyelitis
MMR vaccine for measles, mumps, rubella

(b) ***Killed vaccines***
TAB for enteric fever
Neural and non-neural vaccines for rabies
Hepatitis B vaccine
Salk vaccine for poliomyelitis
Killed cholera vaccine

(c) ***Bacterial products***
Tetanus toxoid for tetanus
Diphtheria toxoid for diphtheria

B. Passive Immunity

Passive immunity is subdivided into two types: Natural and Artificial.

Natural—Through transplacental maternal IgG antibodies.

Artificial—Through antiserum injection.

Passive immunity is induced in an individual by preformed antibodies (generally in the form of antiserum) against infective agent or toxin. The immune system has no active role in passive immunity. Protection starts immediately after transfer of immune serum. There is no latent period as present in active immunity (Table 7.1). Passive immunity is **short lasting** but is useful **when immunity is required immediately**. Passive immunity is again of two types: natural and artificial.

Natural

It is transferred from the mother to foetus or infant. Transfer of maternal antibodies to foetus transplacentally and to infant through milk (colostrum) protects them till their own immune system matures to function.

Artificial

It is through parenteral administration of antibodies. The agents used for artificial passive immunity are hyperimmune sera of animal or human origin, convalescent sera and pooled human gammaglobulin.

Uses of Passive Immunisation

(i) To provide immediate short term protection in a nonimmune host, faced with the threat of a serious infection.
(ii) For suppression of active immunity which may be injurious. Example is to use Rh immunoglobulins during delivery to prevent immune response to Rh factor in Rh negative mothers with Rh positive babies.
(iii) For treatment of serious infections e.g. diphtheria, gas gangrene.
(iv) Postexposure prophylaxis e.g. rabies.

III. MISCELLANEOUS

A. Combined Immunisation

A combination of active and passive immunisation is employed simultaneously which is known as combined immunisation. Passive immunity provides the protection necessary till the active immunity becomes effective.

B. Local (or Mucosal) Immunity

Local immunity is active at the mucosal surfaces such as intestinal, respiratory or genitourinary mucosa. Natural infection or the live viral vaccine administered orally or intranasally provide local immunity at the site of entry such as gut mucosa and nasal mucosa respectively. A special

Table 7.1: Differentiating Features of Active and Passive Immunity

S. No.	Active Immunity	Passive Immunity
1.	Produced actively by the immune system.	Received passively by the host. The host's immune system does not participate.
2.	Induced by infection or by contact with immunogens.	Conferred by administration of ready-made antibodies.
3.	Long-lasting and effective protection.	Protection short lived and less effective.
4.	Immunity is effective only after a lag period, i.e., time required for generation of antibodies.	Immunity is effective immediately.
5.	Immunological memory present, therefore, subsequent challenge is more effective (booster effect).	No immunological memory. Subsequent administration of antibody is less effective due to immune elimination.
6.	Not applicable in immunodeficient persons.	Applicable in immunodeficient persons.

class of immunoglobulins (IgA) plays an important role in local immunity. One such example is live oral polio vaccine (OPV) in which local immunity is involved.

C. Herd Immunity

It refers to the overall resistance in a community (or herd) towards a pathogen. When herd immunity is low, chances of epidemics increase on introduction of a suitable pathogen. Eradication of any communicable disease depends on development of a high level of herd immunity rather than of immunity in individuals.

KEY POINTS

1. The *Immunity* is defined as resistance exhibited by the host against any foreign antigen including microorganisms.
2. Artificial active immunity may be produced by vaccination.
3. Artificial passive immunity is through parenteral administration of *antibodies* (antiserum).
4. *Herd immunity* refers to the overall resistance in the community.

STUDY QUESTIONS

1. Tabulate the differences between active and passive immunity.
2. Write short notes on:
   (i) Innate immunity (ii) Active immunity (iii) Passive immunity

MULTIPLE CHOICE QUESTIONS (MCQs)

1. Clinical or subclinical infections lead to
   (a) Active natural immunity
   (b) Passive natural immunity
   (c) Active artificial immunity
   (d) Passive artificial immunity
2. Vaccination induces:
   (a) Active natural immunity
   (b) Passive natural immunity
   (c) Active artificial immunity
   (d) Passive artificial immunity
3. Artificial passive immunity may be induced by:
   (a) Antiserum injection
   (b) Vaccination
   (c) Maternal antibodies
   (d) All of the above
4. All of the following are live vaccines except:
   (a) BCG
   (b) Sabin vaccine
   (c) MMR
   (d) TAB vaccine
5. All of the following are killed vaccines except:
   (a) Salk vaccine
   (b) Hepatitis B vaccine
   (c) Non-neural vaccines for rabies
   (d) MMR

ANSWERS (MCQs) ...✓

1. (a) 2. (c) 3. (a) 4. (d) 5. (d)

Antigen

8

An antigen is a substance which, when introduced into a body evokes immune response to produce a specific antibody with which it reacts in an observable manner.

I. TYPES OF ANTIGEN

A. Complete Antigen

These are substances which can induce antibody formation by themselves and can react specifically with these antibodies.

B. Haptens

Haptens are substances which are unable to induce antibody formation on its own but can become immunogenic (capable of inducing antibodies) when covalently linked to proteins called *carrier proteins.*

Antigenic determinant (epitope) is the smallest unit of antigenicity. Antigen possesses a number of these determinants. Each type of determinant induces a specific antibody formation.

II. FACTORS OF ANTIGENICITY

The exact basis of antigenicity is not clear but a number of factors have been implicated which make a substance antigenic. These factors are as follows:

1. Foreignness

An antigen must be foreign to the individual (non-self) to induce an immune response.

2. Size

Larger molecules are highly antigenic whereas low molecular weight is either non-antigenic or weakly antigenic.

3. Chemical Nature

Proteins are more effective antigens.

4. Species Specificity

Tissues of all individuals in a species possess species specific antigens.

5. Isospecificity

A species may be grouped according to the presence of different isoantigens in its members. Blood grouping is one example depending on human erythrocyte antigens (isoantigens).

6. Autospecificity

Self antigens are generally non-antigenic, but there are exceptions.

7. Organ Specificity

Organ specific antigens are confined to a particular organ. Some organs like brain, kidney and lens protein of one species share specificity with that of another species.

8. Heterophile Specificity

The same or closely related antigens present in different tissues of more than one species are known as heterophile antigens. Antibodies to these antigens produced by one species cross react with antigens of other species.

KEY POINTS >>>

1. An *antigen* is a substance which, when introduced into a body evokes immune response to produce a specific antibody with which it reacts in an observable manner.
2. Antigen may be classified as *complete antigen* and *hapten.*

STUDY QUESTION

1. Write short note on Haptens.

MULTIPLE CHOICE QUESTIONS (MCQs)

1. Which is the smallest unit of antigen?
   (a) Haptens
   (b) Epitope
   (c) Isoantigen
   (d) None of the above

ANSWERS (MCQs) ...✓

1. (b)

9 Antibodies—Immunoglobulins

ANTIBODIES

Antibodies or immunoglobulins are specified proteins which are formed by immune system in response to an antigen and react with that antigen specifically.

A. Properties of Antibodies

Chemical nature of antibodies is globulin and they are named as immunoglobulins. Immunoglobulins are mainly synthesised by plasma cells.

B. Structure of Immunoglobulin

An antibody molecule consists of two identical heavy and two identical light chains. The 'heavy' (H) chains are longer and 'light' (L) chains are shorter. Both types of chains are polypeptide in nature. The two heavy chains are held together by disulphide (S—S) bonds. Each light chain is also attached to heavy chain by disulphide bond (Fig. 9.1).

The H chains are structurally and antigenically distinct in different classes of immunoglobulins. Five different classes namely IgG, IgM, IgA, IgD, and IgE are designated depending on presence of heavy chain, gamma (γ), mu (μ), alpha (α), delta (δ) and epsilon (ε) respectively.

The L chains are similar in all classes of immunoglobulins. They are present in two forms: kappa (K) and lambda (L). Each immunoglobulin has either two kappa or two lambda light chains but both (K & L) are never found together in a molecule.

Both L and H chains consist of two portions each, a variable (V) region and a constant (C) region. Antigen combining site is at its aminoterminus which consists of both H and L chains (Fig. 9.1).

C. Immunoglobulin Classes

Characteristics of five immunoglobulins present in human sera are shown in Table 9.1.

1. Immunoglobulin G (IgG) (Fig. 9.2)

(i) IgG is the major serum immunoglobulin (about 80% of the total amount). The normal serum concentration is about 8–16 mg/ml.
(ii) Molecular weight is 150,000 (7S).
(iii) It is the only immunoglobulin that is transported through placenta and provides natural passive immunity to newborn.
(iv) It is distributed equally between the intravascular and extravascular compartments.
(v) IgG appears late but persists for longer period. It appears after the initial immune response which is IgM in nature.
(vi) It participates in precipitation, complement fixation and neutralisation of toxin and viruses.
(vii) It is protective against those microorganisms which are active in the blood and tissues.

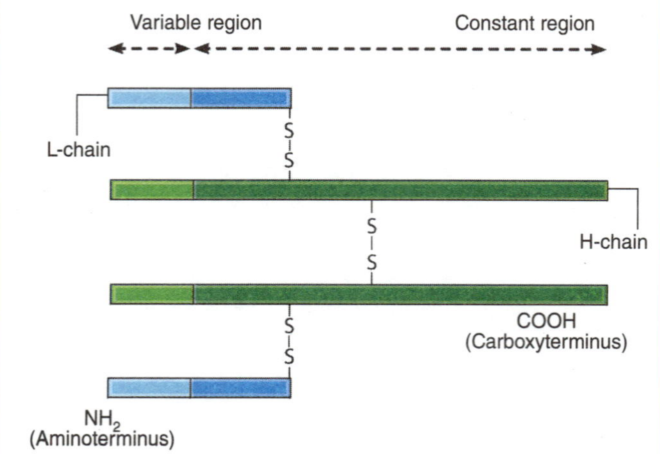

Fig. 9.1 Structure of immunoglobulin

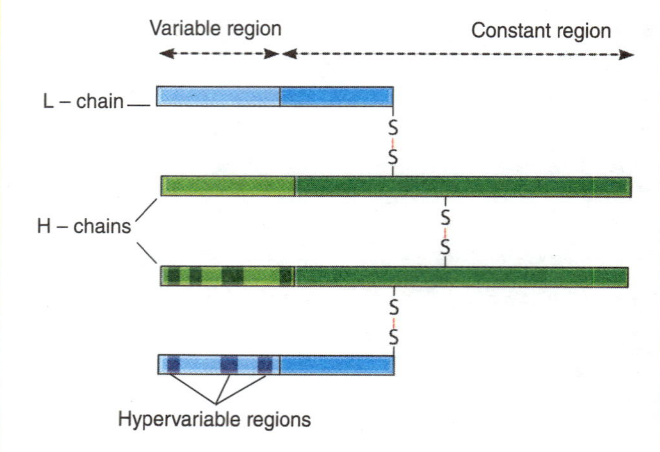

Fig. 9.2 IgG molecule

Table 9.1: Properties of Immunoglobulin Classes

Property	IgG	IgA	IgM	IgD	IgE
Molecular weight	150,000	160,000	900,000	180,000	190,000
Sedimentation coefficient(S)	7	7	19	7	8
Heavy chain	Gamma	Alpha	Mu	Delta	Epsilon
Light chain	K or L	K or L	K or L	K or L	K or L
Serum concentration (mg/ml)	12	2	1.2	0.03	0.00004
Placental transport	+	–	–	–	–
Half life	23 days	6–8 days	5 days	3 days	2–3days
Intravascular distribution(%)	45	42	80	75	50
Present in milk	+	+	–	–	–
Complement fixation					
Classical	++	–	+++	–	–
Alternative	–	+	–	–	–
Selective secretion byseromucous glands	–	+	–	–	–
Heat stability (56°C)	+	+	+	+	–

2. *Immunoglobulin A (IgA)* (Fig. 9.3)

(i) IgA is the second major serum immunoglobulin (about 10–13% of serum immunoglobulins). The normal serum concentration is 0.6–4.2 mg/ml.

(ii) IgA occurs in two forms, serum IgA and secretory IgA.

(iii) Serum IgA is a monomeric 7S molecule (MW 160,000), while IgA found on mucosal surfaces and in secretions (secretory IgA, MW 400,000) is a dimer formed by two monomer units joined together by a glycoprotein named the *J chain* (J for joining).

(iv) Secretory IgA contains another polypeptide called the secretory piece or secretory component.

(v) IgA is the principal immunoglobulin present in secretions such as milk, saliva, tears, sweat, nasal fluids, colostrum and in secretions of respiratory, intestinal and genital systems. It protects the mucous membranes against microorganisms.

(vi) IgA is mainly synthesised locally by plasma cells and little is derived from serum.

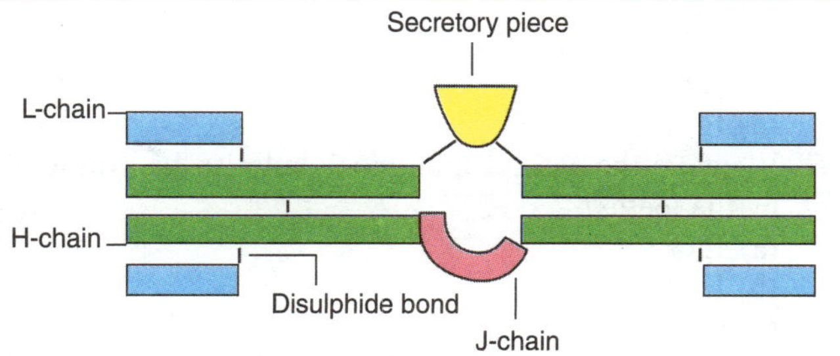

Fig. 9.3 Secretory IgA molecule

3. *Immunoglobulin M (IgM)* (Fig. 9.4)

(i) IgM is a pentamer consisting of 5 immunoglobulin subunits and one molecule of J chain, which joins the Fc region of the basic subunits.

(ii) It constitutes about 5–8 per cent of total serum immunoglobulins. The normal level in serum is 0.5–2 mg/ml.

(iii) It is heavy molecule (19S) with a molecular weight 900,000 to 1,000,000 hence also called the 'millionaire molecule'.

(iv) IgM is mainly distributed intravascularly (80%).

(v) It is the earliest synthesised immunoglobulin by foetus.

(vi) It appears early in response to infection before IgG. IgM antibodies are short lived, and disappear earlier than IgG. Hence, its presence in serum indicates recent infection.

(vii) It cannot cross the placenta, presence of IgM antibody in serum of newborn indicates congenital infection.

(viii) It is very effective antibody in agglutination and complement fixation. It is more efficient than IgG in these reactions.

(ix) IgM provides protection against blood invasion by microorganisms.

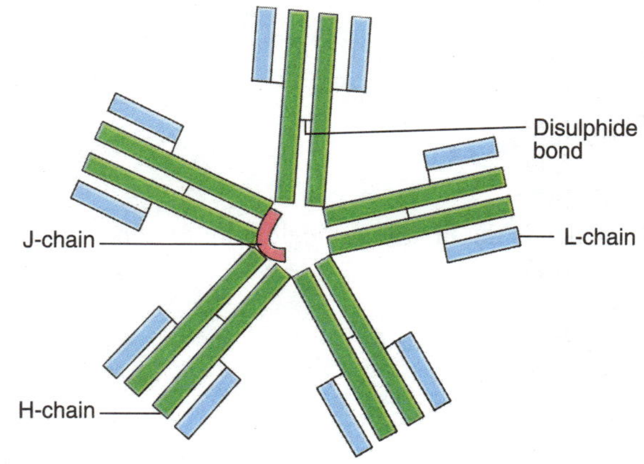

Fig. 9.4 IgM molecule

4. *Immunoglobulin D (IgD)*

(i) IgD resembles IgG structurally.
(ii) IgD is present in a concentration of 3 mg per 100 ml in serum. It is mostly intravascular in distribution.
(iii) Molecular weight is 1,80,000 (7S monomer).

5. *Immunoglobulin E (IgE)*

(i) IgE is mainly produced in the linings of respiratory and intestinal tracts. Serum contains only traces (a few nanograms per ml). It is mostly distributed extravascularly.
(ii) It is also referred to as reagins.
(iii) Molecular weight is 1,90,000 (8S molecule).
(iv) It resembles IgG in structure.
(v) It is heat labile whereas other immunoglobulins are heat stable.
(vi) It has affinity for surface of tissue cells, particularly mast cells of the same species (homocytotropism).
(vii) IgE mediates type I hypersensitivity (atopic) reaction. This is responsible for asthma, hay fever and eczema.
(viii) It cannot cross the placental barrier or fix the complement.
(ix) IgE is responsible for anaphylactic type of reaction.

Role of Different Immunoglobulin Classes

IgG – protects the body fluids
IgA – protects the body surfaces
IgM – protects the blood stream
IgE – mediates reaginic hypersensitivity

KEY POINTS

1. *Antibodies* are substances which are formed in the serum and tissue fluids in response to an antigen and react with that antigen specifically and in some observable manner.
2. There are five different classes of immunoglobulins namely *IgG*, *IgM*, *IgA*, *IgD* and *IgE*.
3. IgG is the major serum immunoglobulin (about 80% of the total amount). It is the only immunoglobulin that is *transported through placenta*.
4. IgA is the principal *immunoglobulin present in secretions* such as milk, saliva, tears, sweat, nasal fluids, colostrum and in secretions of respiratory, intestinal and genital systems.
5. IgM is mainly distributed *intravascularly* (80%). It appears early in response to infection before IgG. It can not cross the placenta, presence of IgM antibody in serum of newborn indicates *congenital infection*.
6. IgE mediates type I *hypersensitivity reactions*.

STUDY QUESTIONS

1. Name the various classes of immunoglobulins. Describe the structure and properties of IgG.
2. Write short notes on:
   (i) IgM (ii) Secretory IgA (iii) IgE.

MULTIPLE CHOICE QUESTIONS (MCQs)

1. Which immunoglobulin class can pass through placenta?
   (a) IgG
   (b) IgM
   (c) IgA
   (d) IgE
2. Which immunoglobulin class is distributed maximum intravascularly?
   (a) IgG
   (b) IgM
   (c) IgA
   (d) IgE
3. J chain is present in:
   (a) IgG
   (b) IgM
   (c) IgD
   (d) IgE
4. Which is the first immunoglobulin to appear in response to an antigen?
   (a) IgG
   (b) IgM
   (c) IgA
   (d) IgE
5. Which immunoglobulin class has maximum concentration in the human body?
   (a) IgG
   (b) IgM
   (c) IgA
   (d) IgE
6. Presence of which immunoglobulin class in serum is a useful indicator for diagnosis of congenital infections?
   (a) IgG
   (b) IgM
   (c) IgA
   (d) IgE
7. Which is the earliest immunoglobulin to be synthesised by the foetus?
   (a) IgG
   (b) IgM
   (c) IgA
   (d) IgE
8. Which immunoglobulin class is involved in type I hypersensitivity reaction?
   (a) IgG
   (b) IgM
   (c) IgA
   (d) IgE

ANSWERS (MCQs)

1. (a) 2. (b) 3. (b) 4. (b) 5. (a) 6. (b) 7. (b) 8. (d)

Antigen-Antibody Reactions 10

I. ANTIGEN-ANTIBODY REACTIONS — *GENERAL FEATURES*

Antigen combines with its specific antibody in an observable manner and the reaction between antigen and antibody is specific.

A. Uses

1. In the Body or in Vivo

(i) It forms the basis of immunity against infectious diseases.

(ii) It may lead to tissue injury in some hypersensitivity reactions and autoimmune diseases.

2. In the Laboratory or in Vitro

(i) For diagnosis of infections

(ii) Detection and quantitation of either antigens or antibodies.

B. Characteristics

1. Reaction is specific, an antigen combines only with its homologous antibody and vice-versa. However, cross reactions may occur due to antigenic similarity.
2. Entire molecules of antigen and antibody react and not the fragments.
3. The reaction is firm, but reversible.

II. TYPES OF ANTIGEN-ANTIBODY REACTIONS

A. Precipitation Reactions

Precipitation

When a soluble antigen reacts with its antibody in the presence of electrolytes (NaCl) at an optimal temperature and pH, the antigen-antibody complex forms an insoluble precipitate and it is called *precipitation*. The precipitate usually sediments at the bottom of the tube.

Flocculation

When instead of sedimenting, the precipitate is suspended as floccules, the reaction is called flocculation. This is a modified form of precipitation.

Prozone Phenomenon

When same amount of antiserum is mixed with increasing quantities of antigen in different tubes, the precipitation takes place in one of the middle tubes, in which antigen and the antibody are present in optimal or equivalent proportion (Zone of equivalence). In the preceding tubes, antibody is in excess and in later tubes, in which antigen is in excess, the precipitation is weak or even absent (Fig. 10.1). Absence of precipitation (false negative) in the presence of excess antibodies is known as prozone phenomenon. This is relevant clinically as these sera should be diluted further to get the proper results of precipitation.

(i) Mechanism of precipitation

Marrack (1934) proposed the lattice hypothesis which is widely accepted. According to this concept, multivalent antigens combine with bivalent antibodies, precipitation occurs only when a large lattice is formed. This occurs in the zone of equivalence. In the zone of antigen excess, the valencies of the antibody are fully satisfied which results in failure to form a large lattice. Similarly, in the zone of antibody excess, the valencies of the antigen are taken up with antibody and results in failure to form a large lattice (Fig. 10.2). This lattice hypothesis holds true for agglutination also.

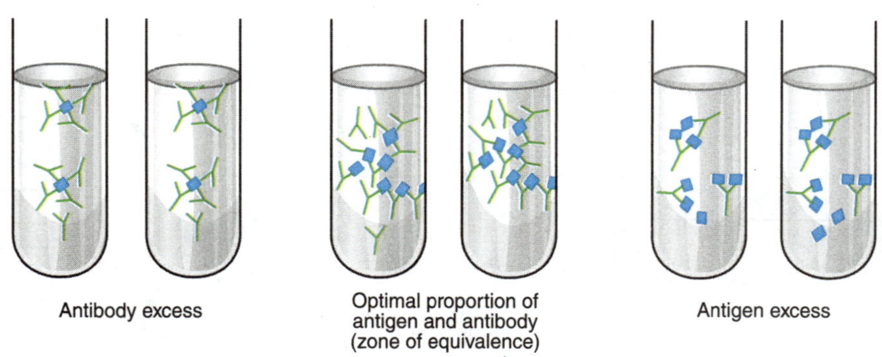

Fig. 10.1 Prozone phenomenon

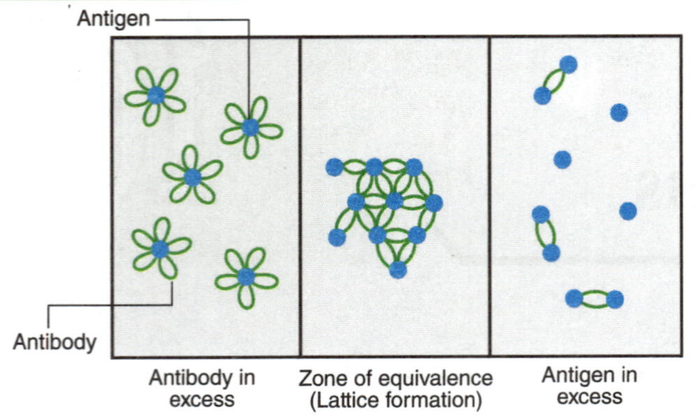

Fig. 10.2 Lattice hypothesis

(ii) Applications of precipitation reaction

Precipitation test has a considerable value in:

1. Identification of bacteria e.g. Lancefield's grouping of *Streptococcus*.
2. Detection of antibody for diagnostic purposes e.g. VDRL in syphilis.

(iii) Types of precipitation reaction

(a) Ring test

Antigen solution is layered over an antiserum in a narrow tube. A precipitate ring appears at the junction of the two liquids. Examples of ring tests are C-reactive protein (CRP) test and streptococcal grouping by the Lancefield technique.

(b) Flocculation test

It can be done in slide and in tube.

Slide test: A drop of antigen solution is added to a drop of inactivated patient's serum on a slide and mixed by shaking, floccules appear. The VDRL test for detection of antibodies against syphilis is an example of slide flocculation test.

Tube test: The Kahn test (tube flocculation) was done previously for diagnosis of syphilis.

(c) Immunodiffusion test

These are precipitation tests in gel. Immunodiffusion is generally done in 1% agar gel.

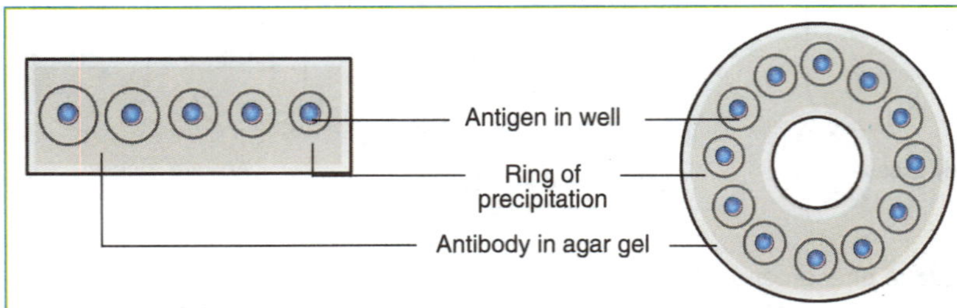

Fig. 10.3 Single diffusion in two dimensions

Various Immunodiffusion Tests

1. Radial Immunodiffusion

The antiserum (antibody) is incorporated in agar gel on a slide or petridish. The wells are cut on the surface of gel. Antigen is added to the wells. The antigen diffuses radially and ring-shaped bands of precipitation (halos) are formed around the well (Fig. 10.3). The diameter of the ring is directly proportional to the concentration of the antigen.

Uses:

It has been widely employed for estimation of immunoglobulin classes, i.e., IgG, IgM, IgA, in sera.

2. Immunoelectrophoresis

Immunoelectrophoresis combines electrophoresis and immunodiffusion. This is done on a glass slide layered with semisolid agar. A well is cut and antigen is filled. The first step is electrophoresis of antigen for about an hour. Rectangular trough is cut in the agar parallel to the direction of migration of antigen and filled with antibody (antiserum). Diffusion is allowed to proceed for 18-24 hours. Precipitation lines develop with each separated component of the antigen. By this technique, a number of antigens can be identified in human serum. It is particularly useful for detection of normal and abnormal serum proteins like myeloma proteins (Fig. 10.4).

3. Electroimmunodiffusion

Immunodiffusion can be speeded up if antigen and antibody are driven by electricity. It is combination of electrophoresis and diffusion. Of these methods, counterimmunoelectrophoresis (CIE or CIEP) is used frequently.

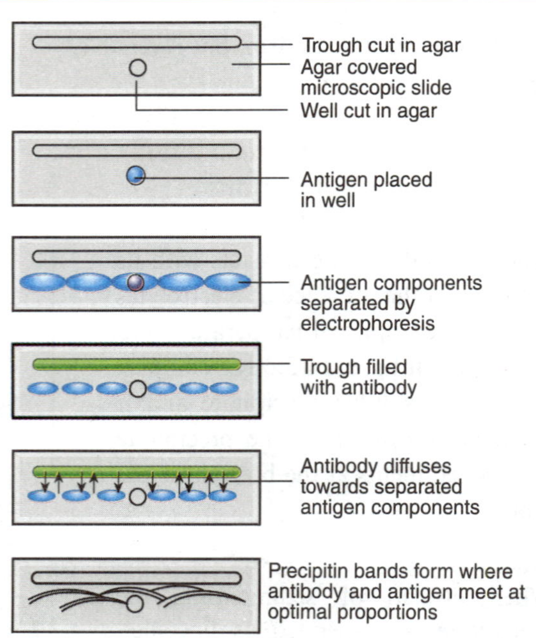

Fig. 10.4 Immunoelectrophoresis

Counterimmunoelectrophoresis (Countercurrent-immunoelectrophoresis, CIE or CIEP)

This test is based on movement of antigen and antibody in opposite direction. This is performed on a glass slide layered with agarose and wells are cut on the surface. One well is filled with antigen and other with antibody. Electric current is passed through the gel. The antigen and antibody move towards each other resulting in a precipitation line at a point between them (Fig. 10.5). It takes about thirty minutes and is more sensitive than standard immunodiffusion technique. It is applied clinically for detecting hepatitis B antigens and antibodies, antigens of cryptococcus in cerebrospinal fluid and in number of other diseases.

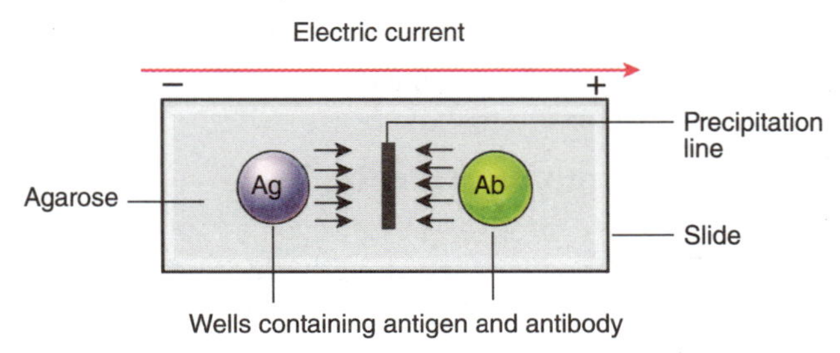

Fig. 10.5 Counterimmunoelectrophoresis

B. Agglutination

It is an antigen-antibody reaction, in which a particulate antigen combines with its antibody in the presence of electrolytes at an optimal temperature and pH, resulting in visible clumping of particles. It differs from precipitation in which soluble antigen is present in contrast to particulate antigen of agglutination. Principles governing agglutination are the same as that of precipitation. Agglutination occurs when antigen and antibody are present in optimal proportions. Lattice formation hypothesis holds good for agglutination too. The zone phenomenon may occur when either an antigen or an antibody is in excess.

Types of Agglutination Reaction

1. Slide Agglutination Test

A uniform suspension of antigen is made in a drop of saline on a slide or tile and a drop of the appropriate antiserum is added. Clumping occurs instantly or within seconds when agglutination test is positive.

Uses:

(i) It is a routine procedure to identify the bacterial strains isolated from clinical specimens. One example is to identify Salmonella species.

(ii) It is also used for blood grouping and cross matching.

2. Tube Agglutination Test

This is a standard quantitative method for determination of antibodies. Serum is diluted serially by doubling dilution in test tubes. An equal volume of a particulate antigen is added to all tubes. The highest dilution of serum at which agglutination occurs is antibody titre. Tube agglutination is routinely employed for antibody detection in diagnosis of typhoid (Widal test), brucellosis and typhus fevers (Weil-Felix reaction).

3. Passive Agglutination Test

A precipitation reaction can be converted into agglutination test by attaching soluble antigens to the surface of carrier particles such as latex particles, bentonite and red blood cells. Such tests are called *passive agglutination* tests. This conversion is done because agglutination tests are more sensitive for detection of antibodies. Passive agglutination tests are very sensitive. When instead of antigen, the antibody is absorbed on the carrier particles for estimation of antigens, it is known as *reversed passive agglutination*.

(i) Latex agglutination test

Polystrene latex particles are employed to adsorb several types of antigens (Fig. 10.6). These tests are very convenient, rapid and specific. These are used for detection of hepatitis B antigen, ASO, CRP, RA factor and many other antigens.

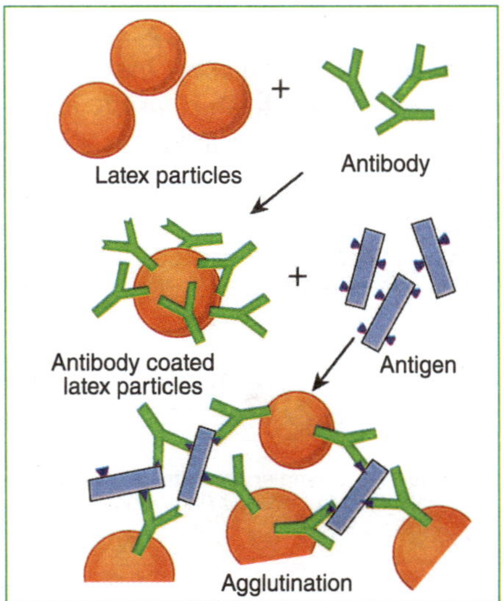

Fig. 10.6 Latex agglutination test

(ii) Haemagglutination test

Instead of latex particles, erythrocytes sensitised with antigen are used for detection of antibodies. It is no longer used.

(iii) Coagglutination

Principle

It is based on the presence of protein A on the surface of some strains of *Staph. aureus* (especially Cowan 1 strain).

Specific IgG immunoglobulin is coated on these Cowan 1 strains of *Staphylococcus aureus*. Fc portion of IgG molecule binds to protein A whereas antigen combining Fab terminal remains free. When the corresponding antigen is mixed with these coated cells, Fab terminal binds to antigen resulting in agglutination (Fig. 10.7). This test was used for detection of bacterial antigens in blood, urine and CSF.

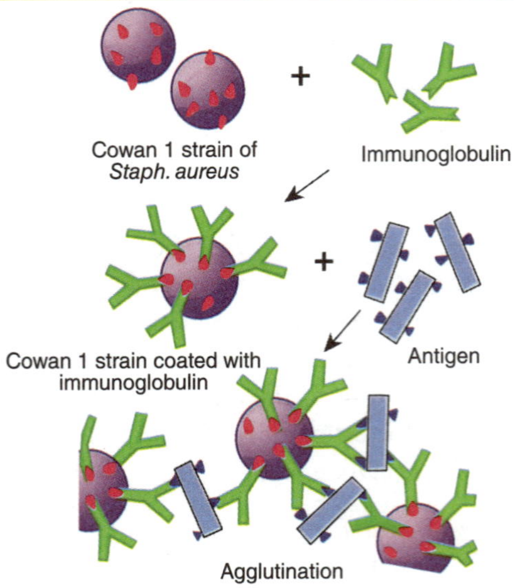

Fig. 10.7 Coagglutination

C. Complement Fixation Test (CFT)

Principle (Fig. 10.8)

The antigen-antibody complexes have ability to 'fix' complement. This reaction has no visible effect. To detect the fixation of complement, an indicator system consisting of sheep erythrocytes coated with amboceptor (rabbit antibody to sheep erythrocytes) is used. Complement can lyse these erythrocytes coated with antibodies. If complement is fixed and utilized in the antigen-antibody reaction, there is no free complement to act on the indicator system and hence no lysis of erythrocytes, which indicates the positive complement fixation test. Lysis of erythrocytes indicates that complement was not fixed in the first step and therefore, the serum is negative for antibodies (negative CFT). Earlier it was commonly used method but is almost not in use now.

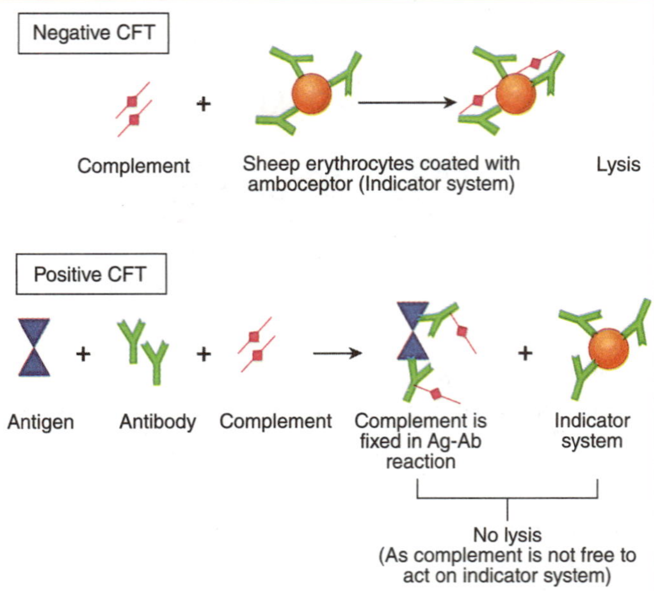

Fig. 10.8 Complement fixation test

D. Immunofluorescence (Fig. 10.9)

Fluorescence is the property of certain dyes which absorb rays of one particular wavelength (ultraviolet light) and emit rays with a different wavelength (visible light). The commonly used fluorescent dyes are *fluorescin isothiocyanate* and *lissamine rhodamine*, exhibiting blue green and orange red fluorescence respectively. Immunofluorescence test is of two types:

1. Direct immunofluorescence test
2. Indirect immunofluorescence test

1. Direct Immunofluorescence Test

Principle

The specific antibodies tagged with fluorescent dye (i.e. labelled antibodies) are used for detection of unknown antigen in a specimen. If antigen is present, it reacts with labelled antibodies and fluorescence can be observed under ultraviolet light of fluorescent microscope (Fig. 10.9).

Uses

1. It is commonly employed for detection of bacteria, viruses or other antigens in blood, CSF, urine, and other specimens.
2. It is a sensitive method to diagnose rabies, by detection of the rabies virus antigens in brain smears.

2. Indirect Immunofluorescence Test

The indirect method is employed for detection of antibodies in serum or other body fluids.

Principle

A known antigen is fixed on a slide. The unknown antibody (serum) is applied to the slide. If antibody (globulin) is present in the serum, it attaches to known antigen on the slide. For detection of this antigen-antibody reaction, fluorescein-tagged antibody to human globulin is added. In positive test, fluorescence occurs under ultraviolet light (Fig. 10.9).

E. Enzyme Linked Immunosorbent Assay (ELISA)

ELISA has been applied widely for detection of a variety of antibodies and antigens. The principle of ELISA is almost the same as that of immunofluorescence, the only

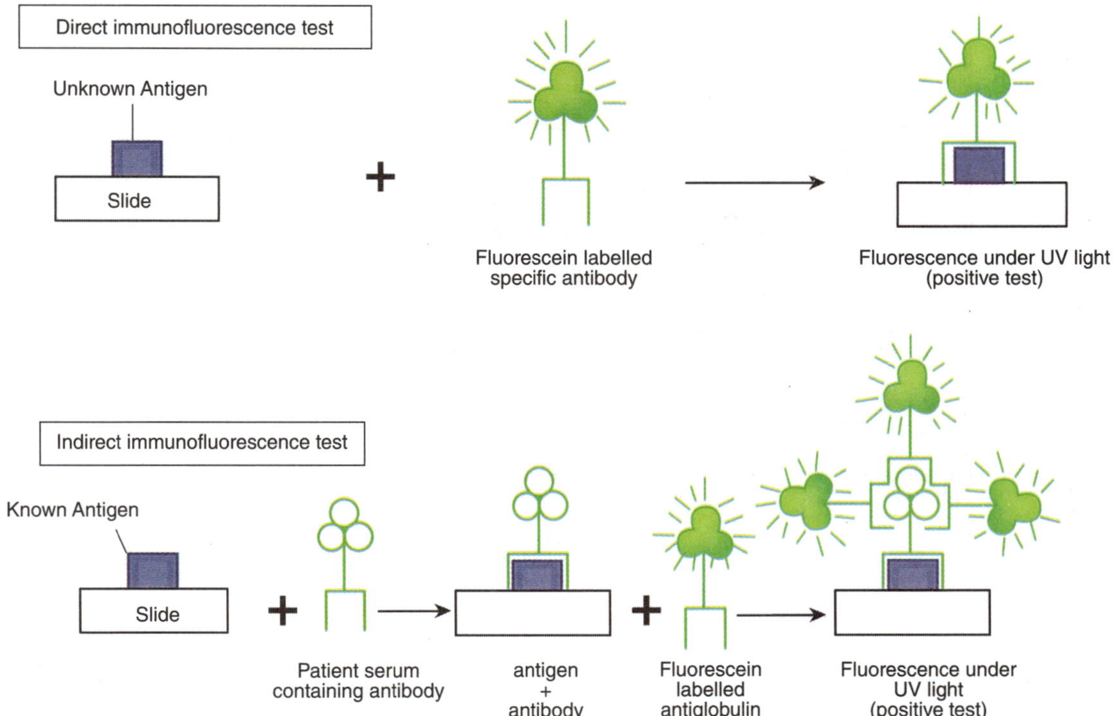

Example :

Treponema pallidum + Serum of syphilis patient (containing anti-treponemal antibodies which is globulin in nature) + Fluorescein labelled antiglobulin → Fluorescence (Positive)

Fig. 10.9 Direct and indirect immunofluorescence tests

difference being, an enzyme is used instead of fluorescent dye. The enzyme acts on substrate to produce a colour in a positive test. The test can be done in polystyrene tubes (macro-ELISA) or polyvinyl microtitre plates (micro-ELISA).

Sandwich ELISA

For antigen detection in a specimen, the wells of microtitre plate are coated with specific antibody against the antigen to be detected. Specimens to be tested are added in coated wells. If antigen is present in specimen, it binds to coated antibody. To detect this antigen-antibody reaction, antiserum (antibody) conjugated with an enzyme is added. This conjugated antiserum binds to an antigen already attached to coated antibody. A substrate is added to know the binding of conjugated antiserum to antigen-antibody complex. In case of binding (positive result), an enzyme acts on substrate to produce colour, intensity of which can be read by spectrophotometer or ELISA reader. Colour detection can also be seen by naked eye. This type of ELISA test is known as sandwich ELISA (Fig. 10.10).

Indirect ELISA

For antibody detection, the wells of microtitre plate are coated with antigen. Sera to be tested are added in these coated wells. If antibody is present in specimen, it binds to coated antigen. To detect this antigen-antibody reaction, a goat antihuman immunoglobulin antibody conjugated with an enzyme is added. Enzyme conjugated antihuman immunoglobulin binds to antibody (immunoglobulin in nature). To detect this binding, a substrate is added and enzyme acts on substrate to produce colour in a positive reaction. This procedure is also named as indirect ELISA (Fig. 10.10). Reading of the test is the same as described in sandwich ELISA.

Competitive ELISA

It has been used for detection of HIV antibodies. Positive result shows no colour whereas appearance of colour indicates a negative test. The microtitre plate wells are coated with HIV antigen. Sera to be tested is added to these wells. If antibodies are present, antigen-antibody reaction occurs. To detect this reaction, enzyme labelled specific HIV antibodies are added. There is no antigen left for these antibodies to act. These antibodies remain free and washed off during washing. Substrate is added but there is no enzyme to act on it. Therefore, positive results show no colour (Fig. 10.10). If serum to be tested is negative for antibodies, antigen is there to combine with enzyme conjugated antibodies and enzyme acts on substrate to produce colour.

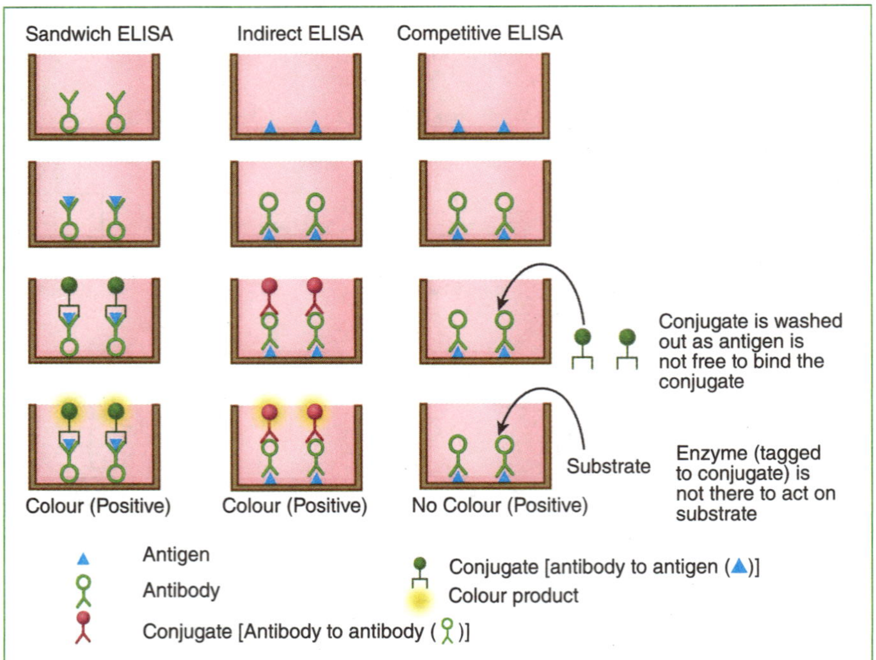

Fig. 10.10 ELISA

Uses of ELISA

It has been used for detection of antigens and antibodies of various microorganisms. Some examples are

(i) Detection of HIV antibodies in serum
(ii) Detection of mycobacterial antibodies in tuberculosis
(iii) Detection of rotavirus in faeces
(iv) Detection of hepatitis B markers in serum.

F. Immunochromatography

Immunochromatography or lateral flow immunoassay is one of the most popular form of rapid immunoassays. It can detect both antigens and antibodies. It has advantage of being a one step test. It can be completed within 30 minute. It is a strip based test. The strip contains a chromatographic pad with three zones: sample pad, conjugate pad and capture line (Fig 10.11). The conjugate pad may be having colloidal gold, dye, or latex beads as conjugate which produces signal. The specimen is applied to the sample pad and flows laterally by capillary action. Upon reaching the conjugate pad, it may bind to conjugate if antigen or antibody is present in the specimen and forms antigen antibody complex. This complex then flow laterally to reach capture line. Here it is captured by antigen or second antibody present in the capture line. The presence of colour line is a positive test. There is a positive control line also to check that the test was properly performed.

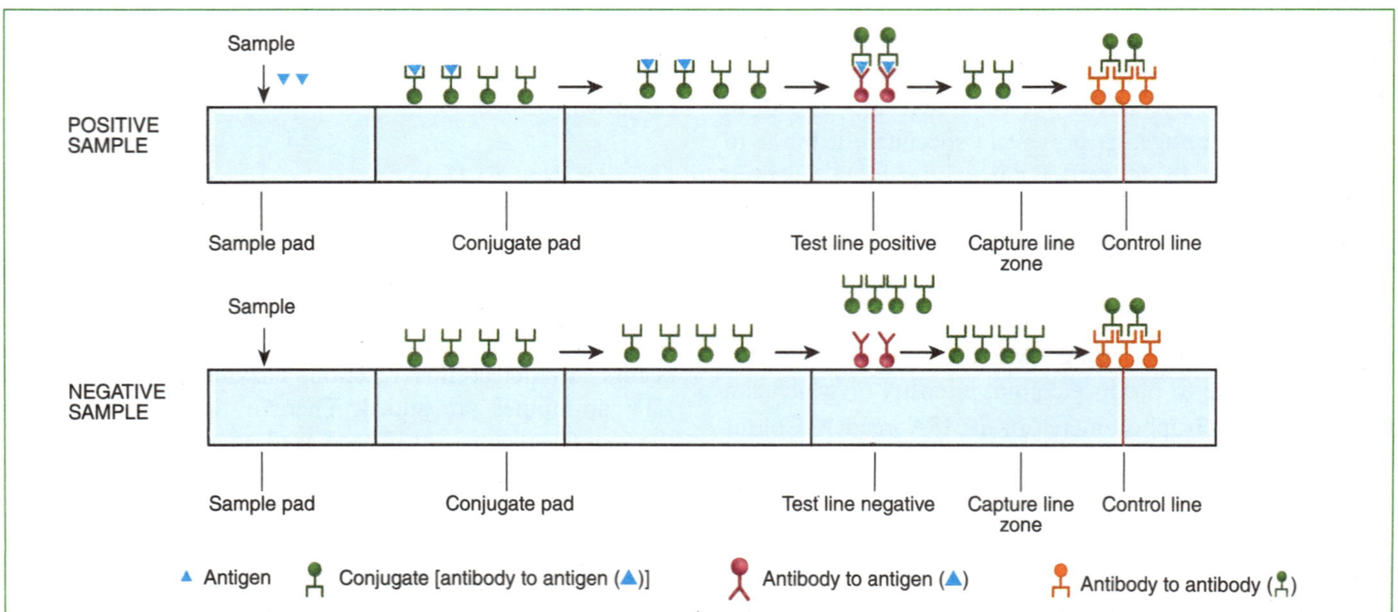

Fig. 10.11 Immunochromatography strip for antigen detection in sample

KEY POINTS

1. There are various types of antigen-antibody reactions. Some of these include *precipitation, agglutination, complement fixation test, immunofluorescence* and *enzyme linked immunosorbent assay (ELISA).*
2. When a soluble antigen reacts with its antibody in the presence of electrolytes (NaCl) at an optimal temperature and pH, the antigen-antibody complex forms an insoluble precipitate and it is called *precipitation.* When instead of sedimenting, the precipitate is suspended as floccules, the reaction is called *flocculation.* This is a modified form of precipitation.
3. *Agglutination* is an antigen-antibody reaction, in which a particulate antigen combines with its antibody in the presence of electrolytes at an optimal temperature and pH, resulting in visible clumping of particles. It differs from precipitation in which soluble antigen is present in contrast to particulate antigen of agglutination.
4. *Passive agglutination reaction* is a precipitation reaction which has been converted into agglutination test by attaching soluble antigens to the surface of carrier particles such as *latex particles*, and *red blood cells.*
5. Immunofluorescence test is of two types: *direct immunofluorescence test* and *indirect immunofluorescence test.* The antibodies tagged with fluorescent dye (i.e., labelled antibodies) are used in these tests.
6. Enzyme linked immunosorbent assay (ELISA) has been applied widely for detection of a variety of antibodies and antigens.

STUDY QUESTIONS

1. Name various antigen-antibody reactions and describe the principle and application of precipitation reactions.
2. Define agglutination reaction. Discuss the principle and application of agglutination reactions.
3. Write short notes on:
   (i) CIEP (ii) Latex agglutination test (iii) CFT.
4. Discuss briefly about:
   (i) Immunofluorescence tests (ii) ELISA.

MULTIPLE CHOICE QUESTIONS (MCQs)

1. Which immunoglobulin class is the most efficient to produce agglutination reaction?
   (a) IgG
   (b) IgM
   (c) IgA
   (d) IgE
2. Which immunoglobulin class is the most efficient to produce precipitation reaction?
   (a) IgG
   (b) IgM
   (c) IgA
   (d) IgE
3. VDRL test is an example of:
   (a) Agglutination test
   (b) Flocculation test
   (c) Immunofluorescence
   (d) All of the above
4. Counterimmunoelectrophoresis is used for detecting:
   (a) Hepatitis B antigens
   (b) Cryptococcal antigens
   (c) *Neisseria meningitidis*
   (d) All of the above
5. Tube agglutination test is used for serological diagnosis of:
   (a) Enteric fever
   (b) Infectious mononucleosis
   (c) Typhus fever
   (d) All of the above
6. Which of the following is/are example/s of passive agglutination test?
   (a) Latex agglutination test
   (b) Haemagglutination test
   (c) Coagglutination
   (d) All of the above
7. Which of the following is/are example/s of neutralisation test?
   (a) Schick test
   (b) Antistreptolysin 'O' test
   (c) Nagler reaction
   (d) All of the above
8. ELISA can be used for detection of antigens and / or antibodies in:
   (a) HIV
   (b) Rotavirus
   (c) Hepatitis B virus
   (d) All of the above

ANSWERS (MCQs)

1. (b) 2. (a) 3. (b) 4. (d) 5. (d) 6. (d) 7. (d) 8. (d)

11 Complement System

COMPLEMENT

The 'complement' (C) refers to a system of some non-specific proteins present in normal human and animal serum, which are activated characteristically by antigen-antibody reaction and subsequently lead to a number of biologically significant consequences. C ordinarily does not combine with either free antigen or antibody, but only with antigen-antibody complex.

A. Components of Complement

There are nine components of complement called C1 to C9. The component C1 is made up of three protein subunits named C1q, C1r and C1s.

Complement is normally present in circulation in inactive form, but when its activity is induced by antigen-antibody reaction or other stimuli, complement components react in a specific sequence as a cascade either through the classical or alternative pathway. Both the pathways have same result i.e. lysis or damage of target cell.

B. Classical Pathway

Complement components react in a specific sequence, following activation by antigen-antibody complex, and results in immune cytolysis. This is known as the classical pathway of complement (Fig. 11.1).

The traditional model used to explain C activity for immune cytolysis is the lysis of erythrocytes sensitised by its antibodies. The erythrocyte (E)-antibody (A) complex is named EA and later on, when C components are attached to EA, it is called EAC.

Immune cytolysis is initiated by the binding of component C1 to EA. C1q is the recognition unit of C1, hence, C1q reacts with the Fc piece of bound antibody molecule (IgM or IgG) in EA. The binding of C1q in the presence of calcium ions leads to activation of C1r and C1s. The activated C1s is an esterase which splits C4 into C4a and C4b, of which C4b joins the cascade. C14b in presence of magnesium ions act on C2 and forms C2a and C2b. The larger fragment C2a attaches to C4 to form (C42) which has enzymatic activity and is called *C3 convertase*. The other C2 fragments possess kinin like activity and increase vascular permeability. C$\overline{42}$ splits C3 into C3a and C3b, of which, C3b joins the cascade. C3a has chemotactic and anaphylatoxic properties. C$\overline{14b2a3b}$ has enzymatic activity and is referred to as *C5 convertase*. It acts on C5, to split it into C5a (anaphylatoxic and chemotactic) and C5b which joins the cascade. C6 and C7 join to form C567, some of which binds to cell membrane and prepares the cell for lysis by C8 and C9. Most of C$\overline{567}$ absorb to unsensitised 'bystander' cells and making them susceptible to lysis by C8 and C9. In this way, C567 serves to amplify the reaction. The unbound C$\overline{567}$complex has chemotactic and leucocyte activating properties. The lysis is done by producing 'holes' approximately 100°A in diameter on cell membrane. This disrupts the osmotic integrity of the cell membrane which results into release of the contents of the cell.

C. Alternative Pathway of Complement Activation

The activation of C3 has the major role in the complement cascade. In the classical pathway, C3 activation occurs by classical C3 convertase (C$\overline{142}$). This activation of C3 without help of C142, is known as the 'alternative pathway'.

The alternative pathway contributes to antimicrobial defence without requiring specific antibodies. A wide range of substances (activators) are known to activate alternative pathway. These include bacterial endotoxins, yeast cell walls, IgA and the cobra venom factor. The binding of C3b to an activator is the first step in the alternative pathway. Although C3b is present in the circulation but in the free state it is rapidly inactivated by the serum protein factors H and I. However, bound C3b is protected from such inactivation.

The bound C3b, in the presence of Mg^{++}, interacts with plasma protein factor B forming C3bB. The factor B portion of C3bB complex is split by factor D into Ba and Bb. Bb fragment binds to C3b forming C3bBb. This C3bBb is C3 convertase of alternative pathway (Fig. 11.2). This enzyme is extremely labile. The properdin or factor P helps to stabilise the enzyme C3 convertase. C3 convertase splits more C3 to C3a and C3b. C3b fragment binds to $\overline{\text{C3bBb}}$ to form $\overline{\text{C3bBb3b}}$ which is C5 convertase. The newly formed C3b also binds more factor B. The alternative pathway then proceeds from C5 convertase to C9 in the similar way as that occurs in the classical pathway.

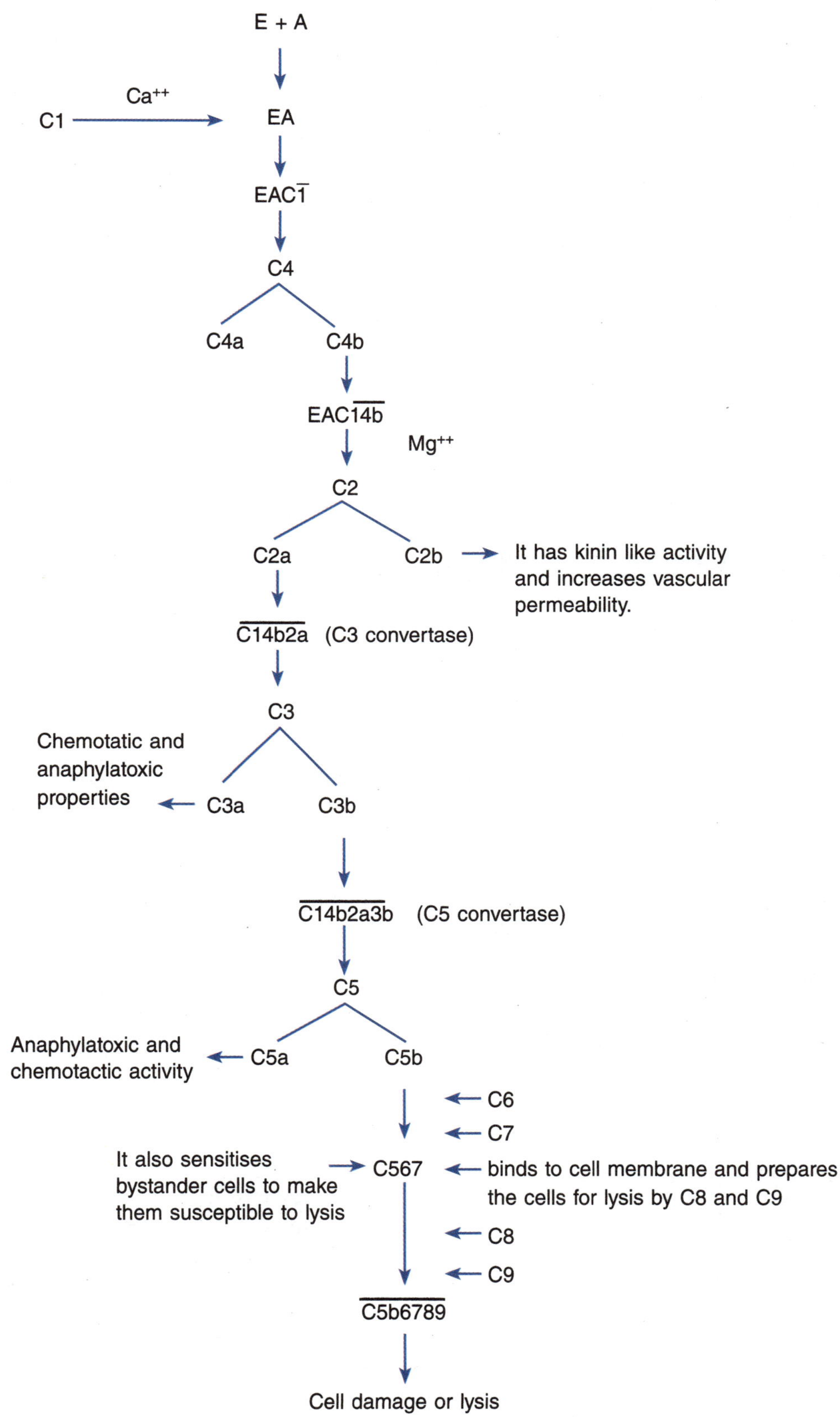

Fig. 11.1 The classical pathway of complement

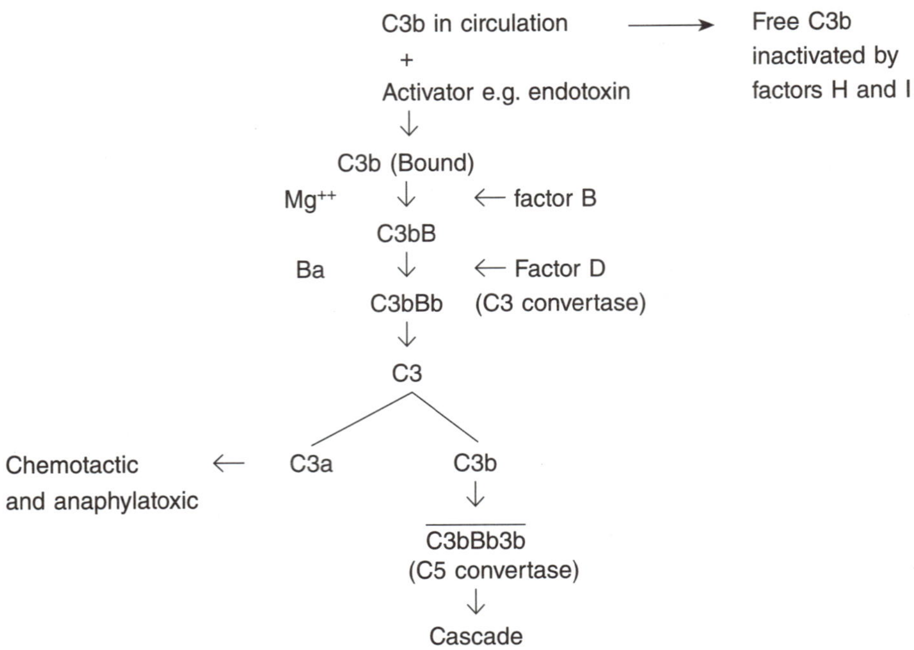

After this, remaining reaction (C5 convertase) is the same as that in the classical pathway (Fig. 11.1).

Fig. 11.2 Alternative pathway of complement

KEY POINTS

1. Complement components react in a specific sequence as a cascade either through the *classical* or *alternative pathway*.
2. Classical pathway is triggered by specific antigen-antibody complex; the alternative pathway can be initiated by *bacterial endotoxin*, *IgA* or *yeast cell wall*.

STUDY QUESTIONS

1. Discuss briefly the classical pathway of complement activation.
2. Write short note on alternative pathway of complement.

MULTIPLE CHOICE QUESTIONS (MCQs)

1. Classical pathway of the complement is activated by:
   (a) Antigen
   (b) Antibody
   (c) Antigen-Antibody complex
   (d) None of the above
2. The alternative pathway of the complement is initiated by:
   (a) Endotoxins
   (b) Lipopolysaccharides
   (c) Yeast cell walls
   (d) All of the above
3. First component of complement which binds to antigen-antibody complex in classical pathway is:
   (a) C1q
   (b) C1r
   (c) C1s
   (d) C3
4. Which component of complement is present in the highest concentration in the serum?
   (a) C1
   (b) C2
   (c) C3
   (d) C5

ANSWERS (MCQs)

1. (c) 2. (d) 3. (a) 4. (c)

Structure and Functions of Immune System

12

The lymphoreticular system is responsible for immune response and it consists of lymphoid and reticuloendothelial components. The lymphoid cells (lymphocytes and plasma cells) are responsible for specific immunity. The phagocytic cells (polymorpho-nuclear leucocytes and macrophages) which are part of reticuloendothelial system, are mainly concerned with scavenger functions, of eliminating micro-organisms and other foreign particles from blood and tissue, thus contributing to non-specific immunity.

I. THE LYMPHOID SYSTEM

Lymphoid cells
- e.g. Lymphocytes
  - Plasma cells

Lymphoid organs

A. Central (Primary) lymphoid organs
- e.g. Thymus
  - Bursa of Fabricius in birds
  - Bone marrow in mammals

B. Peripheral (Secondary) lymphoid organs
- e.g. Spleen
  - Lymph nodes
  - Mucosa associated lymphoid tissue (MALT)
  - Lymphoid tissues in gut, lungs, liver, bone marrow

Types of Immune Response

The specific immune response to an antigen can be of two types:

1. The humoral or antibody mediated immunity (HMI or AMI)
   It is mediated by antibodies which are produced by plasma cells.
2. The cell-mediated immunity (CMI)
   It is mediated by sensitised lymphocytes.

The central lymphoid organs are structures in which precursor lymphocytes proliferate, develop and become immunologically competent. After acquiring immunological capabilities, the lymphocytes migrate to peripheral lymphoid organs, where appropriate immune response occurs when exposed to an antigen.

Cells of Lymphoreticular System

These consist of structural cells (reticulum cells, endothelial cells and fibroblasts) and immunologically competent cells (lymphocytes, plasma cells and macrophages). In the circulating blood, about 70% lymphocytes are T-lymphocytes ('T' for thumus dependent), 20% B-lymphocytes ('B' for Bursa or Bone marrow) and 10% Null Cells.

Lymphocytes which are 'educated' by the central lymphoid organs become *immunologically competent cells* (ICCs). They are fully equipped to deal against an antigen. They serve the following functions:

1. Recognition of antigens ('R' for recognition).
2. Storage of immunological memory ('R' for remembrance or memory).
3. Immune response to antigens ('R' for response).

The nature of immune response depends on the type of cells stimulated by an antigen. Stimulated T-cells produce certain activation products (lymphokines) and induce CMI, while stimulated B-cells divide and transform into plasma cells which synthesise antibodies and induce HMI.

1. Lymphocytes

(i) T-lymphocytes

T-lymphocytes can be classified into different *subpopulations* or *subsets* as follows:

T helper (CD4) cells

T helper cells facilitate B cell response to produce immunoglobulins. Balanced activity of helper and suppressor T-cells produces optimum immune response. Helper cells are about 65 per cent and suppressor cells about 35 percent of circulating T-lymphocytes.

Cytotoxic T (Tc) cells

These cells can lyse specific target cells whose surface antigens are recognised by them e.g. virally infected cells, tumour cells. Cytotoxic T cells possess membrane glycoprotein CD8.

Regulatory T cells

Regulatory T cells (T reg cells) formerly known as suppressor T cells which regulate the immune response by their action on T helper or B cells. These cells also provide tolerance to self antigen and thus prevent development of autoimmune diseases.

(ii) Null Cells

The small proportion of lymphocytes which are neither T-cells nor B-cells are known as *null cells*. Among the null cells, killer cells (K cells) and natural killer (NK) cells are recognised. K cells are now classified with NK cells.

(a) Killer Cells (K Cells)

These cells are capable of killing target cells sensitised with IgG antibodies. They do not require complement for such lysis or killing. These are responsible for antibody dependent cell mediated cytotoxicity (ADCC). This antibody dependent cell mediated cytotoxicity differs from the action of cytotoxic T lymphocytes, which is independent of antibody.

(b) Natural Killer Cells (NK Cells)

Action of NK cells is independent of antibody in contrast to K cells which are dependent on antibody. Their activity is 'natural' or 'nonimmune' as it does not require sensitisation by prior antigenic contact. It is believed that NK cells play an important role in antiviral and antitumour immunity.

(iii) B-Lymphocytes and Plasma Cells

Antigenically stimulated B-lymphocytes undergo blast transformation to become plasma cells. A plasma cell can synthesise an antibody of single specificity, of a single immunoglobulin class (IgM or IgG or IgA). An exception is seen in primary immune response, when a plasma cell synthesising IgM initially, may later switch over to IgG production.

2. Phagocytic Cells

The phagocytic cells are the mononuclear macrophages (of blood and tissues) and the polymorphonuclear microphages.

(i) Macrophages

Tissue macrophages (histiocytes) are named as alveolar macrophages in the lungs and Kupffer cells in the liver.

Functions

(1) Phagocytosis

The primary function of macrophages is phagocytosis.

(2) Specific immune response

(i) They trap and process bacterial antigens and present them in optimal concentration to the lymphocytes for induction of specific immune response.

(ii) Activated macrophages secrete IL-1 which induces T-cells to synthesise IL-2. IL-2 facilitates T-cell activation and thus initiate CMI. Activated T-cells also help B-cells to form antibodies.

(ii) Microphages

The microphages contain polymorphonuclear leucocytes (neutrophils, eosinophils and basophils) of blood.

(a) Neutrophils

They have non-specific phagocytic property. They play a prominent role in acute inflammation.

(b) Eosinophils

Eosinophils are less phagocytic than neutrophils. They are found in large numbers in allergic inflammation and parasitic infections.

(c) Basophils

They are present in blood and tissues (mast cells). Degranulation of mast cells release pharmacologically active agents resulting in anaphylaxis and atopic allergy.

II. MAJOR HISTOCOMPATIBILITY COMPLEX (MHC)

The major histocompatibility complex (MHC) in humans is known as the human leucocyte antigen (HLA) complex.

The HLA Complex

Histocompatibility antigens mean cell surface antigens that evoke immune response to an incompatible host resulting in allograft rejection. These alloantigens are present on surface of leucocytes in man and are called human leucocyte antigens (HLA) and the set of genes coding for them is named the *HLA Complex*.

The HLA complex of genes is grouped in three classes.

Class I — HLA-A, HLA-B and HLA-C

Class II — HLA-DR, HLA-DQ and HLA-DP (All of these are present within HLA-D region of HLA complex.)

Class III — Complement loci encode for C2, C4 and Factor B of complement system and tumour necrosis factors (TNF) alpha and beta.

1. Class I MHC Antigens (A, B, C)

The MHC class I antigens are present on the surface of all nucleated cells. They are involved in graft rejection and cell mediated cytolysis. The cytotoxic T cells (CD8) recognise MHC class I antigens for their action.

2. Class II MHC Antigens (DR, DQ and DP)

They have a very limited distribution and are principally

found on the surface of macrophages, monocytes, activated T-lymphocytes (CD4) and B-lymphocytes. They are primarily responsible for the graft-versus-host response.

3. Class III MHC Antigens

Class III genes encode C2, C4 complement components of the classical pathway and properdin factor B of the alternative pathway.

KEY POINTS »»

1. The nature of immune response depends on the type of cells stimulated by an antigen. Stimulated *T-cells* produce certain activation products (lymphokines) and induce cell mediated immunity (CMI), while stimulated B-cells divide and transform into plasma cells which synthesise antibodies and induce humoral immunity.
2. On the basis of functions, T cells can be classified into *T helper (CD4)* cells and *T suppressor (CD8) cells.*

STUDY QUESTION

1. Write short notes on:
   (i) T-lymphocytes
   (ii) Major histocompatibility complex.

MULTIPLE CHOICE QUESTIONS (MCQs)

1. CD4 antigen is present on:
   (a) T-helper cells
   (b) Macrophages
   (c) Monocytes
   (d) All of the above
2. CD8 antigen is present on:
   (a) T helper cells
   (b) T suppressor cells
   (c) Both of the above
   (d) None of the above
3. Natural killer cells play an important role in:
   (a) Antiviral activity
   (b) Antitumour activity
   (c) Allograft rejection
   (d) All of the above

ANSWERS (MCQs) ...✓

1. (d) 2. (b) 3. (d)

13 Immune Response

INTRODUCTION

The specific reactivity induced in a host following an antigen stimulus is known as the immune response. It is of two types:

1. *Humoral or antibody mediated immunity*
2. *Cell-mediated Immunity.*

Antibody mediated immunity (AMI) provides primary defence against most extracellular bacteria and helps in defence against viruses those infect through respiratory or intestinal tracts. AMI also participates in the pathogenesis of **immediate (type I, II and III) hypersensitivity** and certain autoimmune diseases. Cell mediated immunity (CMI) protects against fungi, viruses and intracellular bacteria like *M. tuberculosis*, *M. leprae* and parasites such as *Leishmania* and trypanosomes. It plays an important role in pathogenesis of **delayed (type IV) hypersensitivity** and certain autoimmune diseases. It also provides immunity against cancer. Both AMI and CMI usually develop together, though at times one or other may be the predominant type.

I. HUMORAL IMMUNE RESPONSE

Antibody production follows a characteristic pattern (Fig. 13.1) which consists of:

1. ***a lag phase***—The immediate stage following antigenic stimulation when no antibody is detectable in circulation.
2. ***a log phase***—There is steady rise in titre of antibodies.
3. ***a plateau***—There is an equilibrium between antibody synthesis and catabolism.
4. ***the phase of decline***—Catabolism exceeds the production and the titre falls.

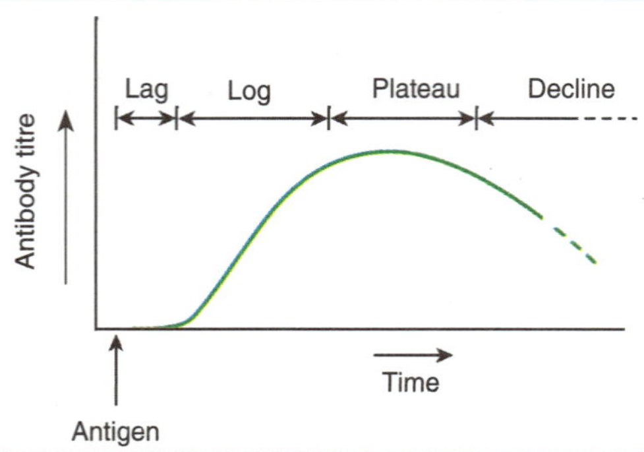

Fig. 13.1 Primary humoral response

A. Primary and Secondary Humoral Responses

The primary humoral response has a long lag phase and low titre of antibodies that do not persist for long. In contrast, the secondary humoral response has a short or negligible lag phase and a much higher level of antibodies that last for long periods. (Fig. 13.2). The antibody formed in the primary humoral response is predominantly IgM and in secondary humoral response IgG.

B. Production of Antibodies

B cells undergo clonal proliferation and differentiate into plasma cells that synthesise and secrete antibodies. B cells carry surface receptors which consist of IgM or other immunoglobulin classes. Depending upon these receptors, a plasma cell secretes an antibody of a single specificity of a single antibody class (IgM, IgG or any other single class). However, in primary humoral response, plasma cells initially secrete IgM and later switching over to form IgG. Following antigenic stimulus, not all B-lymphocytes get converted into plasma cells. A small proportion of them develop into 'memory cells' which have a long lifespan and can recognise the same antigen on subsequent exposure. The increased antibody response during secondary antigenic

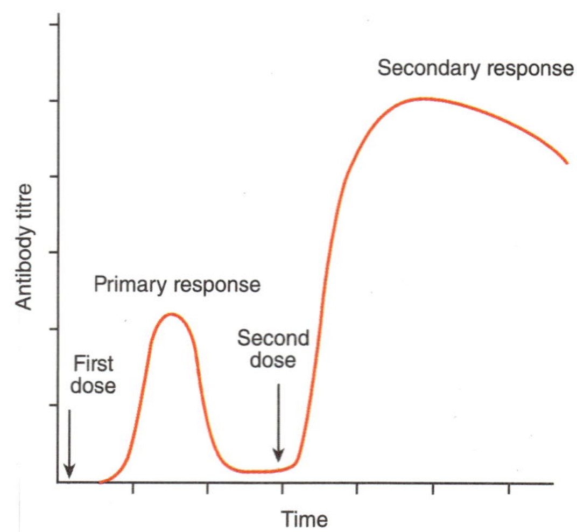

Fig. 13.2 Primary and secondary humoral response

stimulus is due to the memory cells induced by the primary contact with the antigen.

Antibody production by B lymphocytes is regulated by T cells. Helper T cells (TH) stimulate and suppressor T cells (TS) inhibit antibody production. Optimum antibody response depends on the balanced activity of these TS and TH cells.

C. Theories of Antibody Formation

There are two broad groups:

1. Instructive theories
2. Selective theories.

The instructive theories postulate that an immunocompetent cell (ICC) is capable of synthesising antibodies of all specificity. The antigen instructs ICC to produce the complementary antibody. Selective theories, on the contrary, postulate that ICCs have only a restricted immunological range. The antigen selects the appropriate ICC to synthesise an antibody. The most accepted theory is 'clonal salection theory'.

Clonal selection theory

This theory was proposed by Burnet (1957). The theory states that during foetal development a large number of clones of immunological competent cells (ICCs) bearing specific antibody patterns are produced by a process of somatic mutation of ICCs against all possible antigens. Clones of cells with immunological reactivity with self antigens are eliminated during embryonic life. Such clones are known as 'forbidden clones'. Persistence of forbidden clones or their development in later life by somatic mutation lead to autoimmune processes. Each ICC is capable of reacting with one antigen or a small number of antigens. Contact with specific antigen leads to cellular proliferation to form clones synthesising the antibody. The clonal selection theory is widely accepted nowadays.

D. Monoclonal Antibodies

1. *Principle*

Antibodies that are usually produced in response to a single antigen are heterogenous as they are synthesised by several different clones of cells, i.e., polyclonal. A single antibody forming cell or clone produces antibodies directed against a single antigen or antigenic determinant only and such antibodies are called monoclonal antibodies.

Antibody forming spleen cells are fused with myeloma cells to produce hybrid cells (hybridomas). The resultant hybridoma retains the antibody producing capacity of the spleen cells and the ability of myeloma cells to multiply indefinitely.

2. *Applications*

(i) ***Diagnostic Use:*** Many commercial diagnostic systems use monoclonal antibodies for identification of bacterial, viral and other antigens. Direct fluorescence and enzyme-linked assays utilise monoclonal antibody conjugates.

(ii) ***Pure antibody:*** Large amount of pure antibody of defined class can be prepared.

II. CELL MEDIATED IMMUNE RESPONSES

The term cell mediated immunity refers to specific acquired immune responses mediated by sensitised T cells. This form of immunity can be transferred from donor to recipient with intact lymphocytes, but not with antisera, hence it is called *cell mediated immune reaction*. Cell mediated immunity (CMI) plays an important role in the following immunological functions:

1. delayed hypersensitivity (type IV hypersensitivity)
2. immunity in infectious diseases caused by intracellular organisms
3. immunological surveillance and immunity against cancer
4. pathogenesis of certain autoimmune diseases e.g. thyroiditis

A. Induction of CMI

Foreign antigen is presented by antigen presenting cells (APCs) to T-lymphocytes. These sensitised T-lymphocytes undergo blast transformation, clonal proliferation and differentiation into memory cells and effector cells (Th, Tc, Td and Ts). The activated lymphocytes release biologically active products (lymphokines) which are responsible for various manifestations of CMI.

B. Cytokines

These are biologically active substances secreted by monocytes, lymphocytes and other cells. They are named lymphokines if they are derived from lymphocytes and monokines if they are derived from monocytes and macrophages. Interleukins are chemical substances that function primarily as growth and differentiating factors. They exert a regulatory influence on other cells. All these biologically active substances (lymphokines, monokines interleukins) are collectively known as cytokines. They are not specific for antigens.

III. IMMUNOLOGICAL TOLERANCE

Immunological tolerance is defined as a state in which contact with an antigen specifically abolishes the capacity to mount an immune response against that particular antigen when it is administered subsequently, the immune reactivity to other antigens being unaffected.

KEY POINTS »»

1. The specific reactivity induced in a host following an antigen stimulus is known as the *immune response*.
2. *Immune response* is of two types: *humoral immunity* and *cell mediated immunity*.
3. Humoral immunity is due to *antibody* production while cell immunity is because of sensitised T cells.
4. *Hybridoma* technique is used to produce monoclonal antibodies.

STUDY QUESTION

1. Write short notes on:
   (i) Humoral immune response
   (ii) Monoclonal antibodies.

MULTIPLE CHOICE QUESTIONS (MCQs)

1. The widely accepted theory of antibody formation is:
   (a) Direct template theory
   (b) Indirect template theory
   (c) Natural selection theory
   (d) Clonal selection theory
2. The animal used for monoclonal antibodies production is:
   (a) Mouse
   (b) Guinea pig
   (c) Rabbit
   (d) None of the above
3. The technique used for monoclonal antibodies production is called:
   (a) Hybridoma
   (b) Rosette formation
   (c) Opsonisation
   (d) Immunofluorescence

ANSWERS (MCQs) ...✓

1. (d) 2. (a) 3. (a)

Hypersensitivity

14

Immune response is generally a protective process but it may sometimes be injurious to the host. Hypersensitivity refers to a condition in which immune response results in excessive reactions leading to tissue damage, disease or even death in the sensitised host.

I. CLASSIFICATION

Hypersensitivity reactions are classified into two main types, 'immediate' and 'delayed' types. The major differences between the two hypersensitivity reactions are shown in Table 14.1.

Coomb and Gel (1963) classified hypersensitivity reactions into four major types, types I to IV.

Type I (Anaphylactic)
Type II (Cytotoxic)
Type III (Immune complex)
Type IV (Delayed or cell mediated).

Type I, II and III depend on the interaction of antigen with humoral antibodies and are known as immediate type reactions. Type IV reaction is mediated by T-lymphocytes. Reaction develops in 24 to 72 hours and is called delayed hypersensitivity reaction.

Type I (Anaphylactic) Hypersensitivity Reaction

Type I hypersensitivity reactions occur in two forms—the acute, potentially fatal, **systemic form** called **anaphylaxis** and the recurrent non-fatal **localised form** called **atopy**.

1. Mechanism of Anaphylaxis

Anaphylaxis occurs when a sensitised individual comes in contact with a shocking dose of antigen. An interval of 2-3 weeks is required between sensitising and shocking dose, during which antibody IgE (previously known as reagnic antibody) produced against the antigen attaches to surface receptors of mast cells and basophils. When a shocking dose of the same or immunologically related antigen is given, the antigen combines with cell bound IgE antibody on mast cells rapidly. The antigen-antibody complex stimulates mast cells and basophils to release mediators that cause clinical manifestations of anaphylaxis (Fig. 14.1).

2. Chemical Mediators

The chemical mediators are of two types—*primary* mediators which are the preformed contents of mast cell and basophil granules and the *secondary* mediators which are newly formed upon stimulation of mast cells, basophils and other leucocytes.

(i) Primary mediators:

(a) **Histamine:** This is the most important in human anaphylaxis. It causes vasodilatation, increased capillary permeability and contraction of smooth muscle.
(b) **Serotonin:** It causes vasoconstriction, increased capillary permeability and smooth muscle contraction.
(c) **Eosinophil chemotactic factor of anaphylaxis (ECF-A)**

Table 14.1: Distinguishing Features of Immediate and Delayed Type of Hypersensitivity

Feature	Immediate type	Delayed type
1. Onset and duration	Appears and recedes rapidly	Appears slowly in 24-72 hours and lasts longer
2. Immune response	Antibody mediated	Cell mediated (T-lymphocytes)
3. Passive transfer	Possible with serum	Cannot be transferred with serum but possible with lymphocytes or transfer factor
4. Desensitisation	Easy but short lived	Difficult but long lasting
5. Induction	Antigens or haptens, by any route	By antigen injected intradermally or with Freund's adjuvant or by skin contact

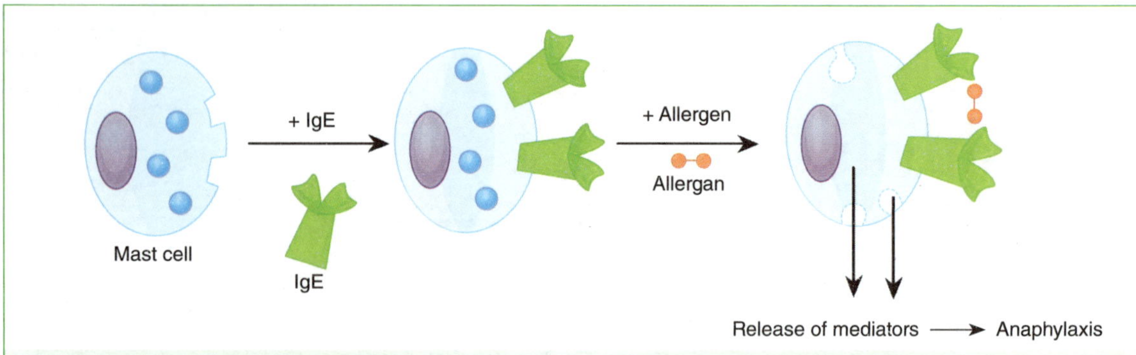

Fig. 14.1 Type I (anaphylactic) hypersensitivity

These are released from mast cell granules and are strongly chemotactic for eosinophils.

(ii) Secondary mediators

(a) **Slow reacting substance of anaphylaxis (SRS-A)**
These are much more potent bronchoconstrictors than histamine. They cause sustained contraction of smooth muscles.

(b) **Prostaglandins and thromboxane**
They are bronchoconstrictors.

(c) **Platelet activating factor (PAF)**
It causes aggregation of platelets and release of their vasoactive amines.

3. Atopy

It is typified by hay fever and asthma. The antigens commonly involved in atopy are pollens, house dust and foods. These atopens induce IgE antibodies.

Mechanism of atopy

The atopen combines with the cell bound IgE antibodies fixed on the surfaces of mast cells and the basophils and this antigen-antibody complex stimulates these cells to release the mediators resulting in clinical features of atopy.

Examples

1. Food allergy e.g. egg, mushroom.
2. Dust allergy e.g. pollens, house dust.

Type II (Cytotoxic) Reaction

Cytotoxic reaction is mediated by IgG (or rarely IgM) antibodies directed against antigens on the surface of cells resulting in cell damage. Antibodies bind to an antigen on the cell surface and cause (*i*) phagocytosis of the cell through opsonic or immune adherence (*ii*) cytotoxicity by natural killer (NK) cells (*iii*) lysis through activation of complement system (Fig. 14.2).

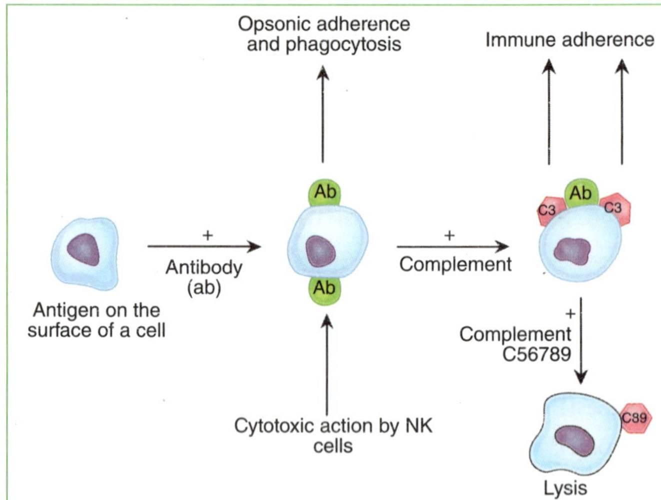

Fig. 14.2 Type II (cytotoxic) hypersensitivity

Examples

1. **Autoimmune anaemias and haemolytic disease of the newborn**
Lysis of red cells occur due to formation of antierythrocyte antibodies.
2. **Drug reactions**
Sedormid purpura is a classical example. A sedative drug sedormid (not used nowadays) combines with platelets and antibodies are formed against these sedormid coated platelets. On subsequent exposure to drug, antibodies attack the platelets leading to thrombocytopenic purpura.

Type III (Immune Complex) Reaction

It is characterised by deposition of antigen-antibody complexes in tissues, activation of complement and infiltration of polymorphonuclear leuococytes leading to tissue damage. Type III reactions differ fom type II reactions because its antigens are not attached to the surface of a cell. The interaction of these antigens with antibodies produce free floating complexes which can be depicted in the tissues leading to *immune complex reaction*.

Two typical type III reactions include *Arthus reaction*

(localised) due to relative antibody excess and *serum sickness* (generalised) because of relative antigen excess.

1. Arthus Reaction

The tissue damage is due to antigen-antibody complexes formed at **equivalence** or **slight antibody excess**. The antigen-antibody complexes are deposited on the walls of blood vessels. These complexes activate complement and attract neutrophils at the local site. Leucocyte-platelet thrombi are formed which reduce the blood supply and cause tissue necrosis.

2. Serum Sickness

It is a systemic form of type III hypersensitivity reaction. It appears following a single injection of high concentration of foreign serum. Antibodies to foreign serum reach high enough titres by 7-12 days but still some **excess antigen** remains in the circulating blood. Immune complexes get deposited on the endothelial lining of blood vessels in various parts of the body, causing inflammatory infiltration. Immune complexes damage the tissue in the same way as that in Arthus reaction. Some important immune complex diseases are post-streptococcal glomerulonephritis, and dengue haemorrhagic fever.

Type IV (Delayed or Cell Mediated) Reaction

The reaction is mediated by sensitised T-lymphocytes which, on contact with specific antigen, release lymphokines that cause biological effects on macrophages, leucocytes and tissue cells. In contrast, all other hypersensitivity reactions are induced by circulating antibodies. Type IV or delayed type of hypersensitivity occurs within 48-72 hours of antigen challenge. As it is not antibody mediated, it cannot be passively transferred by serum, but can be transferred by lymphocytes or the transfer factor. Two types of delayed hypersensitivity reactions are well recognised, the tuberculin (infection) type and the contact dermatitis type.

1. Tuberculin (Infection) Type

When a small dose of tuberculin is injected intradermally in an individual sensitised to tuberculoprotein by prior infection or immunisation, an erythema and swelling (induration) occurs at the site of injection within 48-72 hours. The injection site is infiltrated by large number of lymphocytes and about 10-12% macrophages. Purified protein derivative (PPD) which is the active material of tubercle bacilli, is used in tuberculin test.

The tuberculin test is a useful indicator for delayed hypersensitivity (cell mediated immunity) to the bacillus. Cell mediated hypersensitivity reaction develops in many infections with bacteria (*M. tuberculosis*, *M. leprae*), fungi and parasites.

2. Contact Dermatitis Type

Delayed hypersensitivity may sometimes develop as a result of skin contact with a range of sensitising materials—metals such as nickel, drugs such as penicillin or other antibiotics in ointments, simple chemicals like hair dyes, cosmetics and soaps.

KEY POINTS >>>

1. Hypersensitivity reactions are mainly of four types: *type I (anaphylactic)*, *type II (cytotoxic)*, *type III (immune complex)* and *type IV (delayed or cell mediated)*.
2. Type I, II and III depends on the interaction of antigen with *humoral antibodies* and are known as *immediate* type reactions. Type IV reaction is mediated by *T-lymphocytes*.

STUDY QUESTIONS

1. Classify hypersensitivity reactions. Describe in detail about type I hypersensitivity reactions.
2. Write short notes on:
   - (i) Arthus reaction
   - (ii) Serum sickness
   - (iii) Delayed hypersensitivity reaction
   - (iv) Atopy
   - (v) Anaphylaxis
   - (vi) Type II hypersensitivity reactions.

MULTIPLE CHOICE QUESTIONS (MCQs)

1. Which of the following hypersensitivity reactions has cell mediated immune response?
   (a) Type I
   (b) Type II
   (c) Type III
   (d) Type IV
2. Which class of immunoglobulin mediates type I hypersensitivity reactions?
   (a) IgG
   (b) IgM
   (c) IgA
   (d) IgE
3. Chemical mediators released during type I hypersensitivity reactions may be:
   (a) Histamine
   (b) Serotonin
   (c) Eosinophil chemotactic factors of anaphylaxis
   (d) All of the above
4. Arthus reaction is an example of:
   (a) Type I hypersensitivity reaction
   (b) Type II hypersensitivity reaction
   (c) Type III hypersensitivity reaction
   (d) Type IV hypersensitivity reaction
5. Delayed hypersensitivity reaction is mediated by:
   (a) T lymphocytes
   (b) B lymphocytes
   (c) Macrophages
   (d) All of the above

ANSWERS (MCQs) ...✓

1. (d) 2. (d) 3. (d) 4. (c) 5. (a)

Autoimmunity

15

I. INTRODUCTION

Normally an animal's immune system recognises its own tissue antigens as 'self' and therefore it does not produce antibodies against these self antigens. Autoimmunity is a condition when the body produces autoantibodies and immunologically competent T-lymphocytes against its own tissues. This leads to structural or functional damage of tissues.

II. MECHANISMS OF AUTOIMMUNITY

Autoimmunisation can occur under the following conditions:

A. Hidden or Sequestered Antigens

Certain hidden or 'sequestered' antigens are not recognised as self antigens. When these antigens are released into circulation, they may evoke an immune response. Examples are lens antigen of eye, sperm and thyroglobulin. These self antigens are present in closed system and have no access to the immune apparatus. The lens protein is enclosed in its capsule and has no contact with blood circulation. Hence immunological tolerance against lens protein is not developed during foetal life. When this antigen leaks out, following cataract surgery or injury, it may elicit an immune response which results in damage to the lens of the other eye. As spermatozoa develop only during puberty, the tolerance against this antigen is not induced during foetal life. Following mumps, the virus damages the basement membrane of seminiferous tubules which leads to leakage of sperms and therefore induce an immune response resulting in orchitis.

B. Antigen Alteration

Tissue antigens may be altered by physical, chemical or biological factors and these new cell surface antigens are called 'neo-antigens'. These neoantigens are no longer recognised as 'self' and may elicit an immune response.

C. Cross Reacting Foreign Antigens

Sharing of antigens by different organisms is the basis of 'cross reacting antigen' theory. Streptococcus (M proteins) and heart muscle share antigenic characteristics. Repeated streptococcal infection can therefore induce the immune response which damages the heart.

D. Forbidden Clones

According to clonal selection theory an innumerable number of clones of immunologically competent cells (ICCs) bearing specific antibody patterns are produced against all possible antigens. Any clone of cells carrying a pattern reactive against self antigens is destroyed during embryonic life. Such clones are known as 'forbidden clones'. At the time of birth only cells against non-self persist. Persistence of forbidden clones or development in later life by somatic mutation could lead to autoimmune diseases.

KEY POINTS

1. *Autoimmunity* is a condition when the body produces autoantibodies and immunologically competent T-lymphocytes against its own tissues.
2. Autoimmunity can occur in certain conditions such as *hidden* or *sequestered antigens*, *antigen alteration*, *cross reacting foreign antigens* and *forbidden clones*.

STUDY QUESTION

1. What is autoimmunity? Discuss the various mechanisms of autoimmunity.

MULTIPLE CHOICE QUESTIONS (MCQs)

1. Lens protein of eye is an example of:
   (a) Sequestered antigen
   (b) Neoantigen
   (c) Cross-reacting foreign antigen
   (d) None of the above

ANSWERS (MCQs)

1. (a)

Unit III

SYSTEMIC BACTERIOLOGY

16 Staphylococcus

Staphylococci are Gram positive cocci arranged in grape-like clusters. They are the commonest cause of suppuration. The genus *Staphylococcus* contains various species but the medically important species are *Staphylococcus aureus*, *Staphylococcus epidermidis*, *Staphylococcus saprophyticus*.

I. STAPHYLOCOCCUS AUREUS

A. Morphology

They are Gram positive cocci arranged in grape-like clusters, non-motile, non-sporing, approximately 1 μm in diameter (Fig. 16.1). Cluster formation is due to sequential division of bacteria in three perpendicular planes with daughter cells remaining in close proximity.

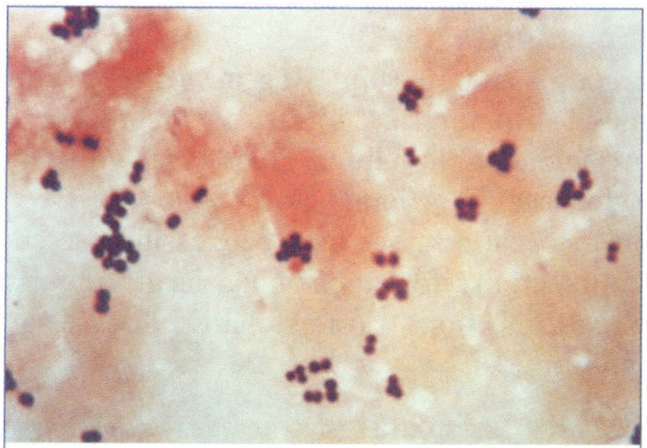

Fig. 16.1 Staphylococcus aureus on Gram staining

B. Culture

They grow readily on ordinary culture media within a temperature range of 10–42°C, the optimal temperature being 37°C and pH 7.4–7.6. They are aerobes and facultative anaerobes.

1. Nutrient Agar

After overnight or 24 hours incubation, the colonies are 2–4 mm in diameter, circular, smooth, convex, opaque and easily emulsifiable. Most of the strains produce golden yellow pigment. The pigment is not diffusable into the medium.

2. Blood Agar

Colonies are similar to those on nutrient agar and in addition a **beta type of haemolysis** is seen.

3. MacConkey's Agar

Colonies are very small and pink due to lactose fermentation.

4. Mannitol Salt Agar

This is both a **selective** and an **indicator medium**. It contains nutrient agar with 1% mannitol, 7.5% sodium chloride and phenol red as indicator. Yellow coloured colonies are seen on this medium due to fermentation of mannitol by most strains of *Staph. aureus*.

5. Liquid Medium

Uniform turbidity is produced in peptone water or nutrient broth.

C. Biochemical Reactions

Staph. aureus is catalase positive (unlike streptococci) and oxidase negative. It ferments a number of sugars producing acid without gas.

The following characteristics help to distinguish a **pathogenic strain of staphylococcus** (*Staph. aureus*) from other **non-pathogenic strains** (e.g. *Staph. epidermidis*).

1. Beta type of haemolysis on blood agar
2. Production of a golden yellow pigment
3. Coagulase production
4. Mannitol fermentation
5. Gelatin liquefaction
6. Phosphatase production
7. Production of enzyme deoxyribonuclease
8. Tellurite reduction.

D. Resistance

Staphylococci are more resistant among the non-sporing bacteria. They survive in dried pus for 2–3 months. Most of the staphylococci are killed at 62°C for 30 minutes but some may require 80°C for one hour.

E. Antigenic Structure (Fig. 16.2)

1. Capsule

Some strains of *Staph. aureus* possess capsule and inhibit phagocytosis. The capsule is composed of polysaccharide. Capsulated strains tend to be more virulent.

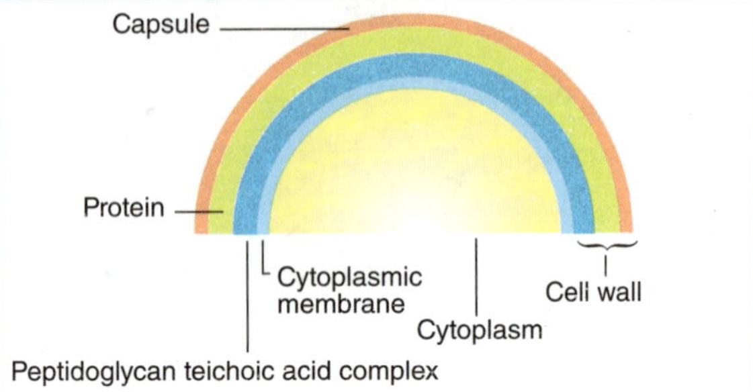

Fig. 16.2 Antigenic structure of Staphylococcus aureus

2. Peptidoglycan

Peptidoglycan is a polysaccharide polymer that provides rigidity to the cell wall.

3. Teichoic Acid

It is a major antigenic determinant of all strains of *Staph. aureus*.

4. Protein A

It is a cell wall component of most strains of *Staph. aureus* (especially Cowan I strain).

F. Toxins and Enzymes

Staph. aureus forms a number of toxins and enzymes. They are important virulence factors of the organism for producing a disease in the host.

1. Toxins

(i) Haemolysins
Four antigenically distinct types called alpha, beta, gamma and delta haemolysins are produced by staphylococci. These are exotoxins.

(ii) Leucocidin

(iii) Enterotoxin
The toxin is responsible for staphylococcal food poisoning.

(iv) Toxic shock syndrome toxin (TSST)

(v) Exfoliative (epidermolytic) toxin

2. Enzymes

Staph. aureus produces a number of enzymes, coagulase, phosphatase and deoxyribonuclease which are related to virulence of the bacteria.

Staph. aureus produces an enzyme coagulase. It has a property to clot human or rabbit plasma. Coagulase is secreted free into the culture medium. It requires a plasma factor **(coagulase reacting factor, CRF)** for its clotting action. Coagulase converts fibrinogen into fibrin.

Clumping factor (also called **bound coagulase**) reacts directly with the fibrinogen and causes clumping of cocci due to the precipitation of fibrin on the cell surface.

The test for coagulase is done by the slide and the tube method. It is done to differentiate pathogenic (*Staph. aureus*) strain from non-pathogenic strains.

(i) Slide coagulase test

Slide coagulase test detects **bound coagulase**. A few colonies of bacteria are emulsified in a drop of normal saline on a clean glass slide and mixed with a drop of undiluted rabbit or human plasma. Prompt clumping of the suspension occurs with coagulase positive strains.

(ii) Tube coagulase test

Tube coagulase test is done for detection of extracellular **free coagulase**. 0.1 ml of an overnight broth culture or an agar culture suspension of the organism is mixed with 0.5 ml of a 1 in 5 dilution of human or rabbit plasma. Diluted plasma alone in a second tube serves as a control. The tubes are incubated in a water bath at 37°C for three to six hours. In case of a positive test, the plasma clots and does not flow when the tube is inverted.

False positive

Citrated plasma should not be used because some contaminated (e.g. Pseudomonas) bacteria may utilize the citrate and produce false positive reaction.

G. Pathogenesis

Staph. aureus is an important **pyogenic organism** and lesions are **localised** in nature in contrast to streptococcal lesions which are spreading in nature. Thick creamy pus is formed in staphylococcal infections.

Staphylococcal diseases may be classified as cutaneous and deep infections; food poisoning, healthcare associated (nosocomial) infections, skin exfoliative diseases and toxic shock syndrome.

1. Cutaneous Infections

Superficial infections include pustules, boils, carbuncles, abscesses, styes, impetigo, pemphigus neonatorum, wound and burn infections.

2. Deep Infections

These include osteomyelitis, tonsillitis, pharyngitis, sinusitis, pneumonitis, empyema, endocarditis, meningitis, bacteriaemia septicaemia and pyaemia.

3. Food Poisoning

Staphylococcal food poisoning may follow 2–6 hours after the ingestion of contaminated food which contains preformed enterotoxin of *Staph. aureus*.

4. Healthcare Associated (Nosocomial) Infections

They are important cause of hospital acquired infections.

5. Skin Exfoliative Diseases

These diseases are produced by the strains of *Staph. aureus* that produce exfoliative toxin. Stripping of the superficial layers of the skin from the underlying tissue occurs in the various exfoliative syndromes caused by staphylococci (bullous impetigo, pemphigus neonatorum, Ritter's disease). Staphylococcal scalded skin syndrome (SSSS) is one example of exfoliative diseases in which toxin spreads systemically.

6. Toxic Shock Syndrome (TSS)

It is caused by toxin shock syndrome toxin (TSST-1). Although TSS became widely known in association with the use of tampons by menstruating women, it occurs in other situations also.

H. Typing Methods

Typing methods may be done for epidemiological purposes.

1. Bacteriophage Typing

Strains of *Staph. aureus* may be distinguished by their susceptibility to different bacteriophages. An internationally accepted set of phages is used. A set of 23 bacteriophages is employed. The strain to be typed is grown on nutrient agar to produce a lawn culture. After drying, the phages of basic set are applied in a fixed dose (routine test dose, RTD). After overnight incubation, the culture will be observed for lysis by the phages. The phage type is designated according to the phages capable of lysing the bacterial strain (Fig. 16.3). Thus a strain of phage type 52/80/94 is the one that is lysed only by phages 52, 80 and 94. Phage typing is important in epidemiological studies of staphylococcal infections.

The reference centre for staphylococcal phage typing in India is located in the Department of Microbiology, Maulana Azad Medical College, New Delhi.

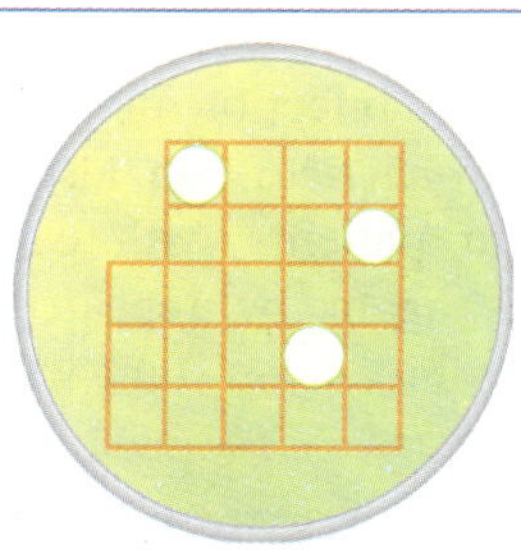

Fig. 16.3 Bacteriophage typing of staphylococci

2. Molecular Typing Methods

Molecular typing methods such as **DNA fingerprinting**, **ribotyping** and **polymerase chain reaction (PCR)** are used.

I. Antibiotic Sensitivity

Most of the strains of ***Staph. aureus*** were sensitive to penicillin originally. Soon after penicillin came to be used clinically, resistant strains began to emerge. Penicillin resistance in staphylococci is due to:

1. Production of ***beta lactamase (penicillinase)*** which is plasmid coded and transmitted by transduction or conjugation. Beta lactamase inactivates penicillin by splitting the beta lactam ring. This type of drug resistance can be overcome by addition of betalactamase inhibitors (e.g. clavulanc acid).
2. **Methicillin resistant staphylococci:** There is reduction in affinity of penicillin binding proteins of the staphylococcal cell wall for β-lactam antibiotics. This change is normally chromosomal in nature. This type of resistance also occurs in beta lactamase resistant penicillins such as methicillin, nafcillin and oxacillin. They may cause outbreaks of hospital infection. These strains are called **methicillin resistant Staph. aureus (MRSA)**. These are important causes of postoperative wound infections and other hospital acquired infections. They may also cause epidemics of hospital cross infection. Vancomycin or teicoplanin is used for treatment of infections with MRSA. Although predominantly a hospital pathogen, MRSA is becoming more common in community. These MRSA strains are named community acquired MRSA strains (CA–MRSA). Hospital personnel harbouring MRSA have been implicated as the chief source of healthcare associated infections.

J. Laboratory Diagnosis

1. Specimens

These are collected according to the nature of lesion as follows:

Pus — suppurative lesions
Sputum — respiratory infections
Blood — septicaemia or PUO
Urine — urinary tract infection
CSF — meningitis
Faeces — food poisoning
Food or vomit — food poisoning

2. Collection and Transport

Specimens should be collected in sterile containers under all aseptic conditions. In case of urine, midstream urine should be collected. Blood should be collected in blood culture bottles comprising of glucose broth and taurocholate broth.

Specimens should be transported immediately to the laboratory and processed.

3. Direct Microscopy

Direct microscopy with Gram-stained smears of pus or wound exudate is useful, where Gram positive cocci in clusters may be seen (Fig. 16.4). This is of no value for specimens where mixed bacterial flora are normally present e.g. sputum.

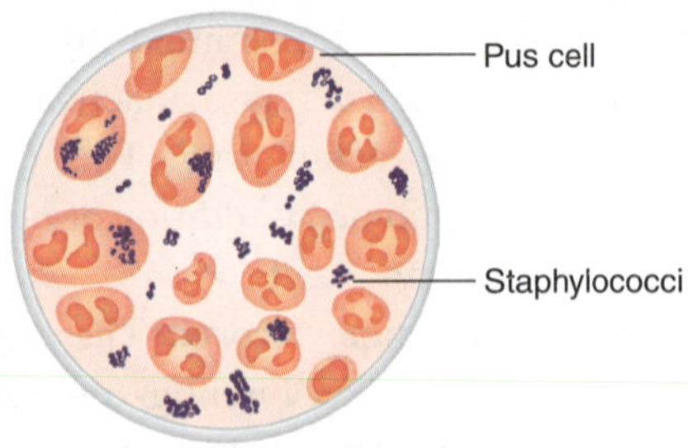

Fig. 16.4 Staphylococci in stained smear of pus

4. Culture

The specimens are inoculated on following media:

- Blood agar
- Peptone Water

Specimens where staphylococci are expected to be scanty or outnumbered by other bacteria (e.g. faeces), are inoculated on selective media.

The inoculated media are incubated at 37°C for 18–24 hours. Next day, culture plates are examined for morphology of bacterial colonies and other characters. Uniform turbidity is produced in liquid medium such as peptone water. Gram staining from colony on blood agar and hanging drop preparation from peptone water are done to further characterise the bacteria.

5. Colony Morphology and Gram Staining

On blood agar, colonies are 2–4 mm in diameter, circular, raised, opaque and produce golden yellow pigment. Beta haemolysis is seen around these colonies (Fig. 16.5).

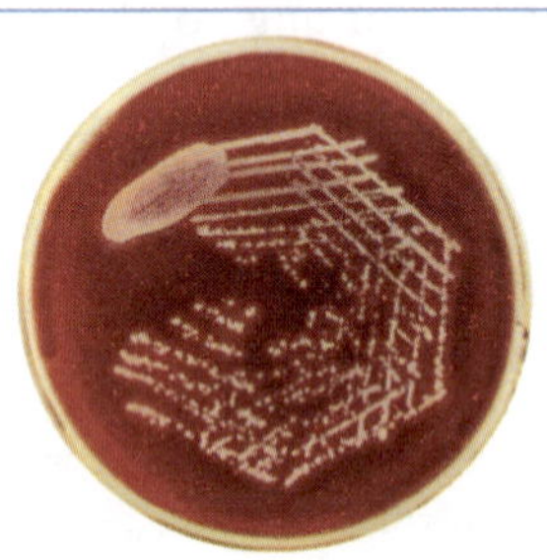

Fig. 16.5 Staphylococcus aureus on blood agar

On Gram staining, they are Gram positive cocci (1 μm in diameter) arranged in grape like clusters.

Non-motile cocci in clusters are seen in hanging drop preparation.

6. Biochemical Reactions

(i) Catalase test: All staphylococci (pathogenic and non-pathogenic) are catalase positive. This test distinguishes Staphylococcus from Streptococcus which is catalase negative.

(ii) Coagulase test: It is positive in *Staph. aureus* but negative in other staphylococci. This test has been described in detail on page no. 62 of this chapter.

Other tests which are positive in pathogenic strain (*Staph. aureus*) and distinguish it from non-pathogenic staphylococci are described on page no. 61.

7. Antibiotic Susceptibility

Antibiotic sensitivity can be determined by Stokes method or Kirby-Bauer method.

K. Treatment

Benzyl penicillin is the most effective antibiotic in sensitive strains. Cloxacillins are used against beta-lactamase producing strains. Vancomycin is used in treatment of infections with MRSA strains. For mild superficial lesions, topical applications of bacitrain or chlorhexidine may be sufficient.

II. COAGULASE NEGATIVE STAPHYLOCOCCI (CONs)

Coagulase negative staphylococci (CONs) form the part of the normal flora of the skin. They are opportunistic pathogens which cause infection in debilitated or immunocompromised patients.

A. Staphylococcus epidermidis

It is a skin commensal and acts as opportunistic pathogen in prosthetic devices e.g. prosthetic heart valves, intraperitoneal catheters, orthopaedic prostheses and vascular grafts. It may cause septicaemia and subacute bacterial endocarditis. It may produce stitch abscess. It mainly acts as pathogen in immunocompromised individual. Their aetiological role may be proved by repeated isolation.

B. Staphylococcus saprophyticus

It acts as an opportunistic pathogen. It is an important cause of urinary tract infection in young, sexually active females. *Staph. saprophyticus* can also cause septicaemia and endocarditis in patients with cardiac surgery. The aetiological role is again by repeated isolation. *Staph. saprophyticus* is novobiocin resistant which distinguishes it from *Staph. epidermidis*.

Differentiating features of *Staph. aureus, Staph. epidermidis* and *Staph. saprophyticus* are shown in Table 16.1.

III. MICROCOCCI

Micrococci are free living in the environment. These are Gram positive cocci, catalase positive, coagulase negative, arranged in clusters which differ from staphylococci in attacking sugars oxidatively. They may appear in irregular clusters, groups of four or eight. They are often larger than staphylococci. Colonies are generally white in colour. Their staining is often not uniform (Table 16.2). They are saprophytes and commensals. They may rarely cause opportunistic infection.

Table 16.1: Differentiating Features of Three Species of Staphylococcus

Feature	Staph. aureus	Staph. epidermidis	Staph. saprophyticus
Coagulase test	+	–	–
Mannitol fermentation	+	–	–
Production of DNAase	+	–	–
Phosphatase	+	–/weak +	–
α–lysin	+	–	–
Protein A in the cell wall	+	–	–
Novobiocin resistance	–	–	+
Pathogenicity	Primary	Opportunistic	Opportunistic

Table 16.2: Distinguishing Characters of Staphylococcus aureus and Micrococcus

Character	Staphylococcus aureus	Micrococcus
Gram staining	Gram positive Grape like clusters Uniform staining 1 μm in size	Gram positive, darkly stained Present in groups of four (tetrad) or eight Often staining is not uniform Larger than staphylococcus
Colony characters	Colonies are golden yellow in colour	Colonies are generally white in colour
Coagulase test	Positive	Negative
Breakdown of carbohydrates (O/F test)	Fermentatively	Oxidatively

KEY POINTS

1. Staphylococci are Gram positive cocci arranged in grape-like clusters. They are the commonest cause of suppuration.
2. Staphylococcus aureus is a pathogenic staphylococcus.
3. Based on production of enzyme coagulase staphylococci are classified as coagulase positive (e.g. Staph. aureus) and coagulase negative (e.g. Staph. epidermidis, Staph. saprophyticus).
4. The test for coagulase is done by the slide and the tube method. It is done to differentiate pathogenic (Staph. aureus) strain from non-pathogenic strains.
5. Staph. aureus is an important pyogenic organism and lesions are localised in nature. They may also cause food poisoning, nosocomial infections, scalded skin syndrome and toxic shock syndrome.
6. Penicillin resistance in staphylococci may be due to production of beta lactamase (penicillinase) which is plasmid coded and transmitted by transduction.
7. Methicillin resistant Staph. aureus (MRSA) may cause outbreaks of hospital infection.
8. Coagulase negative staphylococci form the part of the normal flora of the skin. They are opportunistic pathogens, which cause infection in debilitated or immunocompromised patients.
9. Micrococci are saprophytes and commensals. They may rarely cause opportunistic infections.

STUDY QUESTIONS

1. Describe the laboratory diagnosis of infections caused by *Staph. aureus.*
2. Write short notes on:
   (i) Toxins and enzymes produced by *Staph. aureus*
   (ii) Coagulase test.
3. Write briefly about:
   (i) Micrococci
   (ii) Antigenic structure of *Staph. aureus.*

MULTIPLE CHOICE QUESTIONS (MCQs)

1. Which of the following characteristics help to distinguish *Staphylococcus aureus* from non-pathogenic strains of Staphylococcus?
   (a) Beta type of haemolysis on blood agar
   (b) Production of a golden yellow-pigment
   (c) Coagulase production
   (d) All of the above
2. Protein A is a cell wall component of:
   (a) *Staphylococcus aureus*
   (b) Coagulase negative staphylococci
   (c) Micrococci
   (d) None of the above
3. Which of the following toxins is responsible for Staphylococcal scalded skin syndrome?
   (a) Enterotoxin
   (b) Leucocidin
   (c) Haemolysin
   (d) Exfoliative toxin
4. Slide coagulase test detects:
   (a) Free coagulase
   (b) Bound coagulase
   (c) Both of the above
   (d) None of the above
5. Tube coagulase test detects:
   (a) Free coagulase
   (b) Bound coagulase
   (c) Both of the above
   (d) None of the above
6. Which of the following bacteria produce coagulase enzyme?
   (a) *Staphylococcus aureus*
   (b) *Staph. epidermidis*
   (c) *Staph. saprophyticus*
   (d) None of the above

ANSWERS (MCQs) ...✓

1. (d) 2. (d) 3. (d) 4. (b) 5. (a) 6. (a)

17 Streptococcus and Enterococcus

Streptococci are Gram positive cocci which are arranged in chains. They are part of the normal human flora. Some of them are important human pathogens causing pyogenic infections.

I. CLASSIFICATION (Fig. 17.1)

The streptococci are divided into aerobic streptococci, obligate anaerobes and facultative anaerobes. Obligate anaerobic streptococci are described in chapter on 'Nonsporing anaerobes' (Chapter 23). Aerobic and facultative anaerobic streptococci are classified on the basis of their haemolytic properties. Three types of haemolytic reactions (α, β and γ) are observed on blood agar medium.

A. Alpha (α) Haemolytic Streptococci

They produce a greenish discolouration around the colonies. This is due to partial haemolysis. The zone of lysis is small (1 or 2 mm wide) with presence of unlysed erythrocytes. Alpha haemolysis is seen with viridans group of streptococci and pneumococcus.

B. Beta (β) Haemolytic Streptococci

These streptococci produce a clear, colourless zone of complete haemolysis (2–4 mm wide) around the colonies, within which erythrocytes are completely lysed. The lysis of erythrocytes is due to the production of two types of streptolysin by the organisms: *streptolysin O and streptolysin S*. Most of the pathogenic streptococci fall into this group. *Streptococcus pyogenes* is the most important and is responsible for many important human infections.

C. Gamma (γ) or Non-Haemolytic Streptococci

They produce no haemolysis and *Str. faecalis* is a typical example.

The beta haemolytic streptococci were classified by *Lancefield* (1933) serologically into a number of broad

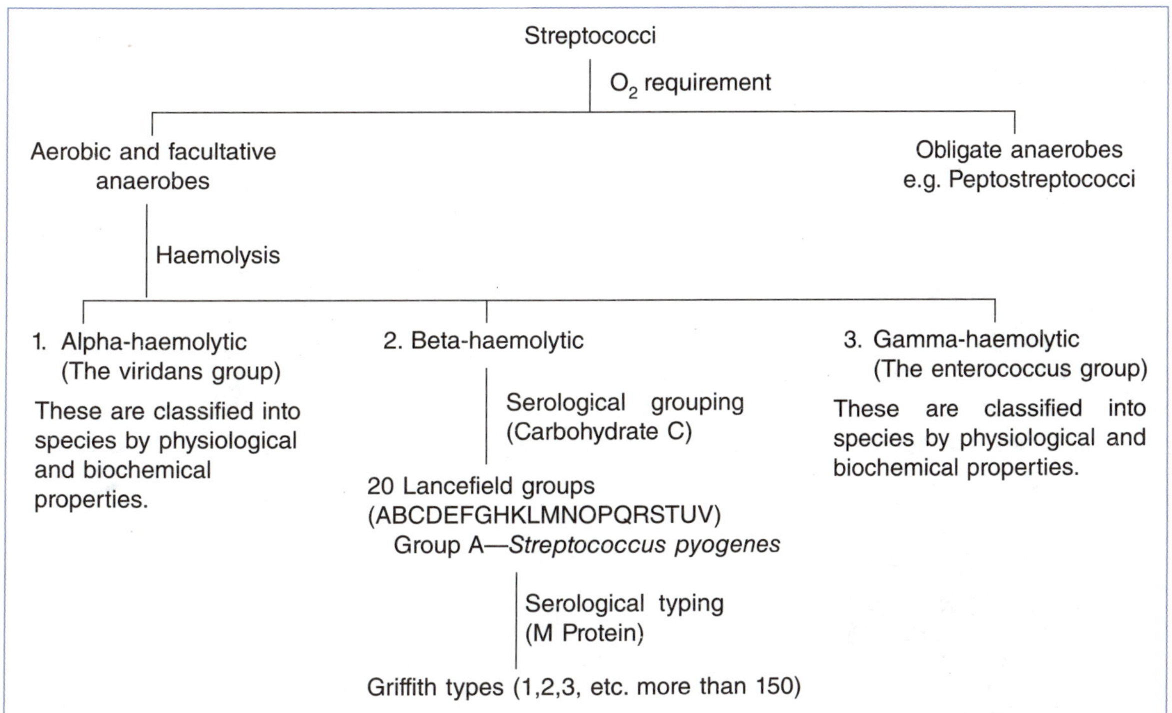

Fig. 17.1 Classification of streptococci

groups based on the nature of a carbohydrate (C) antigen on the cell wall. These are known as *Lancefield groups*, 20 of which have been identified, named A–V (without I and J) by precipitation reaction performed with appropriate sera. Majority of streptococci that produce human infections belong to group A named as *Streptococcus pyogenes*. These are further subdivided by type specific antisera into approximately 80 Griffith serotypes (type 1, 2 etc.) based on their surface proteins (M, T and R).

II. STREPTOCOCCUS PYOGENES

A. Morphology

The individual cocci are spherical or oval, 0.5 to 1.0 µm in diameter and are arranged in chains. Chain formation is due to successive cell divisions occurring in one plane only and daughter cells failing to separate completely (Figs. 17.2 and 17.3).

Streptococci are Gram positive, non-motile and non-sporing. Some strains of *Streptococcus pyogenes* have capsules composed of hyaluronic acid.

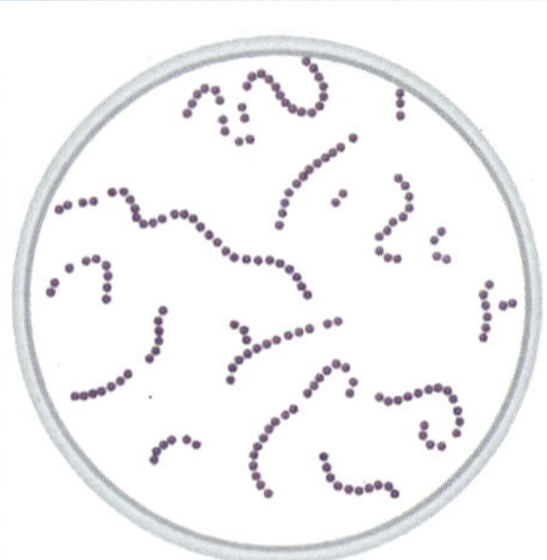

Fig. 17.2 Streptococci

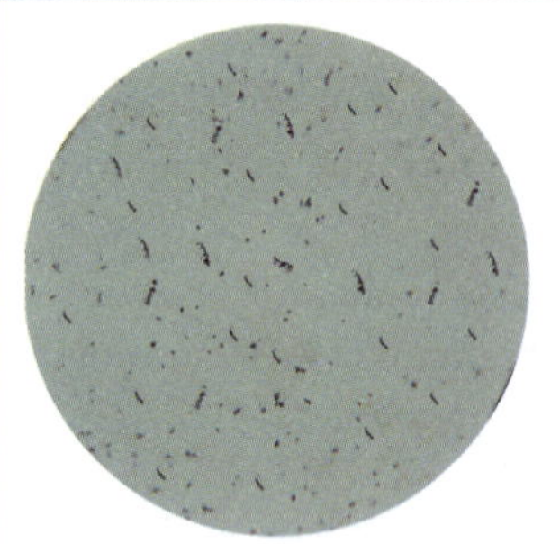

Fig. 17.3 Streptococcus pyogenes

B. Culture

They are aerobes and facultative anaerobes, growing best at a temperature of 37°C (range 22–42°C). These are most exacting in nutritive requirements, growth occurring only in media containing blood, serum or sugars. On blood agar, after overnight incubation, the colonies are small (0.5–1.0 mm, pin point), circular, semitransparent, low convex with a wide zone of β-haemolysis around them (Fig. 17.4). Growth and haemolysis are promoted by presence of 10% CO_2 in the environment. Selective media containing 1:500,000 crystal violet (crystal violet blood agar) permit growth of streptococci but inhibit other bacteria especially staphylococci.

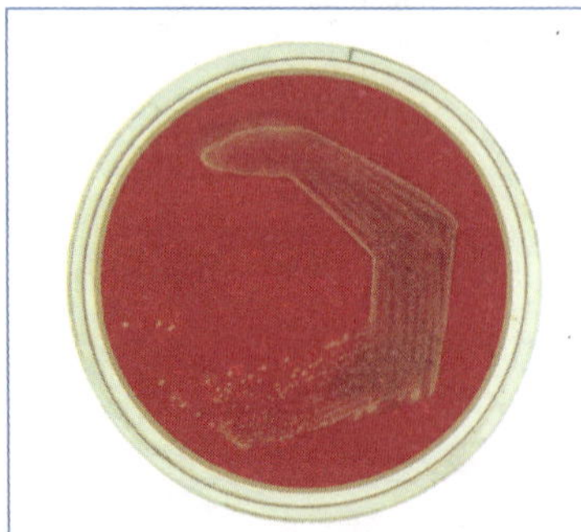

Fig. 17.4 Streptococcus pyogenes

In liquid media, such as glucose broth, growth occurs as a granular turbidity with a powdery deposit. Bacterial chains being heavier settle down as deposit.

C. Biochemical Reactions

Streptococci are catalase negative, unlike staphylococci which are catalase positive.

D. Antigenic Structure

1. *Capsular Hyaluronic Acid*

Capsule may be present on groups A and C streptococci. The capsule when present inhibits phagocytosis.

2. *Group Specific Polysaccharide Antigen*

The cell wall is composed of an outer layer of protein (fimbria containing protein) and lipoteichoic acid, a middle layer of group-specific C carbohydrate and inner layer of peptidoglycan (mucoprotein) (Fig. 17.5). The peptidoglycan is responsible for cell wall rigidity.

3. *Type Specific Antigen*

The outer part of the cell wall contains protein antigens. *Str. pyogenes* is further subdivided on the basis of their surface proteins M, T and R.

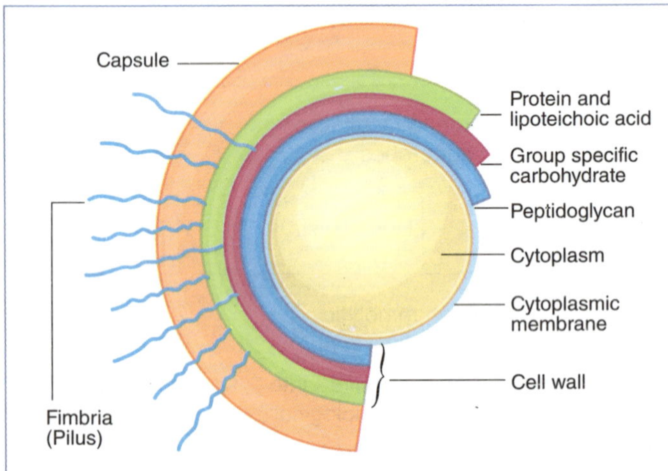

Fig. 17.5 Antigenic structure of Streptococcus pyogenes

E. Toxins and Enzymes

Str. pyogenes produces several exotoxins and enzymes which contribute to its virulence.

1. *Toxins*

(i) Haemolysins

Streptococci produce two types of haemolysins, *streptolysin 'O'* and *'S'*.

Streptolysin 'O'

Streptolysin 'O' is so named because it is oxygen labile. It is inactivated in the presence of oxygen. It lyses red cells and is also cytotoxic for neutrophils, platelets and cardiac tissue. It is antigenic and antistreptolysin 'O' (ASO) regularly appears in sera following streptococcal infection.

Streptolysin 'S'

Streptolysin 'S' is an oxygen stable haemolysin and is responsible for the haemolysis seen around colonies of streptococci on the surface of blood agar plates.

(ii) Streptococcal pyrogenic exotoxin (Spe)

This toxin is responsible for streptococcal toxic shock syndrome and scarlet fever. Spe is also called erythrogenic toxin.

This toxin is responsible for Dick test and Schultz Charlton reaction. When the toxin is injected intradermally into the skin of a susceptible child, a localised erythematous reaction appears. This is called the *Dick test*. In scarlet fever, when homologous antitoxin is injected locally into the rash, blanching of the rash occurs, it is named as *Schultz Charlton reaction*. These tests are now only of historical importance as scarlet fever is now rarely seen.

2. Enzymes

(i) Streptokinase (fibrinolysin)

Streptokinase facilitates the spread of infection by breaking down the fibrin barrier around the lesions.

(ii) Deoxyribonucleases (streptodornase)

Group A streptococci elaborate four antigenically distinct deoxyribonucleases (DNAases), A, B ,C, and D, of which, type B is the most antigenic in man.

(iii) Nicotinamide adenine dinucleotidase (NADase)

NADase acts on the coenzyme NAD and liberates nicotinamide from the molecule. It is believed to be leucotoxic.

(iv) Hyaluronidase

It breaks down hyaluronic acid of the tissues and favours spread of streptococcal lesion along intercellular spaces (spreading factor).

F. Pathogenesis (Table 17.1)

Str. pyogenes produces pyogenic infections with a tendency to spread locally. Non-suppurative sequelae of local infections include acute glomerulonephritis and rheumatic fever.

Table 17.1: Streptococcal Diseases

Streptococcus	Lesions
Str. pyogenes	
(i) Pyogenic infections	
Respiratory tract	Acute tonsillitis or pharyngitis (sore throat), scarlet fever
Skin infections	Infections of wounds, burns and skin lesions (eczema), erysipelas, impetigo
Genital infections	Puerperal sepsis
Streptococcal toxin shock syndrome	Bacteraemia, necrotizing fascitis
Deep infections	Bone and joint infections, lymphadenitis, septicaemia, abscess in internal organs
(ii) Non-suppurative complications	Rheumatic fever, acute glomerulonephritis
Group B Streptococci	Neonatal infections (septicaemia and meningitis)
Str. faecalis	Urinary tract infection, endocarditis
Viridans Streptococci	Endocarditis, dental caries

1. Pyogenic Infections

(i) Respiratory infections

Sore throat (acute tonsillitis and/ or pharyngitis) is the most common of streptococcal diseases.

Scarlet fever

It consists of a combination of sore throat and a generalised erythematous rash. It is caused by a strain producing the erythrogenic toxin.

(ii) Skin infections

Str. pyogenes causes suppurative infections of the skin with a predilection to produce lymphangitis and **cellulitis**.

The two typical streptococcal skin infections are **erysipelas** and **impetigo**. These skin infections are the main cause leading to acute glomerulonephritis in children in the tropics.

(iii) Streptococcal toxic shock syndrome

Streptococcal toxic shock syndrome (TSS) is a condition in which the entire organ system collapses, leading to death. Streptococcal TSS resembles Staphylococcal TSS. Patients are often bacteraemic and have necrotizing fascitis.

(iv) Other pyogenic infections

(a) Puerperal sepsis: *Str. pyogenes* was an important cause of puerperal sepsis. It used to take a heavy toll of life before antibiotics became available.

(b) Sepsis: Infections of skin lesions (eczema, psoriasis, scabies), wounds and burns.

(c) Pyaemia, septicaemia, abscess in internal organs (brain, lung, liver and kidney).

2. Non-Suppurative Complications

Str. pyogenes infections are sometimes followed by two important non-suppurative sequelae, **acute rheumatic fever** and **acute glomerulonephritis**. These complications occur one to four weeks after the acute infection. *Str. pyogenes* is no longer detectable when these complications set in. The latent period suggests an immune response. Rheumatic fever is often preceded by sore throat while acute glomerulonephritis by the skin infection. These sequelae or complications are believed to be the result of hypersensitivity to some streptococcal components. Rheumatic fever may follow infection with any serotype of *Str. pyogenes* while acute glomerulonephritis is caused by only a few nephritogenic types.

G. Laboratory Diagnosis

Diagnosis of acute suppurative infections is made by culture, while in the non-suppurative complications, diagnosis is mainly based on the demonstration of antibodies.

1. Acute Suppurative Infections

(i) Specimens

Specimen is collected according to the site of lesion, such as swab, pus/pus swab, or blood.

(ii) Collection and Transport

Specimens should be collected in sterile containers under all aseptic conditions. These should be plated immediately or sent to the laboratory in Pike's transport medium (blood agar containing 1 in 1,000,000 crystal violet and 1 in 16,000 sodium azide).

(iii) Gram Staining of Smears

Gram positive cocci (0.5–1.0 µm in diameter) in chains is indicative of streptococcal infection. Smears are of no value where streptococci are present as part of the resident flora such as in infections of the throat and genitalia. Smear examination is important in specimens such as pus.

(iv) Culture

The specimen is inoculated on blood agar medium and incubated at 37°C for 18-24 hours. Haemolysis develops better under anaerobic conditions or in the presence of 5–10% carbon dioxide.

Crystal violet blood agar is a selective medium for *Str. pyogenes*.

(v) Colony Morphology and Staining

The colonies of streptococci are small 0.5-1.0 mm (size of pinpoint as compared to pinhead size of staphylococci), circular, low convex with a zone of β-haemolysis around them.

In liquid medium, such as glucose broth, growth occurs as a granular turbidity with a powdery deposit.

Gram staining from colonies show Gram positive cocci in chains. Hanging drop preparation from liquid medium shows non-motile cocci.

(vi) Biochemical Reactions

Streptococci are catalase negative which is an important test to differentiate streptococci from staphylococci.

(vii) Identification of Various Groups of Streptococci

Str. pyogenes **(group A)** is more **sensitive to bacitracin** (0.04 units/disc). **Group 'B'** streptococci may be identified by the **CAMP test** (Christie, Atkins and Munch-Peterson). **Group 'D'** can be isolated by performing **heat resistance test**. Details of these tests are described in respective streptococci group.

(viii) Lancefield Grouping

Haemolytic streptococci are grouped serologically by the Lancefield technique. It is done for definite classification.

(ix) Antigen Detection Tests

ELISA and agglutination tests are used to demonstrate group A streptococcal antigen from throat swab.

(x) Molecular Methods

DNA probes and polymerase chain reaction (PCR) are now available. These are more sensitive methods but are costly.

2. Non-Suppurative Complications

In rheumatic fever and glomerulonephritis, serological tests provide retrospective evidence of streptococcal infection. The routine test done is **antistreptolysin O (ASO)** titration. A titre of 200 units or more is significant in **rheumatic fever** and is indicative of prior streptococcal infection.

ASO test is a neutralisation reaction where antibodies to streptolysin 'O' (ASO) are neutralised with streptolysin 'O' antigen. ASO titre is usually found in high levels in rheumatic fever but in **glomerulonephritis**, titres tend to be low, therefore, **anti-deoxyribonuclease B (anti-DNAase B)** estimation is more reliable. Titres higher than 300 or 350 are significant. This test is very useful for retrospective diagnosis of streptococcal pyoderma, for which ASO is of less value.

H. Treatment

Penicillin G is the drug of choice. In patients allergic to penicillin, erythromycin or cephalexin is used.

III. OTHER HAEMOLYTIC STREPTOCOCCI

A. Group B Streptococci (GBS)

Str. agalactiae is an important pathogen of bovine mastitis in cattle. In recent years, it has been recognised as the single most important pathogen in neonates causing **neonatal septicaemia** and **meningitis**. It may also cause septic abortion and puerperal sepsis. *Str. agalactiae* is a commensal of female genital tract from where bacterial infection in neonates occur. Other Group B infections in neonates include osteomyelitis, arthritis, conjunctivitis, respiratory infections, endocarditis and peritonitis.

The presumptive identification depends on their ability to hydrolyse hippurate. Another test to identify group B is the **CAMP test** (Christie, Atkins and Munch-Peterson), which can be demonstrated by the production of accentuated zone of haemolysis (as butterfly appearance) when Group B streptococci are inoculated perpendicular to a streak of *Staph. aureus* grown on blood agar (Fig. 17.6). Group B streptococci produce a CAMP factor that enhances the lysis of sheep erythrocytes by staphylococcal β-lysin.

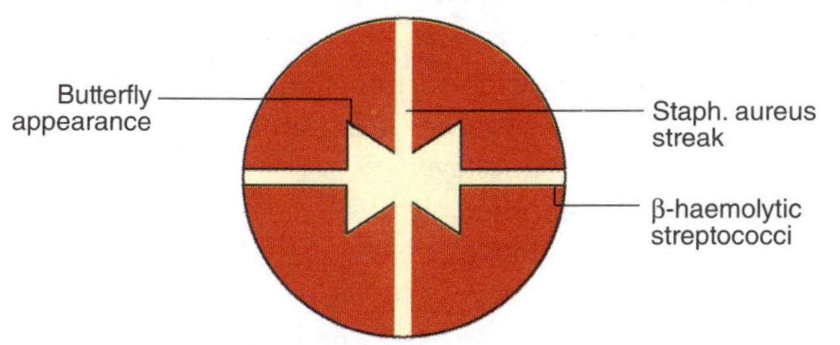

Fig. 17.6 CAMP test

B. Group D Streptococci

Streptococci belonging to group 'D' are classified as enterococci (faecal streptococci) and non-enterococci (non-faecal streptococci). They are usually non-haemolytic while some strains may be alpha or beta haemolytic. The enterococci group has been reclassified as a separate genus called *Enterococcus*. Non-enterococci of group D (*Str. bovis group*) are inhibited by 6.5 per cent sodium chloride. These are now named as Group D streptococci. They may cause genitourinary infection or endocarditis rarely.

IV. ENTEROCOCCUS

Enterococci are normal inhabitants of human intestinal tract and possess some distinctive properties as follows:

1. They are relatively heat resistant and can withstand heat at 60°C for 30 minutes *(heat test or heat resistance test)*.
2. Their ability to grow in the presence of 6.5 per cent sodium chloride.
3. Their ability to grow at 45°C and at pH 9.6.

On MacConkey's medium they grow as tiny deep pink colonies. On Gram's staining, enterococci appear as pairs of oval cocci and short chains. The identification of the species is based on biochemical reactions. *Enterococcus faecalis* is the most commonly isolated enterococcus from human sources.

E. faecalis is frequently isolated from cases of urinary tract infection and wound infection. They may also cause other infections like subacute bacterial endocarditis, septicaemia, peritonitis and infection of biliary tract. Strains resistant to penicillin and other antibiotics occur frequently. Vancomycin is the primary alternative drug to a penicillin for treating enterococcal infections. Vancomycin resistant enterococci (VRE) have also been isolated.

V. VIRIDANS STREPTOCOCCI

This group of streptococci produce alpha haemolysis on blood agar. They are known as viridans streptococci (from *viridis* meaning green) due to greenish discolouration (α-haemolysis) on blood agar. They are commensals of mouth and upper respiratory tract. *Str. viridans* includes *Str. mitis* group, *Str. mutans* group, *Str. bovis* group, *Str. salivarius* group and *Str. anginosus* group.

They are ordinarily non-pathogenic but on occasions cause disease. The viridans streptococci are associated with **dental caries** and **subacute bacterial endocarditis**. They cause endocarditis in persons with predisposing factor such as valvular disease of the heart, congenital heart disease and cardiac surgery. Viridans streptococci are generally penicillin sensitive but some strains may be resistant. Hence, antibiotic sensitivity of these bacteria must be determined for appropriate treatment of endocarditis.

KEY POINTS

1. Streptococci are Gram positive cocci which are arranged in chains.
2. Str. pyogenes produces pyogenic infections with a tendency to spread locally. Sore throat (acute tonsilitis and/or pharyngitis) is the most common of streptococcal diseases. Non-suppurative sequelae of local infections include acute glomerulonephritis and rheumatic fever.
3. Group B streptococci are important pathogens in neonates causing neonatal septicaemia and meningitis. CAMP reaction is used to identify Group B streptococci.

4. Enterococcus faecalis is frequently isolated from cases of urinary tract infection and wound infection. Heat resistance test is positive for E. faecalis.
5. Viridans streptococci produce alpha haemolysis on blood agar. They are commensals of mouth and upper respiratory tract. They are ordinarily non-pathogenic but on occasions cause disease. They are associated with dental caries and subacute bacterial endocarditis.

STUDY QUESTIONS

1. Classify streptococci. Describe the laboratory diagnosis of streptococcal sore throat.
2. Write short notes on:
   (i) Antigenic structure of *Str. pyogenes*
   (ii) Toxins and enzymes of *Streptococcus pyogenes*
   (iii) Non-suppurative complications of *Str. pyogenes* infections
   (iv) Lancefield grouping.
3. Write briefly about:
   (i) Group B streptococci
   (ii) Group D streptococci
   (iii) Enterococci
   (iv) Viridans streptococci
   (v) CAMP reaction.

MULTIPLE CHOICE QUESTIONS (MCQs)

1. On blood agar which type of haemolysis is produced by *Streptococcus pyogenes*?
   (a) Alpha haemolysis
   (b) Beta haemolysis
   (c) Gamma haemolysis
   (d) None of the above
2. Which of the following is selective medium for *Streptococcus pyogenes*?
   (a) Blood agar
   (b) Crystal violet blood agar
   (c) Potassium tellurite blood agar
   (d) Chocolate agar
3. Sensitivity to bacitracin can be used to identify:
   (a) *Streptococcus pyogenes*
   (b) *Str. agalactiae*
   (c) *Str. equisimilis*
   (d) *Str. mitis*
4. CAMP test can be used to identify:
   (a) *Streptococcus pyogenes*
   (b) *Str. agalactiae*
   (c) *Str. equisimilis*
   (d) *Str. mitis*
5. The most important bacterial cause of sore throat is:
   (a) *Streptococcus pyogenes*
   (b) *Staphylococcus aureus*
   (c) *Staphylococcus epidermidis*
   (d) *Neisseria gonorrhoeae*
6. Which of the following are non-suppurative complications of *Streptococcus pyogenes* infections?
   (a) Acute rheumatic fever
   (b) Acute glomerulonephritis
   (c) Both of the above
   (d) None of the above
7. Which of the following tests may be used for diagnosis of non-suppurative complications of *Streptococcus pyogenes* infections?
   (a) ASO test
   (b) Anti DNAase B test
   (c) Streptozyme test
   (d) All of the above

ANSWERS (MCQs) ...✓

1. (b) 2. (b) 3. (a) 4. (b) 5. (a) 6. (c) 7. (d)

Pneumococcus

18

Pneumococci are normal commensals of the upper respiratory tract. They are important pathogens of pneumonia and otitis media in children. They are reclassified as *Streptococcus pneumoniae*. They differ form streptococci in their morphology (diplococci), bile solubility, optochin sensitivity and by a specific polysaccharide capsule.

PNEUMOCOCCUS

A. Morphology

Pneumococci are Gram positive, small (1 μm diameter), slightly elongated cocci arranged in pairs (diplococci) with the broad ends in apposition. Each coccus has one end broad or rounded and other pointed (flame shaped or lanceolate appearance) (Fig. 18.1). They are capsulated and the capsule encloses each pair. The capsule may be demonstrated as a clear halo in India ink preparation (Fig. 18.2). They are non-motile and non-sporing.

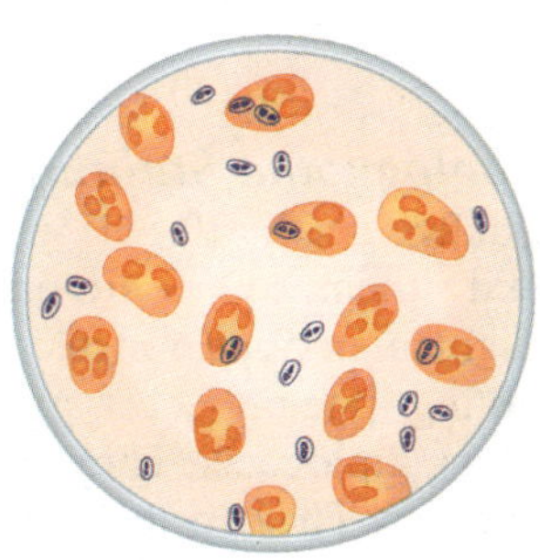

Fig. 18.1 Str. pneumoniae in pus

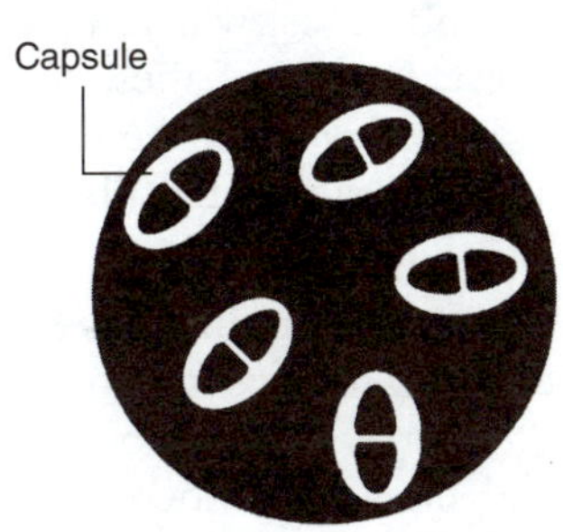

Fig. 18.2 India ink preparation to show pneumococcus capsule

B. Culture

They are aerobes and facultative anaerobes and their growth is improved by 5–10 per cent CO_2. The optimum temperature for growth is 37°C (range 25°C to 42°C) and pH 7.8 (range 6.5–8.3).

On blood agar, after incubation for 18 hours, the colonies are usually small (0.5–1 mm), dome shaped, with an area of greenish discolouration **(alpha haemolysis)** around them. On prolonged incubation, the colonies become flat, with raised edges and central umbonation (due to autolysis occurring at centre) which creates a **draughtsman appearance** (concentric rings are seen when viewed from above).

In liquid medium such as glucose broth, pneumococci produce uniform turbidity.

C. Biochemical Reactions

Pneumococci ferment several sugars with production of acid only. Fermentation is tested in Hiss's serum water. **Fermentation of inulin** by pneumococci is of great value to differentiate them from streptococci.

Bile solubility test

Pneumococci are soluble in bile. When 2% sodium deoxycholate solution is added to a broth culture, the culture clears due to the lysis of the cocci. Alternatively, if a loopful of 10% sodium deoxycholate solution is placed on a pneumococcus colony, lysis of colony occurs within a few minutes. Bile solubility test is an important diagnostic test to differentiate pneumococcus from other streptococci.

Pneumococci are catalase and oxidase negative.

D. Resistance

Pneumococci are delicate organisms and are destroyed at 52°C for 15 minutes. They are more sensitive to usual antiseptics.

Optochin sensitivity test

Pneumococci are sensitive to optochin (ethylhydrocuprein hydrochloride) in a concentration of 1/500,000. When an optochin disc (5 μg) is applied on a blood agar plate inoculated with pneumococci, a wide zone (14 mm or more) of inhibition occurs on incubation. This is very useful test to differentiate pneumococci from other streptococci which do not show zone of inhibition by optochin disc.

E. Antigenic Structure

The most important antigen of the pneumococcus is *capsular polysaccharide.* Other antigens are *somatic M protein* and a group specific *cell wall carbohydrate*.

1. Capsular Polysaccharide

Capsular polysaccharide is type specific. Pneumococci are classified into types based on the nature of the capsular polysaccharide. More than 90 serotypes are recognised. These are named 1, 2, 3, and so on.

Serological typing of pneumococcus is carried out by three methods.

(i) Agglutination of organisms with type specific antiserum.
(ii) Precipitation of capsular polysaccharide with type specific antiserum.
(iii) Quellung reaction or capsule swelling reaction was described by *Neufeld* (1902). In this reaction, a suspension of pneumococci is mixed on a slide with a drop of specific antiserum. In presence of the homologous antiserum, the capsule around pneumococci reveals an apparent swelling, sharply delineated and refractile under the microscope.

2. M Protein

M protein is characteristic for each type of pneumococcus.

3. Cell Wall Carbohydrate (C-Substance)

Pneumococci contain a species specific carbohydrate antigen which is named as C-substance. It is present in all pneumococci. The *C-substance* is precipitated by an abnormal protein (μ-globulin), that appears in the acute phase sera of cases of pneumonia but disappears during convalescence. It is also detected in blood of patients with some other illnesses. This is known as the **C-reactive protein (CRP)**. It is not an antibody of C substance. It is an 'acute phase' substance and its production is stimulated by bacterial infections, malignancies and tissue destruction.

F. Pathogenesis

Str. pneumoniae is one of the most common bacteria causing pneumonia, both lobar and bronchopneumonia. *Str. penumoniae* is the second most important cause of pyogenic meningitis after *N. meningitidis*. This disease is more common in children.

Pneumococcus may also produce empyema, pericarditis, otitis media, sinusitis, conjunctivitis, peritonitis and suppurative arthritis, usually as complications of pneumonia.

G. Laboratory Diagnosis

1. Specimens

Clinical samples, such as sputum, cerebrospinal fluid (CSF), pleural exudate or blood are collected according to the site of lesion. Blood culture is useful in pneumococcal septicaemia.

2. Collection and Transport

All the specimens should be collected in sterile containers under all aseptic conditions. They should be processed immediately. In case of delay, CSF specimen should never be refrigerated but kept at 37°C (*H. influenzae*, another causative agent of pyogenic meningitis, if present, may die at cold temperature).

3. Direct Microscopy

Gram staining of smear reveals a large number of polymorphs and typical organism. In case of meningitis, presumptive diagnosis may be made by finding Gram positive diplococci which may be intracellular as well as extracellular in CSF smear.

4. Antigen Detection

Capsular polysaccharide antigen can be demonstrated in cerebrospinal fluid by latex agglutination or immunochromatographic assay.

5. Culture

Specimen is inoculated on blood agar and incubated at 37°C for 24 hours in the presence of 5–10% CO_2. Typical colonies develop with α–haemolysis. Organisms from the isolated colony are identified by Gram staining and biochemical reactions.

6. Colony Morphology and Staining

Colonies are usually small (0.5–1 mm), with alpha haemolysis around them. On prolonged incubation, colonies have draughtsman appearance.

On Gram staining pneumococci are Gram positive, small (1 μm diameter), diplococci. They are flame shaped or lanceolate in appearance. The capsule may be demonstrated as a clear halo in India ink preparation (Fig. 18.2).

7. Biochemical Reactions

Important biochemical tests are inulin fermentation and bile solubility tests. Another test which has a great value is optochin sensitivity test. Details of these tests have already been described. *Str. pneumoniae* can be differentiated from *Str. viridans* by various characteristics (Table 18.1).

8. Animal Pathogenicity Test

From specimens where organisms are expected to be scanty, intraperitoneal inoculation in mice may be used. Inoculated mice die in 24–48 hours. Heart blood and peritoneal exudate of the animal show pneumococci.

H. Treatment

The antibiotic of choice is parenteral penicillin. Cephalosporin is indicated in case of penicillin resistant strains.

Table 18.1: Differential Characteristics of Str. pneumoniae and Str. viridans

Characteristic	*Str. pneumoniae*	*Str. viridans*
Morphology	Capsulated, lanceolate diplococci (in pairs)	Non-capsulated, oval or round cocci in chains
Colonies on blood agar	Initially dome shaped with α-haemolysis, later 'draughtsman' colonies	Dome shaped with α-haemolysis
Colonies in liquid medium	Uniform turbidity	Granular turbidity, powdery deposit
Bile solubility	Positive	Negative
Inulin fermentation	Positive	Negative
Optochin sensitivity	Positive	Negative
Animal pathogenicity (Intraperitoneal inoculation in mice)	Fatal infection	Non-pathogenic

KEY POINTS

1. Pneumococci are Gram positive, small, slightly elongated cocci arranged in pairs (diplococci) with broad ends in apposition. Each coccus has one end broad or rounded and other pointed (flame shaped or lanceolate appearance). They are capsulated.
2. Pneumococci differ from streptococci in their morphology (diplococci), bile solubility and optochin sensitivity. They may cause pneumonia, meningitis, empyema, otitis media etc.

STUDY QUESTIONS

1. Describe the laboratory diagnosis of pneumococcal infections.
2. Differentiate between *Str. pneumoniae* and *Str. viridans* in a tabulated form.

MULTIPLE CHOICE QUESTIONS (MCQs)

1. Draughtsman colony is a characteristic feature of:
   (a) *Streptococcus pyogenes*
   (b) *Strep. pneumoniae*
   (c) *Enterococcus faecalis*
   (d) Viridans streptococci
2. Capsule of *Streptococcus pneumoniae* can be demonstrated by:
   (a) India ink staining
   (b) Quellung reaction
   (c) Both of the above
   (d) None of the above
3. *Streptococcus pneumoniae* may cause:
   (a) Lobar pneumonia
   (b) Bronchopneumonia
   (c) Meningitis
   (d) All of the above
4. Which of the following tests can be useful to identify *Streptococcus pneumoniae*?
   (a) Bile solubility test
   (b) Inulin fermentation
   (c) Optochin sensitivity test
   (d) All of the above

ANSWERS (MCQs)

1. (b) 2. (c) 3. (d) 4. (d)

Neisseria

19

The genus *Neisseria* consists of Gram negative, aerobic, oxidase positive, nonmotile diplococci (arranged in pairs). They may be classified into pathogenic and non-pathogenic (commensals). The two pathogenic species are *N. meningitidis* (causes pyogenic meningitis) and *N. gonorrhoeae* (causes gonorrhoea). The non-pathogenic species include *N. flavescens*, *N. sicca*, *N. subflava* and other species.

I. NEISSERIA MENINGITIDIS (MENINGOCOCCUS)

A. Morphology

They are Gram negative, spherical or oval cocci, 0.6–0.8 µm in size, arranged in pairs with the adjacent sides flattened (Fig. 19.1). They are non-motile. The cocci are generally intracellular when isolated from lesions.

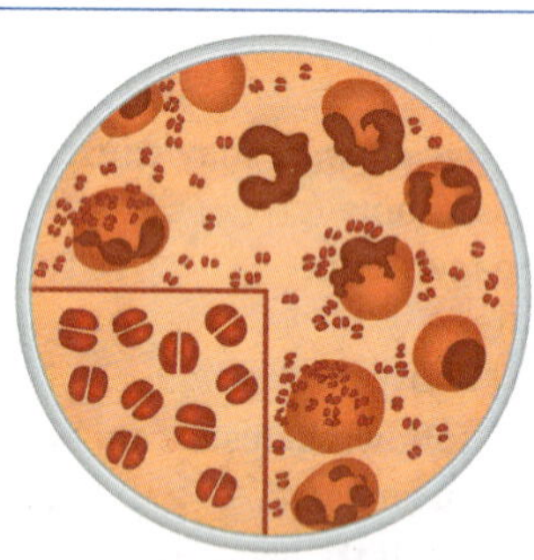

Fig. 19.1 N. meningitidis in cerebrospinal fluid. Inset—enlarged view showing flat adjacent sides of cocci.

B. Culture

They do not grow on ordinary media but have exacting growth requirements. Growth occurs on media enriched with blood or serum. Blood agar, chocolate agar and Mueller-Hinton agar are commonly used media. Thayer-Martin medium with antibiotics (vancomycin, colistin, nystatin and trimethoprim) is selective media used for its isolation.

They are strict aerobes and cannot grow anaerobically. The optimum temperature and pH for growth are 35–36°C and 7.4–7.6 respectively. A moist environment with 5–10% CO_2 is must for growth to occur.

On solid media, the colonies are small (1 mm in diameter), round, convex, grey, translucent and with entire edges. In liquid media, it produces a granular turbidity.

C. Biochemical Reactions

N. meningitidis is catalase and oxidase positive. The prompt oxidase reaction helps to identify neisseria (both meningococci and gonococci) in mixed cultures. Glucose and maltose are fermented with acid production but no gas (gonococci ferment glucose but not maltose). They do not ferment lactose or sucrose. Indole and H_2S are not produced and nitrates are not reduced.

Oxidase test

When freshly prepared oxidase reagent (1% tetramethyl paraphenylene diamine hydrochloride) is poured on the culture plate, neisseria colonies become deep purple. These colonies can be picked up for subcultures immediately, as the organism dies on prolonged exposure to the reagent. The test may also be performed by rubbing bacterial growth with a coverslip on a filter paper strip moistened with the oxidase reagent (***Kovac's method***). A deep purple colour is a positive reaction.

D. Antigenic Structure

N. meningitidis has been divided into 12 serogroups on the basis of immunological specificity of the capsular polysaccharide. These serogroups are A, B, C, X, Y, Z, W (formerly W-135), 29E, H, I, K and L. Groups A, B and C are the most important.

E. Resistance

These are very delicate organisms, being highly susceptible to heat, desiccation and to disinfectants. They are susceptible to penicillin, ampicillin, chloramphenicol, macrolides and ciprofloxacin. Strains resistant to penicillin have now been reported from several countries.

F. Pathogenesis

N. meningitidis causes pyogenic meningitis in all ages, but is most common in children (3 months to 5 years) and young adults (15 to 25 years).

Meningococci are strict human pathogens. The infection is acquired by droplet spread via the carriers and the cases. Human nasopharynx is the reservoir of *N. meningitidis*. The incubation period of the disease is about 3 days.

Meningococcaemia presents as acute fever with petechial rash. A few develop fulminant meningo-coccaemia (***Waterhouse Friderichsen syndrome***) characterised by shock, disseminated intravascular coagulation and multisystem failure. It is usually a fatal condition.

G. Laboratory Diagnosis

1. *Specimens*

The following specimens are collected depending on the clinical presentation.

- CSF
- Blood
- Petechial lesions specimen
- Nasopharyngeal swab—especially to detect carriers.

2. *Collection and Transport*

Collection of specimen is done under sterile conditions by lumbar puncture for CSF and by venepuncture for blood. Blood is injected into blood culture bottles (glucose broth and sodium taurocholate broth) through the hole in the bottle cap. Nasopharyngeal specimen is collected by using a sterile swab. All the specimens must be transported immediately. CSF should never be refrigerated as *H. influenzae* (another common causative agent of meningitis) may die at the cold temperature. The nasopharyngeal swab should be held in a transport medium (e.g. Stuart's) until it is inoculated on a culture medium.

3. *Direct Microscopy and Antigen Detection*

CSF is divided into three portions. **One portion** is centrifuged and smear is prepared from the deposit for Gram staining. Meningococci are seen as Gram negative diplococci present mainly inside polymorphs (intracellular), but may also be present extracellularly. A large number of pus cells are also seen. The supernatant fluid may be used for detection of meningococcal antigen (capsular polysaccharide) by rapid tests, such as latex agglutination test.

The **second portion** of the CSF is used for direct culture while the **third portion** of the CSF is incubated overnight after adding an equal volume of glucose broth and then subcultured on blood agar or chocolate agar. Culture of third portion of CSF may sometimes succeed when direct culture fails.

4. *Culture*

(i) CSF

Centrifuged deposit is inoculated on blood agar or chocolate agar. The plate is incubated at 35–36°C under 5–10% CO_2. Colonies appear after 18–24 hours. These are identified by colony morphology, Gram staining and biochemical reactions.

(ii) Blood

Blood culture is often positive in meningococcaemia and in early cases of meningitis. Blood culture bottles (glucose broth and sodium taurocholate broth) or BHI broth bottle are incubated at 35–36°C for 24 hours. Subcultures are made from these broths on to blood agar and chocolate agar. These plates are again incubated at 35–36°C under 5–10% CO_2 for 18–24 hours. Identification of organism is done by colony morphology, Gram staining and biochemical reactions.

(iii) Other specimens

Other specimens (petechial lesions, nasopharyngeal swab, autopsy specimens) are inoculated on blood agar and chocolate agar and are processed in similar way as described for CSF.

5. *Colony Morphology and Gram Staining*

On solid media, colonies are small (1 mm in diameter), round, convex, grey, translucent and with entire edges. Smear is prepared from the suspected colony and Gram staining is done. On Gram staining, they are Gram negative, spherical or oval cocci, 0.6–0.8 µm in size, arranged in pairs (diplococci) with the adjacent sides flattened (Fig. 19.1).

6. *Biochemical Reactions*

N. meningitidis is catalase and oxidase positive. Glucose and maltose are catabolised with acid production but no gas. The breakdown of glucose and maltose occurs by oxidation and not by fermentation.

7. *Slide Agglutination*

Direct slide agglutination of the organism may be done with specific antisera.

H. Treatment

A third generation cephalosporin (cefotaxime or ceftriaxone) is the drug of choice. Penicillin G can also be given.

I. Prophylaxis

1. *Chemoprophylaxis*

It is indicated for close contacts of patients for eliminating the bacteria from nasopharynx. Rifampicin or ciprofloxacin are recommended.

2. *Immunoprophylaxis*

Meningococcal vaccines prepared from polysaccharides of serogroups A, C, W and Y are available. Single dose is given intramuscularly. The protection is group specific and lasts for at least three years.

II. NEISSERIA GONORRHOEAE (GONOCOCCUS)

N. gonorrhoeae causes the sexually transmitted disease, gonorrhoea.

A. Morphology

They are Gram negative oval cocci arranged in pairs (diplococci) with adjacent sides concave (pear or bean shaped). In smear from purulent material, they are intracellular within polymorphs, some cells containing as many as a hundred cocci (Figs. 19.2 and 19.3).

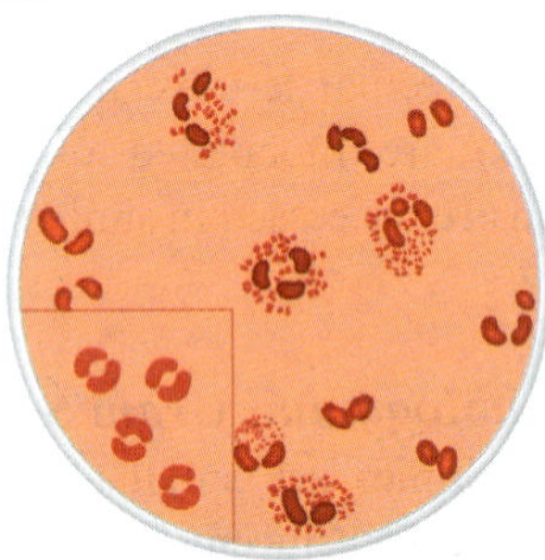

Fig. 19.2 N. gonorrhoeae in urethral pus. Inset—enlarged view showing diplococci with adjacent surfaces concave

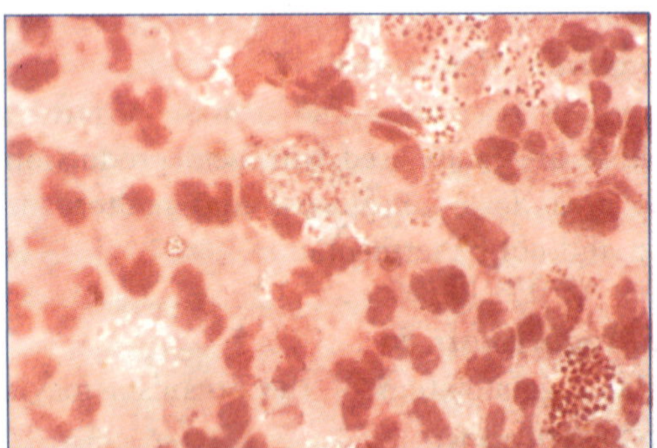

Fig. 19.3 Gram-negative intracellular diplococci (N. gonorrhoeae)

B. Culture

This organism is more difficult to grow than *N. meningitidis*. They are aerobic, but may grow anaerobically as well. They grow best at a temperature of 35–36°C in presence of 5–10% CO_2 and at pH 7.2–7.6. They require an enriched medium like chocolate agar for their growth. A popular selective medium is the ***Thayer-Martin medium*** that contains chocolate agar with antibiotics (vancomycin, colistin, nystatin and trimethoprim) which inhibits most contaminants including commensal neisseria.

Colony morphology

Colonies are small, round, grey, translucent, convex with finely granular surface. They are easily emulsifiable.

C. Biochemical Reactions

N. gonorrhoeae is oxidase positive. Gonococci ferment glucose (with acid production only) and not maltose.

D. Antigenic Structure

The antigenic structure is complex. The surface structures of *N. gonorrhoeae* include the following:

1. Capsule

It is polyphosphate and not polysaccharide.

2. Pili

These are hair like structures extending from the surface. Pili enhance attachment of the organism to host cells and resist phagocytosis. They act as virulence factor. They are made up of pilin proteins.

3. Lipopolysaccharide (LPS)

Toxicity in gonorrhoea is largely due to the endotoxic effects of this component.

4. Proteins

The outer membrane antigens (proteins) are the porins.

E. Resistance

The gonococcus is a very delicate organism. It is strict parasite and dies rapidly outside the human host,

Gonococci are readily killed by heat, drying and antiseptics. Formerly, they were highly susceptible to sulphonamides and penicillin but have steadily developed resistance to many antibiotics. PPNG (penicillinase producing *Neisseria gonorrhoeae*) strains are resistant to penicillin due to production of β lactamase (penicillinase) enzyme by these strains.

F. Pathogenesis

1. Gonococcal Urethritis or Gonorrhoea

It is a sexually transmitted disease involving urethra in both sexes but in females, the endocervix is the primary site of infection. The incubation period is 2–8 days. The disease is an acute urethritis characterised by **purulent urethral discharge**. Asymptomatic infection is common in women. In males, the acute urethritis may extend to the prostate, testes, seminal vesicles and epididymis.

The infection may spread to the periurethral tissues causing abscesses and multiple discharging sinuses (*Watercan perineum*). In females, the primary infection may spread from urethra and cervix to uterus, fallopian tubes, ovaries and may cause pelvic inflammatory disease resulting in sterility.

2. *Ophthalmia Neonatorum*

It is a non-venereal gonococcal conjunctivitis in the newborn through infected birth canal.

3. *Gonococcal Vulvovaginitis*

In adult women the vagina usually is resistant to gonococcal infection because of the acidic pH of the vaginal secretions, but vulvovaginitis can occur in prepubertal girls.

4. *Other Infections*

Sometimes the disease may involve rectum or oropharynx following rectal intercourse or by orogenital contact respectively. Involvement of oropharynx may lead to gonococcal pharyngitis.

G. Laboratory Diagnosis

The diagnosis is readily made in acute stage, as urethral discharge contains large number of gonococci. It is difficult to detect gonococci from chronic cases.

1. *Specimens*

Urethral discharge and cervical discharge (in females) are collected in acute urethritis. In women, cervical swab is collected in addition to urethral discharge. High vaginal swabs are not satisfactory.

In chronic urethritis, urethral discharge is observed only in few cases. In these cases, some exudate obtained after prostatic massage or morning drop of secretion may be examined. Centrifuged deposits of urine is examined in cases where no urethral discharge is available.

2. *Transport*

All the specimens should be transported and processed immediately. If this is not possible, specimens should be collected with charcoal coated swabs and transported to the laboratory in Stuart's transport medium.

3. *Direct Microscopy*

Gram staining of smear provides a presumptive evidence of gonorrhoea in men. Gram negative intracellular diplococci are found in smear of at least 95% cases of acute gonococcal urethritis in males. In females, diagnosis of gonorrhoea by smear examination is unreliable as some of the normal genital flora have similar morphology. Fluorescent antibody tests are more sensitive and specific methods for diagnosis by microscopy especially in females.

4. *Detection of Antigen or Nucleic acid*

The gonococcal antigens can be detected by ELISA in clinical specimens. Nucleic acid can be directly detected in urethral discharge using DNA probe.

5. *Culture*

The specimens should be inoculated directly on preheated plates immediately on collection. Chocolate agar is used for culture of the specimens and incubated at 35°C to 36°C under 5–10% CO_2 for 48 hours. In chronic cases, where mixed infection is usual, selective medium such as Thayer-Martin medium is used.

6. *Colony Morphology and Gram Staining*

On solid medium, colonies are small, round, grey, translucent, convex with finely granular surface. They are easily emulsifiable. Smear is made from the colony and Gram staining is done. Gonococci are Gram negative cocci arranged in pairs (diplococci) with adjacent sides concave (pear or bean shaped).

7. *Biochemical Reactions*

They are oxidase positive. They ferment glucose with acid only. They do not ferment maltose unlike meningococci.

H. Treatment

Currently a single dose of **ceftriaxone intramuscular** or **cefixime orally** is **recommended** for treatment of uncomplicated gonococcal infections.

Coinfection with *C. trachomatis* is common in patients with gonorrhoea therefore dual therapy is frequently recommended. Dual therapy includes ceftriaxone (for gonorrhoea) and azithromycin/doxycycline (for *C. trachomatis*).

I. Prophylaxis

Control of gonorrhoea consists of early detection of cases, tracing of contacts, health education and other general measures. Both partners should be treated. Safe sex practices such as use of condoms should be adopted. Vaccination has no role in prophylaxis.

KEY POINTS

1. The genus *Neisseria* consists of *Gram negative*, *aerobic*, *oxidase positive*, non-motile *diplococci*.
2. The two pathogenic species are *N. meningitidis* (causing pyogenic meningitis) and *N. gonorrhoeae* (causing *gonorrhoea*).
3. *Chocolate agar* is the commonly used medium. *Thayer-Martin* medium is a selective medium used for their isolation.
4. *Meningococcal vaccines* prepared from polysaccharides of serogroups A, C, W-135 and Y are available. Single dose is given intramuscularly.
5. *N. gonorrhoeae* is pear or bean shaped. It can grow on all those culture media used for growth of *N. meningitidis*.
6. Penicillin resistance in *N.gonorrhoeae* may be due to production of enzyme *beta-lactamase (penicillinase)*. It is plasmid coded. These strains are named penicillinase producing *Neisseria gonorrhoeae (PPNG)*.

STUDY QUESTIONS

1. Describe the laboratory diagnosis of meningococcal meningitis.
2. Discuss the laboratory diagnosis of gonorrhoea.

MULTIPLE CHOICE QUESTIONS (MCQs)

1. Which of the following is a selective medium for isolation of *Neisseria gonorrhoeae*?
   (a) Thayer-Martin medium
   (b) Blood agar
   (c) MacConkey's agar
   (d) Potassium tellurite blood agar
2. How many serogroups of *Neisseria meningitidis* are known?
   (a) Nine
   (b) Twelve
   (c) Thirteen
   (d) Fifteen
3. Which of the following rapid tests may be used to detect meningococcal antigen?
   (a) Countercurrent immunoelectropheresis
   (b) Coagglutination test
   (c) Latex agglutination test
   (d) All of the above

ANSWERS (MCQs)

1. (a) 2. (c) 3. (d)

Corynebacterium

20

Corynebacteria are Gram positive, non-acid-fast, non-sporing, non-motile bacilli. They frequently show club-shaped swellings (*coryne* means club shaped). The most important member of the genus is *C. diphtheriae* which causes diphtheria in humans.

I. CORYNEBACTERIUM DIPHTHERIAE

A. Morphology

These are thin, slender, Gram positive bacilli and measure approximately 3–6 µm × 0.6-0.8 µm. They are pleomorphic. They are club-shaped due to the presence of metachromatic granules at one or both ends. With Loeffler's methylene blue stain, granules take up a bluish purple colour and hence they are named ***metachromatic granules***. These granules are also called ***volutin*** *or* ***Babes-Ernst granules***. The bacilli are usually seen in angular fashion resembling the letters V or L. This has been called ***Chinese letter*** or ***cuneiform arrangement*** (Fig. 20.1).

The bacilli look green and metachromatic granules appear bluish black when Albert stain is used. They are non-capsulated, non-acid-fast and non-motile.

B. Cultural Characteristics

C. diphtheriae are grown best on media enriched with blood, serum or egg. Growth is scanty on ordinary media. They are aerobic and facultatively anaerobic. The optimum temperature for growth is 37°C (range 15–40°C) and optimum pH 7.2. The following are the usual media employed for cultivation of diphtheria bacillus.

1. Hiss's Serum Water

This is a liquid medium containing serum. Growth is seen as a turbidity and pellicle formation.

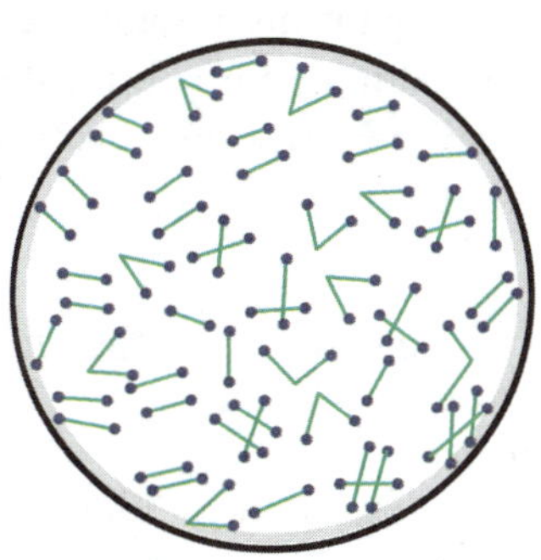

Fig. 20.1 Morphology of C. diphtheriae

2. Loeffler's Serum Slope

Diphtheria bacilli grow on this medium very rapidly. Colonies appear after 6 to 8 hours of incubation, long before other bacteria grow. The colonies are small, circular, white or creamy and glistening.

3. Tellurite Blood Agar Medium

It contains potassium tellurite (0.04%) which inhibits most other bacteria and thus acting as a selective agent. The organisms grow slowly on this medium and form grey or black colonies due to reduction of potassium tellurite to tellurium (Fig. 20.2). The colonies may take two days to appear on this medium. Based on colony morphology on tellurite medium and other properties, three main biotypes of *C. diphtheriae—gravis, intermedius* and *mitis* are distinguished (Table 20.1).

C. Biochemical Reactions

They ferment glucose and maltose with the production of acid but without gas. They do not ferment lactose, mannitol or sucrose. The gravis biotype ferments starch and glycogen while intermedius and mitis have no such action (Table 20.1).

D. Toxin

The pathogenicity is due to production of a very powerful exotoxin by virulent strains of diphtheria bacilli. Avirulent strains are frequent among convalescents, carriers and contacts.

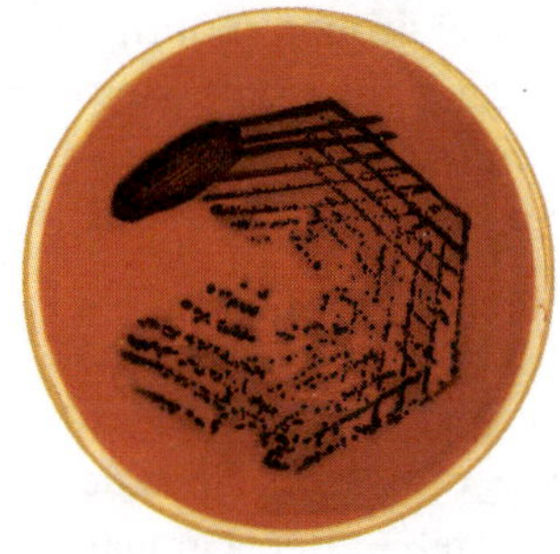

Fig. 20.2 C.diphtheriae on potassium tellurite blood agar

Table 20.1: Type Differentiation of C. diphtheriae Strains

Character	Gravis	Intermedius	Mitis
1. Morphology	Short rods, few metachromatic granules, uniform staining	Long, poor granulation, barred forms with clubbed ends, pleomorphic	Long rods, curved, prominent granules, pleomorphic
2. Colony on tellurite blood agar	In 18 hours, 1–2 mm, grey, raised centre. In 48–72 hours, flat colony with raised centre and crenated edge with radial striation— *daisy head* colony	In 18 hours, 1 mm in size. In 48 hours, no change in size, dull granular centre, more glistening periphery and a lighter ring near the edge—*frog's egg* colony	Size variable, shiny black. In 48–72 hours, flat colony with central elevation— *poached egg* colony
3. Consistency of colonies	Brittle, not easily picked out or emulsifiable, like *cold margarine*	Intermediate between gravis and mitis	Soft, buttery, easily emulsifiable
4. Haemolysis	Variable	Non-haemolytic	Usually haemolytic
5. Growth in broth	Surface pellicle	Turbidity in 24 hours, clearing in 48 hours, with fine granular sediment	Diffuse turbidity
6. Biochemical tests			
Glucose	Acid without gas	Acid without gas	Acid without gas
Glycogen	Acid without gas	Negative	Negative
Starch	Acid without gas	Negative	Negative
7. Virulence	Severe	Moderate	Mild

Mode of Action

It acts by inhibiting protein synthesis. It inhibits polypeptide chain elongation in the presence of nicotinamide adenosine dinucleotide (NAD) by inactivating the elongation factor, EF-2.

E. Pathogenesis

Diphtheria is most commonly seen in children of 2 to 10 years. Infection is confined to humans only. The incubation period is 3 to 4 days, but may on occasion be as short as one day. Infection occurs by way of droplet spread. Diphtheria may be of following clinical types depending upon the site of infection.

1. Faucial
2. Laryngeal
3. Nasal
4. Conjunctival
5. Otitic
6. Vulvovaginal
7. Cutaneous mainly around mouth and nose.

Faucial diphtheria is the commonest type. The toxin has both *local* as well as *systemic* effects.

F. Laboratory Diagnosis

Laboratory confirmation of diphtheria is necessary for control measures and epidemiological studies, but not for the treatment of cases. Specific treatment should be started immediately after clinical diagnosis without waiting for laboratory reports. Any delay may be fatal. Laboratory diagnosis consists of *isolation of organism* and demonstration of its toxicity by *virulence tests*.

1. Isolation of Organism

(i) Collection of specimen

Two swabs from the lesions (throat, nose, larynx, ear, conjunctiva, vagina, or skin) are collected. One swab is used for smear examination and other for culture.

Local lesion is usually in the throat. Swabs are collected prior to start of antibiotics and application of antiseptics in form of gargles. The swabs are rubbed over the affected area and pseudomembrane, if formed, should be scraped with swab. If there is no definite localised lesion, the swabs should be rubbed over tonsils and the posterior pharyngeal wall without touching the mouth parts.

(ii) Direct microscopy

Smears are stained with both Gram and Albert stain. Diphtheria bacilli show beaded slender green rods in typical Chinese letter pattern on Albert's staining. However, they cannot be confidently differentiated from some commensal corynebacteria normally present in the throat. Hence it is reported as "the organisms resembling *C. diphtheriae*" seen in direct smear examination. Gram staining is done to identify Vincent's spirochaetes and fusiform bacilli (other causes of sore throat).

(iii) Culture

The swabs are inoculated on the following culture media:

(a) Loeffler's serum slope
   Growth appears within 6–8 hours on this medium. Subculture from Loeffler's serum slope is made on tellurite blood agar and plate is incubated at 37°C for 48 hours.

(b) Tellurite blood agar
These plates have to be incubated at 37°C for at least 48 hours before declaring these as negative, as growth may sometimes be delayed.

(iv) Colony morphology and staining

On Loeffler's serum slope, the colonies are small, circular, white or creamy. Diphtheria bacilli grow as black or grey coloured colonies on tellurite blood agar.

Smears are prepared from suspected growth from various media. These smears are stained with Albert and Gram stain to confirm the morphology of *C. diphtheriae*. Albert staining shows green bacilli with bluish black metachromatic granules. Gram staining reveals Gram positive bacilli.

(v) Biochemical reactions

Hiss's serum water is used for testing fermentation of carbohydrates.

2. Virulence Tests

These tests demonstrate the production of exotoxin by bacteria isolated on culture. Virulence testing may be done by *in vivo* or *in vitro* methods.

In Vivo Tests

Two types of test are used viz. subcutaneous and intracutaneous.

(a) Subcutaneous test

The growth from an overnight culture on Loeffler's serum slope is emulsified in 2–5 ml broth and 0.8 ml of this emulsion is injected subcutaneously into two guinea pigs, one of which has received an intramuscular injection of 500 units of diphtheria antitoxin 18–24 hours previously (this protected animal acts as a control). If the strain is virulent, the unprotected animal will die within 2 to 3 days with evidence of haemorrhage in the adrenal glands which is the pathognomonic feature.

(b) Intracutaneous test

Two guinea pigs (or rabbits) are injected intracutaneously with 0.1 ml emulsion from growth on Loeffler's serum slope, one of these animals is protected with 500 units antitoxin the previous day (control) and the other is given 50 units of antitoxin intraperitoneally four hours after the skin test, in order to prevent death. If the strain is toxigenic (virulent), the inflammatory reaction at the site of injection progresses to necrosis in 48 to 72 hours in the test animal but there is no change in the control animal. An advantage in the intracutaneous test is that 8 to 10 strains can be tested at a time on a pair of animals and the animals do not die.

In Vitro Test

Elek's gel precipitation test

This is an immunodiffusion test. A rectangular strip of filter paper soaked in diphtheria antitoxin (1000 units per ml) is placed on the surface of a 20% horse serum agar plate while the medium is still fluid. When the agar solidifies, the test strain is streaked at right angle to the filter paper strip. The positive and negative controls are also put up. The plate is incubated at 37°C for 24 to 48 hours. The toxin produced by the bacterial growth diffuses in the agar and produces a line of precipitation where it meets the antitoxin at optimum concentration (Fig. 20.3). Non-toxigenic strains will not produce any precipitation line.

G. Prophylaxis

1. Active Immunisation

Active immunisation is started at 6 weeks of age by toxoid in combination with tetanus toxoid and pertusis vaccine (DPT, Triple vaccine). Three doses of 0.5 ml each are given by intramuscular route at an interval of 4–6 weeks. Booster doses of DPT are given at 18 months and at 5 years.

Pentavalent vaccine contains DPT along with hepatitis B and **Haemophilus influenzae** type b. This vaccine is being used in National Immunisation Programme of India.

2. Passive Immunisation

This is an emergency measure when susceptible persons are exposed to infection, as when a case of diphtheria is admitted to paediatric wards. In such cases 500–1000 units of antitoxin (antidiphtheric serum, ADS) is administered subcutaneously.

H. Schick Test

This test demonstrates immunity or susceptibility of

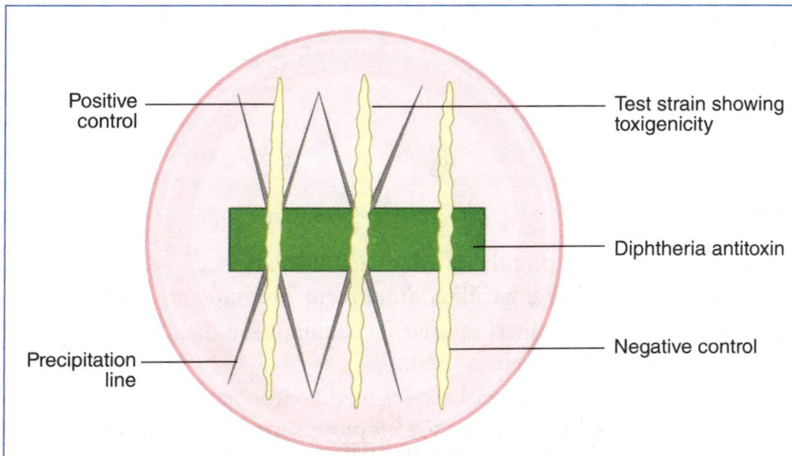

Fig. 20.3 Elek's gel precipitation test

a person against diphtheria and is one example of neutralisation test (toxin-antitoxin).

1. Method

A test dose of 0.2 ml diphtheria toxin is injected intradermally on one forearm and a similar amount of inactivated toxin is injected on another forearm.

2. Results

Results are read after 1, 4 and 7 days. There may be four types of reaction.

(i) Positive reaction

An area of swelling and erythema appears at the site of injection of toxin after 24-48 hours. The control forearm injected with heated toxin will show no reaction. A positive test signifies that the person is susceptible to diphtheria due to either absence or lack of adequate amount of circulating antitoxin.

(ii) Negative reaction

There is absence of any reaction in either forearm (control and test). It indicates that the toxin has been neutralised by sufficient amount of antitoxin present in the blood and that the person is immune to diphtheria.

(iii) Pseudoreaction

There is erythema occurring in both forearms within 6–24 hours and disappearing completely from both forearms within four days. This indicates that the individual is immune to diphtheria and he is also hypersensitive to the components of diphtheria bacilli.

(iv) Combined reaction

The initial reaction is similar to that of pseudoreaction. Erythema disappears in the control forearm within four days but it progresses in the test forearm to a typical positive reaction. It indicates that the individual is susceptible to diphtheria and hypersensitive to bacillus.

Shick test is not used nowadays.

I. Treatment

Treatment should be started immediate when there is clinical suspicion of diphtheria.

C. diphtheriae is sensitive to penicillin, erythromycin and other antibiotics.

The antibiotics are of little value as these cannot inactivate the toxin already present in patient's body. When a case is suspected as diphtheria, antidiphtheric serum should be given immediately as the mortality rate increases with delay in starting antitoxin treatment.

II. DIPHTHEROIDS

Commensal corynebacteria are normally present in the throat, skin, conjunctiva and other areas. These may sometimes be mistaken for *C. diphtheriae* and are called diphtheroids (Table 20.2). The common diptheroids include *C. xerosis* (found in the conjunctival sac) and *C. pseudodiphtheriticum* (*C. hofmannii*) which is found in the throat.

Table 20.2: Distinguishing Features of C. diphtheriae and Diphtheroids

Feature	*C. diphtheriae*	Diphtheroids
1. Morphology	(i) Weakly Gram positive and thin bacilli (ii) Metachromatic granules present (iii) Chinese letter pattern (iv) Pleomorphism present	Strongly Gram positive, short and thick bacilli Few or absent Pallisade arrangement Very little pleomorphism present
2. Culture	Grow on special enriched media	Can grow on ordinary media
3. Biochemical tests	Ferments glucose only and does not ferment sucrose	Ferments both glucose and sucrose
4. Toxin production	Toxic	Non-toxic

KEY POINTS >>>

1. Corynebacterium diphtheriae are bacilli usually seen in angular fashion resembling the letters V or L. This has been called Chinese letter. These bacilli contain metachromatic granules.
2. Special stain like Albert is used for staining the bacilli. The bacilli look green and metachromatic granules appear bluish black when Albert stain is used.
3. C. diphtheriae are grown best on media enriched with blood, serum or egg. Loeffler's serum slope (LSS) and potassium tellurite blood agar medium are employed for cultivation of this bacillus.
4. Potassium tellurite blood agar is a selective medium. The organisms grow slowly on this medium and form grey or black colonies due to reduction of tellurite to tellurium.

5. C. diphtheriae causes diphtheria. The pathogenicity is due to production of a very powerful exotoxin.
6. Virulence tests demonstrate the production of exotoxin by bacteria isolated on culture.
7. Triple vaccine (DPT) is used for active immunisation. This vaccine contains diphtheria toxoid, tetanus toxoid and pertussis vaccine.

STUDY QUESTIONS

1. Discuss in detail the laboratory diagnosis of diphtheria.
2. Write short notes on:
   - (i) Diphtheria toxin
   - (ii) Schick test
   - (iii) Diphtheroids
   - (iv) Toxigenicity of *C. diphtheriae*

MULTIPLE CHOICE QUESTIONS (MCQs)

1. Chinese letter arrangement of bacilli is a characteristic feature of:
   - (a) *Mycobacterium tuberculosis*
   - (b) *M. leprae*
   - (c) *Corynebacterium diphtheriae*
   - (d) *Bacillus cereus*
2. Babes-Ernst granules are present in:
   - (a) *Mycobacterium tuberculosis*
   - (b) *M. laprae*
   - (c) *Corynebacterium diphtheriae*
   - (d) *Bacillus cereus*
3. What is the colour of colonies of *C. diphtheriae* on tellurite blood agar medium?
   - (a) White
   - (b) Golden yellow
   - (c) Grey to black
   - (d) Cream
4. Which is the selective medium used for isolation of *C. diphtheriae*?
   - (a) Tellurite blood agar
   - (b) Loeffler's serum slope
   - (c) Lowenstein-Jensen medium
   - (d) Chocolate agar
5. Production of diphtheria toxin by bacteria can be demonstrated by:
   - (a) Subcutaneous test
   - (b) Intracutaneous test
   - (c) Elek's gel precipitation test
   - (d) All of the above

ANSWERS (MCQs) ...✓

1. (c) 2. (c) 3. (c) 4. (a) 5. (d)

21 Bacillus

Members of the genus *Bacillus* are ubiquitous, present in soil, dust, air and water and are frequently isolated as contaminants in bacteriological culture media. *B. anthracis*, the causative agent of anthrax, is the most important pathogen of the group. *B. cereus* can cause food poisoning. They are generally motile with peritrichous flagella except the anthrax bacillus which is non-motile.

I. BACILLUS ANTHRACIS

It is the causative agent of anthrax, a disease primarily of animals, and man gets infected secondarily.

A. Morphology

Bacillus anthracis is a Gram positive, non-acid-fast, non-motile, large (3–10 µm × 1–1.6 µm), rectangular, spore forming bacillus. The spores are refractile, oval and central in position and are of the same width as the bacillary body so that they do not cause bulging of vegetative cell (Fig. 21.1).

In cultures, the bacilli are arranged end-to-end in long chains. The ends of the bacilli are truncated or often concave and somewhat swollen so that a chain of bacilli presents a *bamboo-stick* appearance.

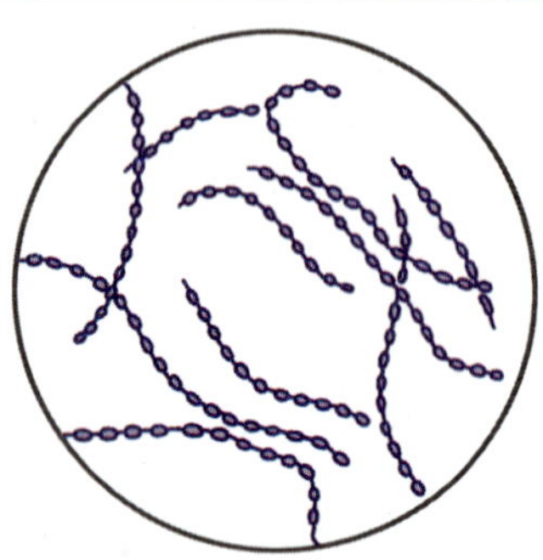

Fig. 21.1 Anthrax bacilli

B. Culture

B. anthracis is an aerobe and facultative anaerobe, with a temperature range for growth being 12–45°C (optimum 35–37°C).

1. Nutrient Agar Media

Colonies are round, 2–3 mm in diameter, raised, opaque and greyish white. Under low power of the microscope, the edge of the colony is found to be composed of long, interlacing chains of bacilli, resembling locks of matted hair, the so called the *Medusa head* appearance (Fig. 21.2).

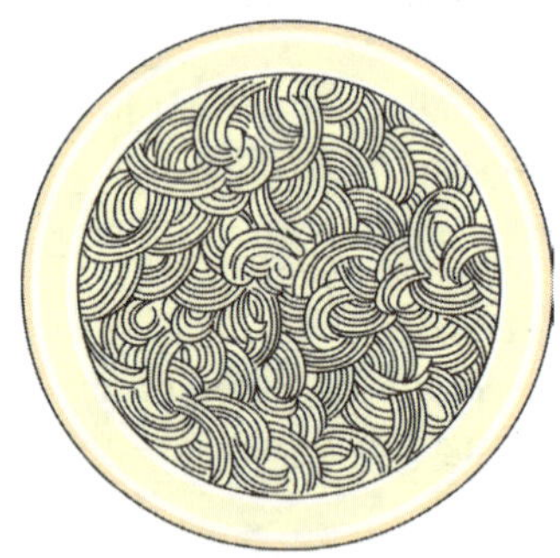

Fig. 21.2 Medusa head appearance of colony on nutrient agar

2. Blood Agar Media

The colonies are non-haemolytic, though occasional strains produce a narrow zone of haemolysis.

3. Selective Medium

A selective medium (PLET medium) consisting of heart infusion agar with polymyxin, lysozyme, ethylene diamine tetracetic acid (EDTA) and thallous acetate has been devised for isolation of *B.anthracis* from mixtures containing other spore-bearing bacilli.

C. Pathogenesis

Anthrax is primarily a disease of animals like cattle and sheep, and less often of horses and swine. Infected animals discharge large number of bacilli from the mouth, nose and rectum. These bacilli sporulate in soil and remains as the source of infection.

Human Anthrax

Humans are occasionally secondarily infected from diseased animals. There are three clinical type of disease based on route of infection—cutaneous, pulmonary and intestinal anthrax. All types lead to septicaemia.

Cutaneous anthrax follows entry of the spores through the abraded skin. This is commonly found in farmers and persons handling carcasses. The cutaneous lesion is also called 'malignant pustule'. Cutaneous anthrax may resolve spontaneously, but may sometimes lead to fatal septicaemia.

Pulmonary anthrax occurs due to inhalation of the dust or filaments of wool from infected animals, particularly in wool factories. This is also called *wool sorter's disease*.

Intestinal anthrax is rare in man and is found in those who consume improperly cooked infected meat.

D. Laboratory Diagnosis

1. Specimens

Swabs, fluid or pus from pustules; sputum and blood from pulmonary and septicaemic anthrax are generally collected.

2. Microscopy

Gram stained smear from the specimen shows often chain of large Gram positive bacilli. Capsule appears as a clear halo around the bacterium by India-ink staining.

3. Culture

Specimen is inoculated on nutrient agar medium and incubated at 37°C for overnight. Medusa head colonies appear on the medium. Smears made from these colonies show typical Gram positive spore bearing bacilli.

4. Animal Inoculation

White mouse or guinea pigs are injected with exudate or culture. Animal dies in 36–48 hours. Smears made from heart blood and sputum show bacilli.

II. ANTHRACOID BACILLI

Aerobic spore bearing bacilli resembling *B. anthracis* are called anthracoid or pseudoanthrax bacilli. Some of them are frequent laboratory contaminants and have to be differentiated from *B. anthracis.* The main differentiating features between anthracoid bacilli and *B. anthracis* are shown in Table 21.1.

III. BACILLUS CEREUS

B. cereus has assumed importance as a cause of food poisoning. It is widely distributed in nature such as soil, vegetables, milk, cereals, spices, meat and poultry. Some spores survive cooking and germinate into vegetative bacilli which produce *enterotoxin* that cause food poisoning.

A. Types of Food Poisoning

1. Short Incubation Period Type (1–5 Hours)

It is characterised by acute nausea and vomiting, 1–5 hours after the meal. Diarrhoea is not common. It is usually associated with consumption of cooked rice, usually fried rice from Chinese restaurants.

2. Long Incubation Period Type (8–16 Hours)

It is characterised by acute abdominal pain and diarrhoea, 8–16 hours after ingestion of contaminated food. Vomiting is rare.

Table 21.1: Differentiating Features of B. anthracis and Anthracoid Bacilli

Feature	*B. anthracis*	Anthracoid Bacilli
1. Motility	Non-motile	Generally motile
2. Capsule	Capsulated	Non-capsulated
3. Chain formation	Long chains	Short chains
4. Colony on nutrient agar	Medusa head colony	Not present
5. Growth in broth	No turbidity	Uniform turbidity
6. Gelatin stab culture	Inverted fir tree appearance and slow gelatin liquefaction	Rapid gelatin liquefaction
7. Haemolysis on blood agar	Absent or weak	Usually well marked
8. Growth in Penicillin agar (10 units/ml)	No growth	Grow usually
9. Growth at 45°C	No growth	Grow usually
10. Susceptibility to gamma phage	Susceptible	Not susceptible
11. Pathogenicity test in animals	Pathogenic	Not pathogenic
12. Ascoli's precipitin test	Positive	Negative
13. Fluorescent antibody test with anthrax antiserum	Positive	Negative

B. Diagnosis

Suspected food, faeces and vomitus are cultured on ordinary media or a special mannitol-egg yolk-phenol red-polymyxin agar (MYPA) medium. Spore bearing Gram positive bacilli may be seen on smear from colonies. *B. cereus* is a motile bacillus, non-capsulated, not susceptible to gamma phage and does not react with fluorescent antibody conjugate.

C. Treatment

Disease is mild and self limiting, requiring no specific treatment.

KEY POINTS

1. Members of the genus Bacillus are ubiquitous, present in soil, dust, air and water. They are sporogenous, rod shaped, aerobic, Gram positive bacteria.
2. *B. anthracis*, the causative agent of anthrax, is the most important pathogen of the bacillus group. *B. cereus* can cause food poisoning.

STUDY QUESTION

1. Write short notes on:
   (i) Anthracoid bacilli
   (ii) *Bacillus cereus* food poisoning.

MULTIPLE CHOICE QUESTIONS (MCQs)

1. 'Medusa head' appearance of colonies is a characteristic feature of:
   (a) *Clostridium perfringens*
   (b) *Bacillus anthracis*
   (c) *Mycoplasma hominis*
   (d) *Ureaplasma urealyticum*
2. 'Malignant pustule' lesion is found in:
   (a) Cutaneous anthrax
   (b) Pulmonary anthrax
   (c) Intestinal anthrax
   (d) None of the above
3. Which of the following characteristics can differentiate *Bacillus cereus* from *Bacillus anthracis*?
   (a) Non-capsulated
   (b) Motile
   (c) Not susceptible to gamma phage
   (d) All of the above

ANSWERS (MCQs) ...✓

1. (b) 2. (a) 3. (d)

Clostridium

22

I. CLASSIFICATION

Clostridia of medical importance may be classified on the basis of diseases they produce:

A. Tetanus	*Cl. tetani*
B. Gas gangrene	
Established pathogens	*Cl. perfringens*
	Cl. novyi
	Cl. septicum
C. Food poisoning	
1. Gastroenteritis	*Cl. perfringens*
2. Necrotising enteritis	*Cl. perfringens*
3. Botulism	*Cl. botulinum*
D. Acute colitis	*Cl. difficile*

II. CLOSTRIDIUM PERFRINGENS (CLOSTRIDIUM WELCHII)

Cl. perfringens is the most important and common aetiological agent of gas gangrene. It also produces food poisoning and necrotising enteritis in man.

Cl. perfringens is a commensal in the large intestines of man and animals. The spores are commonly found in soil and dust.

A. Morphology

It is a large, stout, Gram positive bacillus measuring 4–6 µm × 1 µm with subterminal spore (Fig. 22.1). It is capsulated and non-motile.

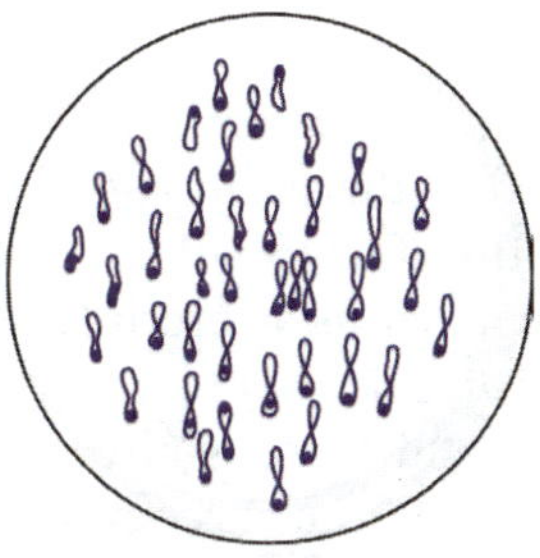

Fig. 22.1 Clostridium perfringens

B. Culture

It grows on blood agar, cooked meat broth (CMB) and thioglycollate broth within 24–48 hours. It is anaerobic and grows over a pH range of 5.5–8.0 and wide temperature range of 20°C–50°C. The optimum temperature for growth is 37°C.

On blood agar, colonies of most strains show a ***target haemolysis***, resulting from a narrow zone of complete haemolysis caused by theta-toxin and a much wider zone of incomplete haemolysis due to alpha toxin. In Robertson cooked meat broth, the meat pieces turn pink but are not digested.

C. Biochemical Reactions

Cl. perfringens is predominantly saccharolytic but also have mild proteolytic action (gelatin liquefaction). It ferments glucose, lactose, sucrose and maltose with the production of acid and gas.

In litmus milk, lactose fermentation leads to formation of acid, which changes the colour of litmus from blue to red. The acid coagulates the casein (acid clot) and the clotted milk is disrupted due to vigorous gas production and this is known as ***stormy fermentation***.

D. Resistance

Spores are usually destroyed within five minutes by boiling but those of the 'food poisoning' strains resist boiling for 1–3 hours. Autoclaving at 121°C for 15 minutes is lethal. Spores are resistant to commonly used antiseptics and disinfectants.

E. Toxins

Cl. perfringens produce at least 12 distinct toxins but four major toxins include *alpha*, *beta*, *epsilon* and *iota*.

Alpha (α) Toxin

It is produced by all types of *Cl. perfringens.* Chemically it is a phospholipidase (lecithinase C) and is responsible for profound toxaemia in gas gangrene.

Nagler reaction

Cl. perfringens is grown on a medium containing 6% agar, 5% Fildes' peptic digest of sheep blood and 20% human serum or 5% egg yolk in a plate. To one half of the plate, antitoxin is spread on the surface. The inoculated culture plate is incubated at 37°C for 24 hours. Colonies on the half plate without the antitoxin will be surrounded by opacity while colonies on the other half with antitoxin shows no opacity, due to specific neutralisation of the alpha toxin (Fig. 22.2). Alpha toxin (lecithinase C) splits lecithin into phosphoryl choline and a diglyceride (lipid). The lipid deposits around the colonies resulting in opacity.

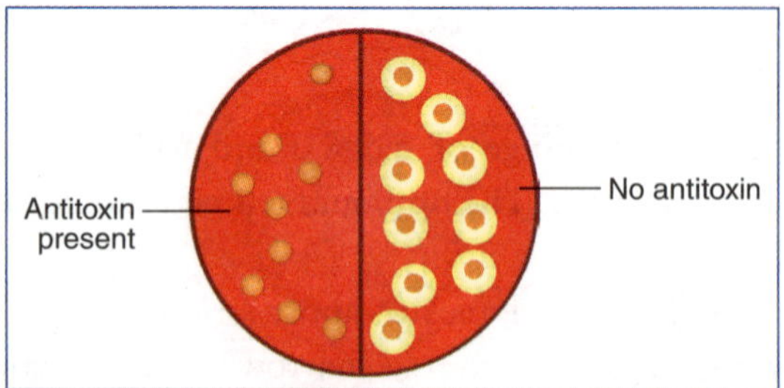

Fig. 22.2 Nagler reaction

Reverse CAMP test

This test is similar to the CAMP test for identifying group B streptococci (refer chapter 17) except that *Clostridium sp.* is inoculated in place of *Staph. aureus* and a known group B streptococcus is used. Although group B streptococci may show some enhanced haemolysis with other clostridia but only *Cl. perfringens* exhibits accentuated zone of haemolysis as butterfly appearance (Fig. 22.3).

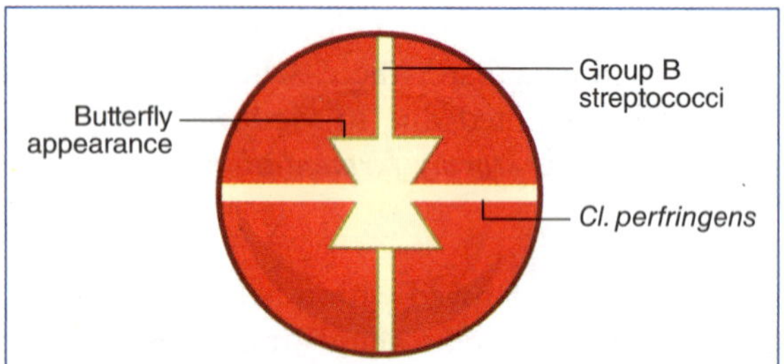

Fig. 22.3 Reverse CAMP test

Other Major Toxins

Beta (β), *epsilon* (ε) and *iota* (ι) toxins have lethal and necrotising properties.

Enterotoxin

Some strains produce enterotoxin which causes diarrhoea and other symptoms of food poisoning.

F. Pathogenesis

Cl. perfringens produces the following human infections:

1. Gas Gangrene
2. Food Poisoning
3. Necrotising Enteritis.

G. Laboratory Diagnosis

The diagnosis of gas gangrene must be made primarily on clinical grounds and the laboratory only confirms the clinical diagnosis. The specimens to be collected are exudates from wound, necrotic tissue and muscle fragments.

1. Direct Microscopy

Gram stained smears give presumptive diagnosis. Large number of Gram positive bacilli without spores is strongly suggestive of *Cl. perfringens*.

2. Culture

The specimens are inoculated on fresh and heated blood agar and cooked meat (CMB) broth. Growth in CMB is subcultured on blood agar plates after 24–48 hours. The blood agar is incubated anaerobically for 48–72 hours. Most strains produce beta haemolysis on blood agar and a few are non-haemolytic. A plate of serum or egg yolk agar is used for **Nagler reaction**. The bacterial isolates are identified by **morphology**, **cultural characteristics** and **biochemical reactions**. Toxigenicity of the strain can be done by animal pathogenicity.

III. CLOSTRIDIUM TETANI

Cl. tetani is the causative agent of tetanus. It is widely distributed in soil and intestine of man and animals.

A. Morphology

It is a Gram positive, slender bacillus (measuring 4–8 μm × 0.5 μm) with spherical, terminal spores giving the bacillus the characteristic *drumstick* appearance (Fig. 22.4). It is non-capsulated and motile (except *Cl. tetani* type VI) with peritrichate flagella.

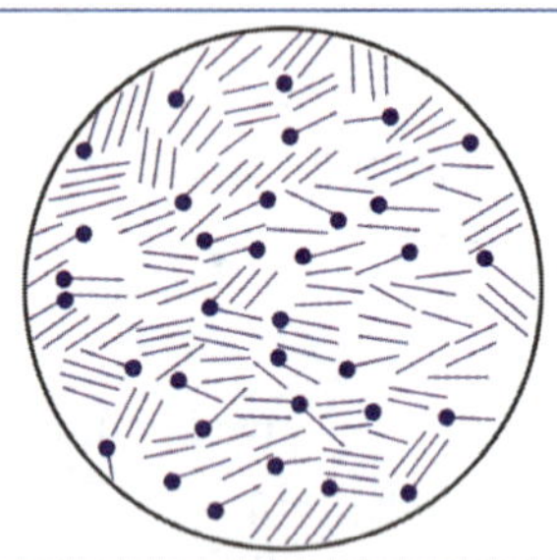

Fig. 22.4 Clostridium tetani

B. Culture

It is an obligate anaerobe which grows on ordinary media. Growth is improved by the addition of blood or serum. The optimum temperature for growth is 37°C and pH 7.4. It can grow well in cooked meat broth (CMB), thioglycollate broth, nutrient agar and blood agar. In CMB, growth occurs as turbidity and there is also some gas formation. The meat is not digested but becomes black on prolonged incubation. The bacilli produce a swarming (thin spreading film) growth on blood agar.

C. Biochemical Reactions

Cl. tetani has slight proteolytic, but no saccharolytic property. Gelatin liquefaction occurs very slowly. It does not ferment any sugar.

D. Resistance

Most of the strains are killed by boiling for 10–15 minutes but some resist boiling for three hours. However, autoclaving (at 121°C for 20 minutes) kills the spores of most strains. The spores may survive in soil for years.

E. Toxins

Cl. tetani produces two distinct toxins—*tetanolysin* (haemolysin) and *tetanospasmin* (neurotoxin).

F. Pathogenesis

Cl. tetani has little invasive power. Tetanus develops following the contamination of wound with *Cl. tetani* spores. The source of infection may be soil, dust, faeces etc. Infection strictly remains localized in the wound. Pathogenic effects are mainly due to tetanospasmin (neurotoxin) of *Cl. tetani.*

G. Laboratory Diagnosis

The diagnosis of tetanus should always be made clinically and laboratory tests are done only to confirm it. Laboratory diagnosis may be made by demonstration of bacilli by microscopy, culture or by animal inoculation. Specimens generally collected are wound swab, exudate or tissue from the wound.

1. Microscopy

Gram staining may show Gram positive bacilli with drumstick appearance.

2. Culture

Specimen is inoculated on freshly prepared blood agar and incubated at 37°C for 24-48 hours under anaerobic conditions. *Cl. tetani* produces a swarming growth. Gram stained smear from culture shows typical Gram positive bacilli with drumstick appearance.

3. Toxigenicity Test

Pathogenicity of the isolated organism is established with demonstration of toxin production. It is best tested in animals.

H. Prophylaxis

The available methods are

1. Surgical
2. Antibiotics
3. Immunisation

1. Surgical

It aims at removal of foreign body, blood clots etc., in order to prevent anaerobic conditions favourable for the bacillus.

2. Antibiotics

Antibiotics destroy or inhibit tetanus bacilli and other pyogenic bacteria in wounds and thus the production of toxin is prevented. Long acting penicillin injection or erythromycin may be given.

3. Immunisation

Tetanus is a preventable disease.

(i) Active immunisation

It is the most effective method of prophylaxis. *Tetanus toxoid* (formol toxoid) is commonly used for active immunisation. Three doses of 0.5 ml tetanus toxoid each are given intramuscularly, with an interval of 4 to 6 weeks between first two doses and 6–12 months between the second and third dose. A full course of three doses confers immunity for a period of at least 10 years. A 'booster dose' of toxoid is recommended after 10 years.

Tetanus toxoid is given along with diphtheria toxoid and pertusis vaccine (DPT) in children. Pertusis vaccine acts as adjuvant. Three doses are given intramuscularly at interval of 4–6 weeks, starting at age as early as 6 weeks. Booster doses are given at age of 18 months and then at five years.

(ii) Passive immunisation

Antitetanus serum (ATS), prepared by immunising horses with toxoid, has been used for preventing tetanus. Being a horse serum, it carries the risk of hypersensitivity reaction.

Homologous serum prepared from humans, human antitetanus immuno–globulins (HTIG), is now being used without the risk of hypersensitivity.

IV. CLOSTRIDIUM BOTULINUM

Clostridium botulinum causes a severe form of food poisoning named botulism. It is a widely distributed saprophyte and is found in soil, animal manure, vegetables and sea mud.

A. Morphology

It is a Gram positive, non-capsulated bacillis about 5 μm × 1 μm, motile by peritrichate flagella and produces subterminal, oval, bulging spores (Fig. 22.5).

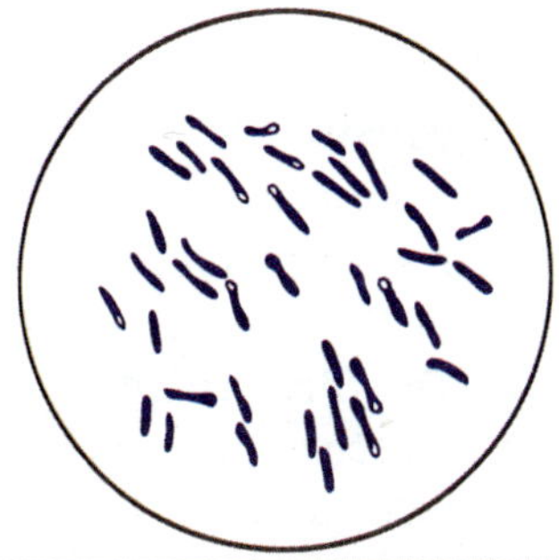

Fig. 22.5 Clostridium botulinum

B. Culture

It is a strict anaerobe and can grow on ordinary media. Optimum temperature is 35°C. Commonly used media are blood agar and cooked meat broth (CMB). Colonies are large, irregular, semitransparent, with fimbriate border. On blood agar, haemolysis around the colonies is observed.

C. Resistance

The spores are highly resistant, and can withstand heat for several hours at 100°C and for upto 10 minutes at 120°C.

D. Toxin

Cl. botulinum forms a powerful exotoxin. The toxin differs from other exotoxins in that it is not released during the life of the bacterium. It is produced intracellularly and appears in the medium on autolysis of the cell. It is a neurotoxin and acts slowly, therefore, takes several hours to kill.

E. Pathogenesis

Cl. botulinum is non-invasive and its pathogenicity is due to the action of preformed toxin, the manifestations of which are collectively called botulism. Botulism is of three types—foodborne, infant and wound botulism.

1. Foodborne Botulism

It is due to preformed toxin in food contaminated with *Cl. botulinum*. The source of botulism is usually various preserved foods—meat, fish, vegetables etc.

The symptoms appear 12–36 hours after ingestion of contaminated food. Vomiting, thirst, constipation, ocular paresis, difficulty in swallowing, speaking and breathing are the common symptoms. Diarrhoea is not a symptom.

2. Infant Botulism

It affects infants, usually below 6 months. It is a disease due to ingestion of food contaminated by spores of *Cl. botulinum*.

3. Wound Botulism

It is a very rare condition which results from wound infection with *Cl. botulinum*.

F. Laboratory Diagnosis

Diagnosis may be confirmed by demonstration of the bacillus or the toxin in suspected residual food or in faeces.

Demonstration of the Organism

Smears made from suspected food or faeces are examined by Gram's staining which may show Gram positive sporing bacilli. Culture is done on blood agar or cooked meat broth (CMB). Growth on culture media may be confirmed by Gram's staining. Presence of bacilli in food or faeces in absence of toxin is of no significance. Hence, toxin in culture fluid must be demonstrated by toxigenicity test in mice.

G. Prophylaxis and Treatment

As botulism follows consumption of canned or preserved food, control may be achieved by proper canning and preservation. By the time symptoms appear, the toxin is fixed to nervous tissue and it can no longer be inactivated by antitoxin. However, if outbreak occurs, prophylactic dose of antitoxin should be given intramuscularly to all who have consumed the suspected food.

V. CLOSTRIDIOIDES DIFFICILE

Cl. difficile was so named due to unusual difficulties involved in its isolation. Taxonomically, it is placed into a separate genus **Clostridioides** and named as **Clostridioides difficile**.

A. Morphology

It is a long, slender, Gram positive bacillus containing oval and terminal spores.

B. Toxins

It produces two toxins, an **enterotoxin (toxin A)** and a **cytotoxin (toxin B)**. The enterotoxin is primarily responsible for diarrhoea.

C. Pathogenesis

The pathogenic role of *Cl. difficile* was established in 1977, when it was found to be responsible for **antibiotic associated colitis**. Many antibiotics have been incriminated but lincomycin and clindamycin are particularly prone to cause **pseudomembranous colitis**. If the condition is not recognised early and properly treated, it terminates fatally.

D. Laboratory Diagnosis

1. Demonstration of Toxin

Toxin can be demonstrated in the faeces by its characteristic effect on human diploid cells and HEp–2. ELISA can also be used for the demonstration of toxin.

2. Nucleic Acid Amplification Tests

Nucleic acid amplification tests (NAATs) which can determine the presence of toxins A and B genes in faeces are becoming the new gold standard for the detection of toxin producing *Cl.difficile*.

3. Isolation of Bacilli

Cl. difficile can be grown from the faeces of patients with subsequent test for toxigenicity.

E. Treatment

Cl. difficile are generally resistant to most antibiotics, but these are susceptible to vancomycin. Clindamycin and lincomycin should be avoided. Metronidazole is the drug of choice.

KEY POINTS

1. The genus *Clostridium* consists of *anaerobic*, *spore forming*, *Gram positive bacilli.*
2. This genus contains bacteria that cause three major diseases of man—*tetanus*, *gas gangrene* and *food poisoning*.
3. Clostridial pathogenicity is mainly due to production of a powerful exotoxin.
4. Clostridia grow well on blood agar medium under *anaerobic* conditions. Liquid media like *cooked meat broth* (*CMB*) is very useful for growing clostridia.
5. *Cl. tetani* produces two distinct toxins—*tetanolysin* (haemolysin) and *tetanospasmin* (neurotoxin). It is the causative agent of *tetanus*.
6. *Tetanus toxoid* is used for prophylaxis of tetanus.
7. As clostridia are toxin producing bacteria, antitoxins are used for passive immunisation in the diseases associated with them. *Anti-gas gangrene* and *human antitetanus immunoglobulins* (*HTIG*) are two examples of antitoxins used in gas gangrene and tetanus respectively.

STUDY QUESTIONS

1. Discuss the laboratory diagnosis of gas gangrene.
2. Write short notes on:
   (i) Nagler reaction
   (ii) Laboratory diagnosis of tetanus
   (iii) Prophylaxis against tetanus
   (iv) Laboratory diagnosis of botulism
   (v) *Clostridioides difficile.*

MULTIPLE CHOICE QUESTIONS (MCQs)

1. All of the following species of *Clostridium* may cause gas gangrene except:
   (a) *Clostridium perfringens*
   (b) *Cl. novyi*
   (c) *Cl. septicum*
   (d) *Cl. difficile*
2. *Clostridium perfringens* may produce the following infections:
   (a) Gas gangrene
   (b) Food poisoning
   (c) Necrotising enteritis
   (d) All of the above
3. Drumstick appearance of spores is a characteristic feature of:
   (a) *Clostrdium perfringens*
   (b) *Cl. tetani*
   (c) *Cl. septicum*
   (d) *Cl. novyi*
4. Stormy fermentation is useful in identification of:
   (a) *Clostridium perfringens*
   (b) *Cl. tetani*
   (c) *Cl. botulinum*
   (d) *Cl. difficile*
5. Botulism is due to
   (a) Preformed toxin of *Clostridium botulinum*
   (b) Invasion of *Cl. botulinum* in the intestine
   (c) Both of the above
   (d) None of the above

ANSWERS (MCQs)

1. (d) 2. (d) 3. (b) 4. (a) 5. (a)

23

Nonsporing Anaerobes

Non-sporing anaerobes have been recognised as an important cause of human and animal infections. Many of these bacteria form commensal flora of man and animals in mouth, oropharynx, gastrointestinal tract and genital tracts. Some of these anaerobic bacteria act as opportunistic pathogens when body resistance is lowered.

I. CLASSIFICATION

A. Cocci

1. Gram positive cocci
   - (i) *Peptococcus*
   - (ii) *Peptostreptococcus*
2. Gram negative cocci
   - (i) *Veillonella*

B. Bacilli

1. Gram positive bacilli
   - (i) *Eubacterium*
   - (ii) *Lactobacillus*
   - (iii) *Bifidobacterium*
   - (iv) *Propionibacterium*
   - (v) *Actinomyces*
   - (vi) *Mobiluncus*
2. Gram negative bacilli
   - (i) *Bacteroides*
   - (ii) *Prevotella*
   - (iii) *Porphyromonas*
   - (iv) *Fusobacterium*
   - (v) *Leptotrichia*

C. Spirochaetes
   - (i) *Treponema*
   - (ii) *Borrelia*

Spirochaetes are described separately in Chapter 32.

II. LABORATORY DIAGNOSIS

As anaerobic bacteria form part of the normal flora of the skin and mucous surfaces, their isolation from clinical specimens has to be interpreted cautiously. The mere presence of an anaerobe does not prove it as a causative agent.

A. Specimens

Specimens are to be collected in such a manner to avoid normal resident flora. For example, material collected by aspiration in case of lung abscess is acceptable but not the sputum. As these anaerobic bacteria die on exposure to oxygen, care has to be taken to minimise contact of specimen with air during collection, transport and handling of specimens. Specimens should be inspected for characteristics that strongly indicate the presence of anaerobes, such as foul odour. Other clues suggestive of anaerobic infection include:

1. Failure to isolate organisms from pus (sterile pus)
2. Deep abscesses.
3. Pus which shows red fluorescence under UV light.
4. Failure to respond to conventional antimicrobial treatment.

B. Direct Microscopy

Examination of a Gram stained smear is very useful. Pus in anaerobic infection shows a variety of organisms and numerous pus cells.

C. Culture

Freshly prepared blood agar is a suitable culture medium. Culture plates are incubated at 37°C in anaerobic jar with 10 per cent CO_2. Anaerobiosis can also be maintained by Gas-Pak system. Plates are examined after 24–48 hours.

Other anaerobic media, such as cooked meat broth (CMB) previously known as Robertson cooked meat (RCM) medium and thioglycollate broth, may also be used for inoculating the specimens.

Definitive identification of the anaerobes depends on colony morphology and various biochemical tests.

KEY POINTS

1. Non-sporing anaerobes form *commensal flora* of man and animals in mouth, oropharynx, gastrointestinal tract and genital tracts. Some of these anaerobic bacteria act as *opportunistic pathogens* when body resistance is lowered.
2. Anaerobic bacteria can be grown on blood agar under anaerobic conditions. *Anaerobic jar* is generally used for producing anaerobiosis. *Cooked meat broth* (CMB) may also be used to grow these bacteria.

STUDY QUESTION

1. Classify non-sporing anaerobes. Discuss the laboratory diagnosis of infections caused by non-sporing anaerobes.

MULTIPLE CHOICE QUESTION (MCQ)

1. Which of the following bacteria are Gram negative cocci?
   (a) *Peptococcus*
   (b) *Peptostreptococcus*
   (c) *Veillonella*
   (d) All of the above

ANSWER (MCQ) ...✓

1. (c)

Enterobacteriaceae

24

Members of the family *Enterobacteriaceae* are aerobic and **facultative anaerobic Gram negative enteric bacilli**. They are **motile by peritrichous flagella** or are **non-motile**. They grow readily on ordinary media, **ferment glucose with production of acid or acid and gas**, reduce nitrates to nitrites, oxidase negative and catalase positive except *Sh. dysentriae* type 1 which is catalase negative and *Plesiomonas sp.* which is oxidase positive. They are non-capsulated and non-sporing.

I. ESCHERICHIA COLI

A. Morphology

Esch. coli is a Gram negative bacillus measuring 1–3 µm × 0.4–0.7 µm. Most strains are motile. It is non-sporing and non-capsulated.

B. Culture

It is an aerobe and facultative anaerobe and grows on ordinary culture medium at optimum temperature of 37°C (temperature range 10–40°C) in 18–24 hours. On MacConkey's medium, colonies are pink due to lactose fermentation **(LF or lactose fermenter colonies)**. In general, colonies are circular, moist, smooth with entire margin and **non-mucoid** unlike colonies of klebsiella which are mucoid. In liquid medium, growth occurs as uniform turbidity.

C. Biochemical Reactions

They ferment most of the sugars (glucose, lactose, mannitol, maltose) with production of acid and gas. Typical strains do not ferment sucrose. Indole and methyl red (MR) reaction are positive but Voges–Proskauer (VP) and citrate utilisation tests are negative (IMViC ++ – –). Urea is not split.

D. Antigenic Structure

Serotyping of *Esch. coli* is based on the presence of O (somatic antigen), K (capsular antigen) and H (flagellar antigen) antigens detected by agglutination reactions. Another antigen present is F (fimbrial) antigen. 173 'O' antigens, 103 K antigens and 53 H antigens have been described.

E. Toxins

Some strains of *Esch. coli* produce *enterotoxins*, *haemolysin* and *Verocytotoxin*.

1. Enterotoxins

Enterotoxigenic strains of *Esch. coli* (ETEC) produce one or both of two enterotoxins, a heat-labile toxin (LT) and a heat-stable toxin (ST).

2. Haemolysin

Some strains of *Esch. coli* produce a haemolysin which can lyse erythrocytes of some species.

3. Verocytotoxin (VT)

It is also called Shiga like toxin (SLT). Biological, physical and antigenic properties of VT are similar to Shiga toxin produced by *Sh. dysentriae* type 1.

F. Pathogenesis

Esch. coli forms a part of normal intestinal flora of man and animal. There are four major types of clinical syndromes which are caused by *Esch. coli:* (1) urinary tract infection (2) diarrhoea (3) pyogenic infections, and (4) septicaemia.

1. Urinary Tract Infection

Esch. coli is the commonest organism responsible for urinary tract infection (UTI). *Esch. coli* that causes UTI often originates in the intestine of the patient.

2. Diarrhoea

Esch. coli causing diarrhoeal diseases are of four groups. They produce diarrhoea with different pathogenic mechanisms.

(i) Enteropathogenic Esch. coli (EPEC)

EPEC adhere tightly to enterocytes, leading to inflammatory reactions and epithelial degenerative changes. EPEC are non invasive and do not produce enterotoxins.

(ii) Enterotoxigenic Esch. coli (ETEC)

These are the strains that form a heat-labile enterotoxin

(LT) or a heat-stable enterotoxin (ST) or both. They are now known to be a major cause of diarrhoea in children in developing countries and are the most important cause of ***travellers diarrhoea***. The name 'travellers' diarrhoea refers to diarrhoea in persons from the developed countries within a few days of their visit to one of the developing countries.

(iii) Enteroinvasive Esch. coli (EIEC)

Some strains of *Esch. coli* invade the intestinal epithelial cells as do dysentery bacilli and produce disease identical to shigella dysentery. These have been named enteroinvasive *Esch. coli* (EIEC). On instillation into the eyes of guinea pigs, EIEC cause keratoconjunctivitis, this diagnostic test for EIEC is called ***Sereny test***. This test is no longer used.

(iv) Enterohaemorrhagic Esch. coli (EHEC) or Verocytotoxin producing Esch. coli (VTEC)

These strains cause **haemorrhagic colitis (HC)** and **haemolytic uraemic syndrome (HUS)**. Toxin responsible is called 'Verotoxin' because of its effect on vero cells in culture.

3. Pyogenic Infections

Esch. coli may cause wound infection, peritonitis, cholecystitis and neonatal meningitis. It is an important cause of neonatal meningitis.

4. Septicaemia

Esch. coli is a very common cause of septicaemia in many hospitals. This condition usually occurs in debilitated patients and mortality is very high.

G. Laboratory Diagnosis

URINARY TRACT INFECTION

Normal urine is sterile, but during voiding may become contaminated with commensals of genital tract.

1. Specimen Collection

(i) Midstream urine specimen (MSU)

It is collected preferably prior to administration of antibiotics. Specimen is collected in a sterile container. Before collecting a sample, genitalia should be cleaned with soap and water and men are instructed to retract the foreskin of glans penis whereas women should keep the labia apart. The first portion of urine is allowed to pass, then without interrupting the urine flow, mid-portion of the stream is collected. The first portion of urine adequately flushes out the normal urethral flora.

(ii) Catheter specimen

Urine should be collected directly from the catheter and not from the collection bag. The catheter should not touch the container. Although a catheter specimen yields excellent results but catheterisation to obtain urine is not justified because of risk of introducing infection.

(iii) Urine specimens from infants

A clean catch specimen after cleansing of genitalia is preferred.

2. Transport

As urine is a good culture medium, specimens after collection should reach the laboratory with minimum delay, if it is not possible, the specimen is to be refrigerated at 4°C.

3. Laboratory Methods

Part of the specimen is used for bacteriological culture and the rest is examined immediately under the microscope.

(i) Microscopy

Urine is centrifuged and deposit is examined under the microscope for detecting pus cells, erythrocytes, epithelial cells and bacteria.

(ii) Culture

Most laboratories use a semiquantitative method (standard loop technique) for culture of urine specimens.

Standard loop technique

A standard calibrated loop is used to culture a fixed volume of uncentrifuged urine. Blood agar and MacConkey's agar are used and incubated at 37°C for 24 hours. Next day, the number of colonies grown is counted and total count per ml is calculated. The blood agar gives a quantitative measurement of bacteriuria, while MacConkey's medium enables the presumptive diagnosis of the bacterium.

Interpretation of results

Kass (1956) gave a criterion for active bacterial infection of urinary tract as follows:

Significant bacteriuria — When bacterial count is more than 10^5/ml of a single species.

Doubtful significance — between 10^4 to 10^5 bacteria per ml. Specimen should be repeated for culture.

No significant growth — $< 10^3$ bacteria per ml and are regarded as contaminant.

(iii) Identification

The organisms are identified by colony characters, Gram's staining, motility, biochemical reactions and slide agglutination test.

(iv) Antibiotic sensitivity test

Esch. coli and other common urinary pathogens develop multiple drug resistance. Antibiotic sensitivity is necessary to administer proper antibiotics.

DIARRHOEA

Laboratory diagnosis of *Esch. coli* diarrhoea has been complex as there is no single test which can identify all strains of *Esch. coli* responsible for diarrhoea. Faeces or rectal swab is plated directly on blood agar and MacConkey's medium. After overnight incubation, growth on culture media is identified by colony morphology, Gram staining, motility and biochemical reactions.

PYOGENIC INFECTIONS

The specimens are usually pus and wound swab. Cultures are made on McConkey's agar and the isolate is identified by colony morphology, staining, motility and biochemical reactions.

SEPTICAEMIA

Diagnosis depends on the isolation of the organism by blood culture and its identification by colony morphology, staining, motility and biochemical reactions.

II. KLEBSIELLA

The genus *Klebsiella* consists of Gram negative, capsulated, non-sporing, non-motile bacilli that grow well on ordinary media, produce pink mucoid colonies on MacConkey's agar.

A. Classification

Klebsiella has been classified into two species namely *K. pneumoniae* and *K. oxytoca*. *K. pneumoniae* is further subdivided into three subspecies namely pneumoniae, ozaenae and rhinoscleromatis.

B. Morphology

These are short, plump, Gram negative, capsulated, non-motile bacilli. They are about 1–2 µm × 0.5–0.8 µm in size.

C. Culture

Klebsiellae grow well on ordinary media at optimum temperature of 37°C in 18-24 hours. On MacConkey's agar, the colonies appear large, mucoid and pink to red in colour. Mucoid nature of colonies is due to accumulation of slime produced by the organism.

D. Biochemical Reactions

They ferment sugars (glucose, lactose, sucrose, mannitol) with production of acid and gas. They are urease positive, indole negative, MR negative, VP positive and citrate positive (IMViC – – ++). These reactions are typical of *K. pneumoniae subsp. pneumoniae*.

E. Antigenic Structure

1. Capsular (K) Antigen

On the basis of capsular (K) antigens, the klebsiellae have been classified into 80 (1-80) serotypes.

2. Somatic (O) Antigen

Klebsiellae contain five (01–05) different somatic or O antigens.

F. Pathogenesis

K. pneumoniae subsp. *pneumoniae* is the second most populous member next to *Esch. coli* of aerobic bacterial flora of intestine of humans. It is responsible for severe bronchopneumonia, urinary tract infections, nosocomial infections, wound infections, septicaemia, meningitis and rarely diarrhoea. *Klebsiella* pneumonia is a serious disease with high case fatality. It is very important pathogen causing nosocomial infections of the lower respiratory tract.

K. pneumoniae subsp. ozaenae has been associated with atrophic rhinitis, a condition known as *ozaena*. *K. pneumoniae subsp. rhinoscleromatis* causes a granulomatous disease of the nose and pharynx called *rhinoscleroma*.

G. Laboratory Diagnosis

Laboratory diagnosis is done by culturing appropriate specimens on blood agar and MacConkey agar. The isolate is identified by colony morphology, Gram staining, test for motility and biochemical reactions.

H. Treatment

Klebsiellae are usually sensitive to cephalosporins, trimethoprim, nitrofurantoin, co-amoxiclav and gentamicin.

III. PROTEUS

The tribe *Proteeae*, in the family *Enterobacteriaceae*, contains three genera: *Proteus, Morganella*, *Providencia*. The single biochemical character, phenyl pyruvic acid test (PPA test), distinguishes this tribe from all other members of *Enterobacteriaceae*. These bacteria are PPA test positive i.e. they contain an enzyme phenyl alanine deaminase which converts phenyl alanine to phenyl pyruvic acid (PPA).

A. Classification

The genus *Proteus* was previously classified into five biotypes namely *Pr. vulgaris, Pr. mirabilis, Pr. morganii, Pr. rettgeri* and *Pr. inconstans*. Recently, *Pr. morganii, Pr. rettgeri* and *Pr. inconstans* are placed under new genera *Morganella* and *Providencia*. *Pr. vulgaris* and *Pr. mirabilis* are included in the genus *Proteus*.

These are motile, Gram negative bacilli, characterised by *swarming* growth on agar.

B. Morphology

These are Gram negative bacilli measuring 1-3 μm × 0.5 μm in size. They are non-capsulated, non-sporing and actively motile.

C. Culture

They are aerobic and facultatively anaerobic. They grow on ordinary media and culture emits a characteristic putrefactive (**fishy** or **seminal**) **odour**. When grown on nutrient agar or blood agar, *Pr. vulgaris* and *Pr. mirabilis* exhibit '**swarming**', but it does not occur with *Morganella* and *Providencia* species. Proteus grows on the culture plate (blood agar) in successive waves to form a thin filmy layer in concentric circles, which is named as 'swarming'. Swarming of *Proteus* appears to be due to vigorous motility of the bacteria although the exact cause is yet not established.

They form smooth, pale or colourless (NLF) colonies on McConkey's agar and do not swarm on this medium. In liquid medium (peptone water), *Proteus* produces uniform turbidity with a slight powdery deposit and an ammonical odour.

D. Biochemical Reactions

The distinctive characters of this genus are:

(*i*) Deamination of phenyl alanine to phenyl pyruvic acid (PPA test)—It is always positive.

(*ii*) Hydrolysis of urea by enzyme urease—It is another characteristic of *Proteus*, but is negative in some Providencia strains.

They ferment glucose by producing acid and gas. Lactose is not fermented. Indole is formed by *Pr. vulgaris* but is negative in *Pr. mirabilis*. H_2S is produced by *Pr. vulgaris* and *Pr. mirabilis*. They are MR positive and VP negative.

E. Antigenic Structure

The bacilli possess 'O' (somatic) and 'H' (flagellar) antigens, based upon which, several serotypes have been recognised.

F. Pathogenesis

Proteus species are saprophytic and widely distributed in nature. They also occur as commensals in the intestine. They are opportunistic pathogens and may cause many types of infections such as **urinary tract infection (UTI)**, pyogenic lesions, infection of ear, respiratory tract infection and **nosocomial infections**.

G. Laboratory Diagnosis

(i) ***Specimens:***

(a) Mid stream urine sample in UTI

(b) Pus in pyogenic lesions

(ii) ***Collection:*** Specimen should be collected in sterile container under all aseptic conditions and transported immediately.

(iii) ***Culture:*** It is cultured on MacConkey agar or blood agar with 6% agar to inhibit swarming. Culture media are incubated at 37°C for 18–24 hours. NLF colony are seen on MacConkey agar. Peptone water is also inoculated.

(iv) ***Gram's staining:*** Gram negative bacilli which are non-capsulated and non-sporing.

(v) ***Hanging drop preparation:*** Actively motile bacilli are observed.

(vi) ***Biochemical reactions:*** Most important are PPA and urease tests. PPA test is positive in all *Proteus* species. Urease test is also positive in all *Proteus* species with exception of *Providencia* which is negative.

(vii) ***Agglutination test:*** Strain may be agglutinated with polyvalent group specific sera to confirm it.

(viii) ***Antibiotic susceptibility test:*** It is important as proteus bacilli are resistant to many of the common antibiotics.

IV. SHIGELLA

The organisms of genus *Shigella* are exclusively parasites of human intestine and other primates and cause bacillary dysentery in man.

A. Morphology

Shigellae are short, Gram negative bacilli measuring about 1–3 μm × 0.5 μm. They are non-motile, non-capsulated and non-sporing.

B. Culture

They are aerobes and facultative anaerobes and can grow on ordinary media. Optimum temperature for growth is 37°C and pH 7.4. They can grow at temperature range of 10-40°C. After overnight incubation, colonies are about 2 mm in diameter, circular, convex, smooth and translucent. Colonies on MacConkey's agar and deoxycholate citrate agar (DCA) are colourless (non-lactose fermenting–NLF) except in case of *Sh. sonnei* which forms pink colonies due to late lactose fermentation. DCA is a useful selective medium to isolate these organisms from faeces.

ENRICHMENT MEDIUM

Selenite F broth: Sodium selenite in this medium inhibits coliform bacilli while permitting salmonellae and shigellae to grow.

C. Classification

Shigellae are divided into four subgroups (A, B, C & D) based on a combination of biochemical and serological specificity. Mannitol fermentation reaction distinguishes subgroup A (mannitol negative) from subgroups B, C, and D (all of them are mannitol positive).

1. Subgroup A (Sh. dysenteriae)

It is divided into 15 serotypes. Serotype 1 is the bacillus originally described by Shiga (*Sh. shigae*). It is the only member of the family that is always catalase negative. Serotype 2 is also known as *Sh. schmitzi*.

2. Subgroup B (Sh. flexneri)

It is antigenically the most complex among shigellae. They have been classified into six serotypes (1–6) based on specific antigens. Each of these is further divided into subtypes (e.g. 1a and 1b). In addition to six serotypes, two antigenic 'variants' (X and Y) are recognised, which do not possess type specific antigens.

3. Subgroup C (Sh. boydii)

It resembles *Sh. flexneri* biochemically but not antigenically. Nineteen serotypes (numbered 1 to 20 except 13) of *Sh. boydii* have been identified.

4. Subgroup D (Sh. sonnei)

It is indole negative but ferments lactose and sucrose late.

D. Toxins

1. Endotoxin

All shigellae release endotoxin after autolysis. Endotoxin has irritating effect on intestinal wall which causes diarrhoea and subsequently intestinal ulcers.

2. Exotoxin

Sh. dysenteriae type 1 produces a powerful exotoxin. It acts as enterotoxin and as well as neurotoxin.

3. Verocytotoxin (VT)

Sh. dysentriae type 1 also produces a cytotoxin which acts on Vero cells and is named *verocytotoxin* or VT.

E. Pathogenesis

Shigellae cause bacillary dysentery. Man is the only natural host of shigellae. The minimum infective dose is as few as 10-100 bacilli. *Sh. dysentriae* type 1 causes most severe form of dysentery usually associated with toxaemia. The infection due to *Sh. flexneri* and *Sh. boydii* are less severe and prevalent in tropical countries including India. *Sh. sonnei* causes the mildest form of the disease and is common in Western countries like Britain. It is more frequently seen in children.

The incubation period of the disease is usually less than 48 hours but varies between 1–7 days. Mode of infection is by ingestion of contaminated food.

The food or drink is contaminated by faeces of cases or of carriers. The organisms tend to remain localised in the gut wall and usually do not lead to bacteraemia.

F. Laboratory Diagnosis

Diagnosis depends upon isolating the bacillus from faeces.

1. Specimens

Fresh stool is collected. Rectal swabs are not satisfactory. The ideal specimen is a direct swab of an ulcer taken under sigmoidoscopic examination.

2. Transport

Specimens should be transported immediately and inoculated without delay. If delay is inevitable, specimens should be transported in a suitable medium.

3. Direct Microscopy

Saline and iodine preparation of faeces show large number of pus cells, erythrocytes and macrophages. Parasitic causes of dysentery may also be excluded by this examination.

4. Culture

Specimen is inoculated on selective media like MacConkey's agar or DCA. Selenite F broth is used as enrichment medium which permits rapid growth of enteric pathogens while inhibiting the growth of normal flora like *Esch. coli* for 6–8 hours. Subculture is done on solid media from selenite F broth. All the solid media are incubated at 37°C for 24 hours.

5. Colony Morphology and Staining

Colourless (NLF) colonies appear on MacConkey's agar which are further confirmed by Gram staining, hanging drop preparation and biochemical reactions. Shigellae are Gram negative bacilli and are non-motile.

6. Slide Agglutination Test

Identification of shigella is confirmed by slide agglutination with polyvalent antisera and monovalent sera.

G. Treatment

Uncomplicated shigellosis is a self limiting condition that usually recovers spontaneously. Dehydration has to be corrected promptly particularly in infants and young children.

Routine antibacterial treatment is not indicated but antibiotics should be reserved for the severe toxic cases. Ciprofloxacin is the drug of choice. Alternative antibiotics ceftriaxone and azithromycin are effective. The wide prevalence in shigellae of R factors confers resistance to multiple antibiotics.

V. SALMONELLA

The salmonellae are primarily intestinal parasites of vertebrates and which infect man, leading to **enteric fever, gastroenteritis** and **septicaemia**. The most important member is *Salmonella* Typhi, the causative agent of typhoid fever.

A. Morphology

Salmonellae are Gram negative bacilli measuring 1–3 µm × 0.5 µm. They are motile, non-sporing and non-capsulated. Motility is due to the presence of peritrichous flagella except *S. gallinarum* and *S. pullorum* which are non-motile.

B. Culture

Salmonellae grow on ordinary culture media at optimum temperature of 37°C (range 15–41°C), pH 6–8 and are aerobic and facultatively anaerobic. They produce colonies of 2–3 mm in diameter, circular, translucent, low convex and smooth. On **MacConkey's agar** and **deoxycholate citrate agar (DCA)**, colonies are colourless due to non-lactose fermentation (NLF). On **Wilson and Blair bismuth sulphite medium** (selective medium for salmonellae), jet black colonies with metallic sheen are formed due to formation of hydrogen sulphide. *S.* Paratyphi A and other species which do not form H_2S produce green colonies. **Xylose lysine deoxycholate (XLD) agar** is another medium used for isolation of this organism. Most strains of salmonellae produce red colonies with black centres, when grown on this medium. H_2S negative serotypes of Salmonella produce red colonies without black centres.

Selenite F broth and **tetrathionate broth (TTB)** are commonly used enrichment media for inoculation of specimens especially faeces.

C. Biochemical Reactions

Salmonellae ferment glucose, mannitol and maltose forming acid and gas except *S.* Typhi which produces only acid and no gas. They do not ferment lactose or sucrose. Indole is not produced. Most salmonellae produce H_2S in triple sugar iron (TSI) agar except *S.* Paratyphi A and *S.* Cholerae-Suis. They utilise citrate (except *S.* Typhi and *S.* Paratyphi A) and are MR positive and VP negative. Urea is not hydrolysed.

D. Resistance

The salmonellae are killed at 60°C in 15 minutes. Boiling, chlorination of water and pasteurisation of milk destroy the bacilli. They survive in water, ice and snow for weeks and months.

E. Antigenic Structure

Salmonellae possess three types of antigens based on which they are classified. These are (1) flagellar antigen 'H', (2) somatic antigen 'O', and (3) a surface antigen 'Vi', found in some species.

F. Pathogenesis

S. Typhi, *S.* Paratyphi A and usually *S.* Paratyphi B are confined to human beings. The majority of other salmonellae are primarily infective for animals and human beings are secondarily infected.

Salmonellae cause three types of clinical syndrome in human beings, enteric fever, septicaemia and gastroenteritis.

1. Enteric Fever

The term enteric fever includes typhoid fever (*S.* Typhi) and paratyphoid fever (*S.* Paratyphi A, B, C). Infections due to *S.* Typhi and *S.* Paratyphi A are prevalent in India.

(i) Typhoid fever

The infection is acquired by ingestion through contaminated food and water. The incubation period is usually 7–14 days.

The clinical course may vary from a mild pyrexia to a fatal fulminating disease. The characteristic features are hepatosplenomegaly, step-ladder pyrexia with relative bradycardia and leucopaenia. Skin rashes known as rose-spots may appear during the second or third week.

(ii) Paratyphoid fever

Paratyphoid fever resembles typhoid fever but is milder. *S.* Paratyphi A, B And C cause paratyphoid fever.

2. Septicaemia

Salmonella septicaemia is commonly caused by *S.* Choleraesuis or *S.* Paratyphi C and occasionally by other salmonellae. There is early invasion of blood stream and it produces local suppuration in different organs.

3. Gastroenteritis

Salmonella gastroenteritis or food poisoning is caused by ingestion of food like meat, milk, egg contaminated by certain salmonellae which are primarily animal pathogens. Eggs and egg products are of great concern. *S.* Typhimurium is the most frequently isolated in food poisoning. The incubation period is 12 to 24 hours.

G. Laboratory Diagnosis

Bacteriological diagnosis of enteric fever consists of

1. Isolation of bacilli
2. Demonstration of antibodies

1. Isolation of Bacilli

This may be done by culture of specimens like blood, faeces, urine, aspirated duodenal fluid etc. Selection of relevant specimen depends upon duration of illness which is very important for the laboratory diagnosis of enteric fever (Table 24.1, Fig. 24.1).

Table 24.1: Relevance of Examination of Different Specimens at Different Phases of Enteric Fever

Duration of disease	Specimen examination	% Positivity
1st Week	Blood culture	90
2nd Week	Blood culture	75
	Faeces culture	50
	Widal test	low titre
3rd Week	Widal test	80–100
	Blood culture	60
	Faeces culture	80

Blood Culture

Blood cultures are positive in approximately 90 per cent of cases in first week of fever, 75 per cent in the second week and 60 per cent in the third week. Positivity rate declines thereafter and blood cultures remain positive in 25 per cent of cases till the subsidence of pyrexia.

10 ml of blood is collected by venepuncture under aseptic conditions and transferred into blood culture bottles (glucose broth and taurocholate broth). Single bottle of brain heart infusion broth (BHI) can be used instead of two bottles of glucose broth and taurocholate broth.

Blood contains substances that inhibit the growth of the bacilli and hence it is essential to dilute out these substances (5 ml blood into the 50 ml culture media, 1:10 dilution). Alternative is addition of liquoid (sodium polyanethol sulphonate) which counteracts the bactericidal action of these substances.

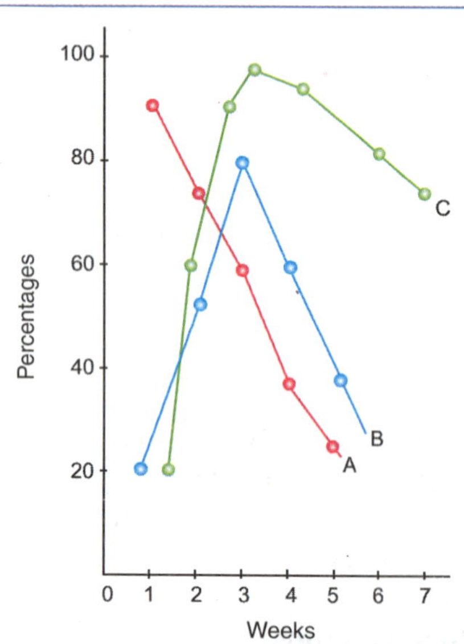

Fig. 24.1 Bacteriological diagnosis in typhoid fever. The approximate percentage of positivity during different weeks of disease A—Blood culture, B—Faeces culture, C—Widal test.

Both blood culture bottles are incubated at 37°C for overnight. In case of BHI broth, subcultunes are made on both blood agar and MacConkey's agar from that bottle after overnight incubation. However in case of two blood culture bottles, the glucose broth is subcultured on blood agar and the taurocholate (bile) broth on MacConkey's agar. Taurocholate broth is inhibitory to Gram positive bacteria, therefore, Gram negative bacilli are selected out. Pale non-lactose fermenting (NLF) colonies appear on MacConkey's agar.

If salmonellae are not obtained from the first subculture from taurocholate broth, subcultures should be done every other day up to ten days before declaring the culture as negative.

Clot Culture

It is an alternative to blood culture. 5 ml of blood is withdrawn aseptically into a sterile container and allowed to clot. The serum is separated and used for the Widal test. The clot is broken up with a sterile glass rod and added to bile broth containing streptokinase (100 units/ml) which digests the clot causing its lysis and thereby the bacteria are released from the clot. Serum used for Widal test may be negative due to the early stage of the disease but it may be useful as baseline titre against which the results of tests performed later may be evaluated.

Faeces Culture

Salmonellae are shed in the faeces throughout the disease and even in convalescence, due to lesions present in the intestine. Hence, faecal cultures may be helpful in patients as well as for the detection of carriers. Faeces cultures are generally positive after the second week of illness.

As normal flora is present in faeces, successful culture will depend on use of enrichment and selective media. Faecal samples are inoculated into one tube each of selenite and tetrathionate broth (both enrichment media) and are also plated directly on MacConkey's agar, DCA, XLD and Wilson-Blair media. Salmonellae appear as pale yellow (NLF) colonies on MacConkey's agar and DCA media. On Wilson-Blair medium, *S. typhi* forms large black colonies with a metallic sheen whereas *S. paratyphi A* produces green colonies due to the absence of H_2S production.

Enrichment media (selenite F and tetrathionate broths) are incubated for 6-8 hours before subculture on to selective media such as MacConkey's agar and DCA. These selective media are then incubated at 37°C for overnight.

Urine Culture

Urine culture is less frequently positive than the culture of blood or faeces. Cultures are generally positive only in the second and third weeks. After third week, only about 25 per cent cases may be positive. Repeated cultures improve the chances of isolation.

Other Specimens for Culture

Bone marrow culture is valuable as it is positive even when blood cultures are negative. Culture of bile is usually positive and may be useful in detection of chronic carriers.

Colony Morphology and Staining

On MacConkey's agar or DCA, salmonellae grow as pale yellow, non-lactose fermenting (NLF) colonies. Gram staining from these colonies show Gram negative bacilli and on hanging drop preparation, these are motile bacilli.

Biochemical Reactions

Salmonellae are catalase positive, oxidase negative, nitrate reduction positive and ferment glucose, mannitol but not lactose or sucrose. *S.* Typhi ferments glucose and mannitol with production of acid only but paratyphoid bacilli (*S.* Paratyphi A, B and C) form acid and gas.

Slide Agglutination Test

A loopful of the growth from a nutrient agar slope is emulsified in two drops of saline on a microscopic slide. One emulsion acts as a control and other as a test. Agglutination is carried out with the antisera. Positive agglutination confirms the isolate at genus and species level.

2. Demonstration of Antibodies

Widal Test

It is an agglutination test for detection of agglutinins (H and O) in patients with enteric fever. Salmonella antibodies start appearing in the serum at the end of first week (Fig. 24.1) and rise sharply during the third week of enteric fever. Two specimens of sera at an interval of 7 to 10 days are preferred to demonstrate a rising antibody titre.

H. Treatment

Chloramphenicol has been the antibiotic of choice for enteric fever. Resistance to chloramphenicol and other antibiotics has been reported. Fluoroquinolones (ciprofloxacin, pefloxacin, ofloxacin) and the third generation cephalosporins (ceftazidime, cefotaxime, ceftrioxone cefoperazone) are useful in such multiresistant cases.

I. Prophylaxis

1. General Measures

Typhoid fever can be effectively controlled by sanitary measures for disposal of sewage, clean water supply and supervision of food processing and handling.

2. Carriers

Carriers should not be engaged in food preparation and should observe strict personal hygiene.

3. Vaccination

Vaccine is indicated for travellers or who live in endemic areas.

(i) TAB vaccine

TAB vaccine is not used nowadays. It was heat-killed whole cell vaccine which contained *S.* Typhi 1,000 million, *S.* Paratyphi A and B, 750 million each per ml and preserved in 0.5 per cent phenol. The vaccine used to be given subcutaneously in two doses of 0.5 ml at an interval of 4–6 weeks followed by booster every three years. It is **no longer used** because of significant side effect.

(ii) Live oral (Ty 21a) typhoid vaccine

Avirulent mutant strain of *S. typhi* (Ty 21a) has been used as a live oral vaccine.

Dose schedule: Four doses are given on alternate days (Days 1, 3, 5 and 7). A better dose is needed every 5 years. It is indicated for those over five years of age. The oral vaccine (*typhoral*) is available in capsule form containing 10^9 viable lyophilised mutant bacilli.

(iii) Vi Capsular polysaccharide vaccine (Vi–CPS)

It contains purified Vi polysaccharide antigen derived from *S.* Typhi strain Ty2.

Dose schedule: It is injected intramuscularly or subcutaneously in a single dose of 25 µg. The efficacy is about 75%.

Vi–CPS vaccine is given to persons aged two years and above. The protection starts after 2 to 3 weeks after administration and lasts for three years. The booster may be given after 3 years.

KEY POINTS

1. Members of family *Enterobacteriaceae* are aerobic and facultative anaerobic *Gram negative* enteric bacilli. They are motile by *peritrichous flagella* or are non-motile. Some important genera of family *Enterobacteriaceae* include *Escherichia, Salmonella, Shigella, Klebsiella, Proteus, Morganella* and *Providencia.*

2. *Urinary tract infection*, *diarrhoea*, *pyogenic infections* and *septicaemia* are the diseases caused by *Esch. coli*.
3. There are two species of proteus, i.e., *Pr. vulgaris* and *Pr. mirabilis*. These species exhibit '*swarming*' when grown on blood agar. They are PPA test positive. Hydrolysis of area by enzyme urease is aother characteristic of Proteus. Proteus may cause *urinary tract infections* (*UTI*), *pyogenic lesions*, *infection of ear*, *respiratory tract infection* and *nosocomial infections*.
4. The organisms of genus *Shigella* cause *bacillary dysentery* in man. They are short, *Gram negative*, *non-motile* bacilli. Shigella has four species, i.e., *Sh. dysenteriae*, *Sh. flexneri*, *Sh. boydii* and *Sh. sonnei*.
5. Salmonellae are Gram negative, motile bacilli. They grow on ordinary culture media. On MacConkey's agar and deoxycholate citrate agar (DCA), colonies are colourless due to non-lactose fermentation (NLF). Salmonellae cause three types of clinical syndrome in human beings, *enteric fever*, *septicaemia* and *gastroenteritis*. Laboratory diagnosis of enteric fever consists of *isolation of bacilli*, *demonstration of antibodies*, and *demonstration of circulating antigen*. Live oral (Ty 21a) typhoid vaccine and Vi capsular polysaccharide vaccine (Vi-CPS) are available for prophylaxis..

STUDY QUESTIONS

1. Discuss the laboratory diagnosis of urinary tract infections caused by *Esch. coli*.
2. Describe in detail the laboratory diagnosis of diarrhoea caused by *Esch. coli*.
3. Write briefly about:
   (i) *Klebsiella pneumoniae* (ii) *Proteus sp*.
4. Discuss the laboratory diagnosis of bacillary dysentery.
5. Describe in detail the laboratory diagnosis of enteric fever.
6. Write briefly about Widal test.

MULTIPLE CHOICE QUESTIONS (MCQs)

1. Travellers diarrhoea is caused by:
   (a) Enteropathogenic *Escherichia coli* (EPEC)
   (b) Enterotoxigenic *Esch. coli* (ETEC)
   (c) Enteroinvasive *Esch. coli* (EIEC)
   (d) Enterohaemorrhagic *Esch. coli* (EHEC)
2. The term 'significant bacteriuria' is used in urinary tract infection when bacterial count is:
   (a) more than 10^5 bacteria per ml
   (b) between 10^4 to 10^5 bacteria per ml
   (c) less than 10^3 bacteria per ml
   (d) None of the above
3. Which of the following has/have positive phenyl pyruvic acid test (PPA test)?
   (a) *Proteus*
   (b) *Morganella*
   (c) *Providencia*
   (d) All of the above
4. Which of the following is used as an enrichment medium for the isolation of *Shigella* from the faeces?
   (a) Selenite F broth
   (b) Alkaline peptone water
   (c) Taurocholate tellurite peptone water
   (d) None of the above
5. Which of the following *Shigella* species does not ferment mannitol?
   (a) *Shigella dysenteriae*
   (b) *Sh. boydii*
   (c) *Sh. sonnei*
   (d) None of the above
6. Which *Shigella* species is late fermenter of lactose and sucrose?
   (a) *Shigella dysenteriae*
   (b) *Sh. flexneri*
   (c) *Sh. boydii*
   (d) *Sh. sonnei*
7. Which of the following disease/s is/are produced by *Salmonella*?
   (a) Enteric fever
   (b) Gastroenteritis
   (c) Septicaemia
   (d) All of the above
8. Bacteriological diagnosis of enteric fever consists of:
   (a) Isolation of bacilli
   (b) Demonstration of antibodies
   (c) Demonstration of antigen
   (d) All of the above
9. The most important specimen for isolation of *Salmonella* Typhi in first week of enteric fever is:
   (a) Blood
   (b) Faeces
   (c) Urine
   (d) Pus
10. What type of test is Widal test?
   (a) Slide agglutination test
   (b) Tube agglutination test
   (c) Co-agglutination test
   (d) Latex agglutination test

ANSWERS (MCQs) ...✓

1. (b) 2. (a) 3. (d) 4. (a) 5. (a) 6. (d) 7. (d) 8. (d) 9. (a) 10. (b)

Vibrio

25

Vibrios are **Gram negative**, **oxidase positive**, short, rigid, **curved rods** that are actively motile by a **polar flagellum**. The most important member of the genus is *Vibrio cholerae*. It is the causative agent of cholera.

I. VIBRIO CHOLERAE

A. Morphology

V. cholerae is a **Gram negative**, **curved** or **comma-shaped rod**, non-sporing, non-capsulated, about 1.5 µm × 0.2–0.4 µm in size (Fig. 25.1). The organism is very actively motile with a single polar flagellum and movement is named as ***darting motility***.

In stained mucus flakes of cholera cases, the vibrios are arranged in parallel rows, described by koch as the '***fish in stream***' appearance.

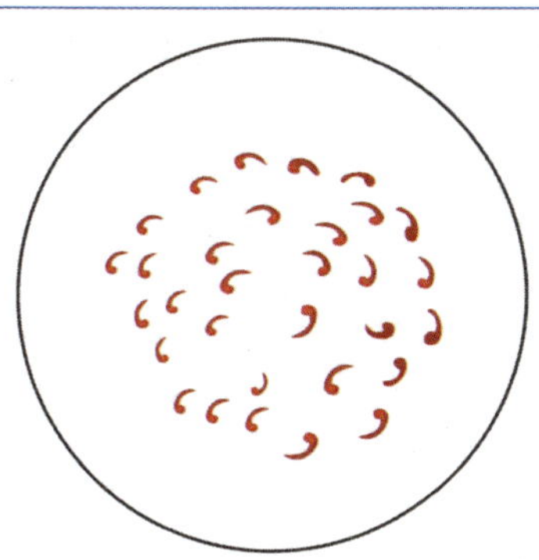

Fig. 25.1 Vibrio cholerae

B. Culture

V. cholerae is strongly aerobic. It grows within a temperature range of 16°–40°C but optimum temperature is 37°C. It grows best in **alkaline media**, the optimum **pH** being **8.2** (pH range 7.4–9.6).

1. Ordinary Media

(i) Nutrient agar

After overnight incubation, the colonies are moist, translucent, round disks, 1–2 mm in diameter, with a bluish tinge in transmitted light.

(ii) MacConkey's agar

The colonies are colourless or pale at first, but becomes reddish or pink on prolonged incubation due to late fermentation of lactose.

(iii) Blood agar

V. cholerae, classical biotype, does not produce hemolysis although some strains produce greenish discolouration around colonies which later becomes clear due to **haemodigestion**.

(iv) Peptone water

It grows as a **surface pellicle** because of its aerobic nature.

2. Special Media

The special media are classified as follows:

(i) Transport or holding media
(ii) Enrichment media
(iii) Plating media.

Transport or Holding Media

Venkatraman-Ramakrishnan (VR) medium

It contains 20 gm common salt and 5 gm peptone in one litre of distilled water and pH is adjusted to 8.6–8.8. Vibrios do not multiply, but remain viable for several weeks.

Cary-Blair medium

This medium is prepared by adding disodium phosphate, sodium thioglycollate, sodium chloride and calcium chloride and pH is adjusted at 8.4.

If a transport medium is not available, **a strip of thick blotting paper** is soaked in the faecal matter, then placed in a sealed plastic bag, and sent to the laboratory.

Enrichment Media

Alkaline peptone water (APW)

It is a peptone water at pH 8.6. Besides enrichment medium, it is also an excellent transport medium.

Monsur's taurocholate tellurite peptone water

It contains peptone, sodium chloride, sodium taurocholate in one litre of distilled water and pH is adjusted at 9.2. To this medium, sterile potassium tellurite solution is added. Like APW, it is not only a good enrichment medium but is transport medium as well.

Plating Media

Alkaline bile salt agar (BSA); pH 8.2

It is modified nutrient agar medium containing 0.5% sodium taurocholate (bile salt). The colonies are similar to those on nutrient agar.

Monsur's gelatin taurocholate trypticase telurite agar (GTTA) medium; pH 8.5

The colonies are small, translucent with a greyish black centre and a turbid halo around the colonies due to hydrolysis of gelatin. The colonies become 3–4 mm in size after 48 hour incubation.

Thiosulphate citrate bile sucrose (TCBS) agar; pH 8.6

It is the most widely used selective medium for isolation of vibrios. It contains sodium thiosulphate, sodium citrate, bile salts, sucrose, bromothymol blue (indicator), yeast extract, peptone, sodium chloride, ferric citrate and water. *Vibrio cholerae* forms yellow colonies due to sucrose fermentation, while non-sucrose fermenters such as *V. parahaemolyticus* produce green colonies.

C. Biochemical Reactions

Carbohydrate breakdown is fermentative, producing acid, but no gas. It is catalase and oxidase positive. It ferments glucose, mannitol, sucrose, maltose and mannose, but not lactose, though lactose may be split very slowly. It is indole positive and reduces nitrates to nitrites. It is methyl red (MR) and urease negative. Gelatin is liquefied. It decarboxylates lysine and ornithine but do not utilise arginine. Voges-Proskauer (VP) reaction and haemolysis of sheep erythrocytes are positive in EL Tor biotype and both these tests are negative in classical biotype.

D. Antigenic Structure

V. cholerae contain somatic 'O' and flagellar 'H' antigens. The 'H' antigen is shared by all the strains. On the basis of O antigen, it is divided into subgroups (now named O serogroups or serovars). Both classical and El Tor biotypes belong to serogroups O1 and are antigenically indistinguishable. These are referred as *V. cholerae O1*. On the basis of minor O antigens (A, B, C), *V. cholerae* O1 are subdivided into three serotypes—Ogawa (AB), Inaba (AC) and Hikojima (ABC) (Table 25.1).

At least 139 (O1 to O139) O serogroups are recognised. Serogroups 02 to O138 are called non-O1 *V. cholerae*. Since these organisms were not agglutinated by O-1 antiserum, they were called non-agglutinating (NAG) vibrios.

Table 25.1: Serotypes of Cholera Vibrios

Serotype	O antigen
Ogawa	AB
Inaba	AC
Hikojima	ABC

E. Toxins

Besides heat stable *endotoxin, V. cholerae* also produces *exotoxin* (enterotoxin). The enterotoxin is also named as **cholera toxin (CT)**.

Enterotoxin

It is a heat labile, protein in nature. It has a molecular weight of 90,000. It has two fractions: one A (*active*) *subunit* and five B (*binding*) *subunits*. The cholera toxin (CT) resembles heat-labile toxin (LT) of *Esch. coli* chemically, antigenically and in its mode of action. CT is more potent than LT of *Esch. coli*.

Mechanism of action

The B subunit binds specifically to the **Gm1, ganglioside receptor** on the intestinal epithelial cell. The active A *subunit* then enters the cell and is cleaved to its fragments, A1 and A2. The A2 fragment links the active A1 to the B subunit and thus the A1 fragment **stimulates adenyl cyclase activity** of the epithelial cell. This in turn, **converts ATP into cAMP**. The cAMP concentration within the cells causes (i) hypersecretion of water and electrolytes (Na, K, HCO_3^-) within the intestinal lumen and (ii) inhibition of reabsorption of sodium and chloride by cells, which results in purging diarrhoea of *rice water stool*.

EL TOR VIBRIOS

Antigenically *El Tor Vibrio* is identical to classical cholera vibrio and is now proved to be biotype of *V. cholerae–O1*. The Differentiating tests used for identification of El Tor biotype are listed below (Table 25.2).

Table 25.2: Differentiating Features of Classical and El Tor Vibrios

Test	Classical	El Tor
Haemolysis of sheep erythrocytes	–	+
Agglutination of chick erythrocytes	–	+
Voges-Proskauer (VP) reaction	–	+
Polymyxin B sensitivity	+	–
Susceptibility to Mukherjee Phage IV	+	–

NON-AGGLUTINATING VIBRIOS (NON-01 V. CHOLERAE)

The somatic antigen O1 is specific to the *classical* and El Tor biotypes of *V. cholerae*, while vibrios containing antigen other than O1 are called non-agglutinating (NAG) or non-cholera vibrios (NCV) or Non-01 *V. cholerae*. There are 139 serogroups containing O antigen, O1 to O139. Serogroup O1 and O139 contain *V. cholerae*, while O2 to O138 are NAG vibrios. It is extremely difficult to distinguish most of the NAG vibrios from *V. cholerae* by means of culture and biochemical reactions. They are not agglutinable by O1 antiserum, therefore, named as non-agglutinable (NAG) vibrios. However, they are readily agglutinable by their homologous antiserum.

F. Pathogenesis

V. cholerae (both O1 and O139) causes an acute diarrhoeal disease known as **cholera** and it occurs only in man. The human infection occurs by ingestion of contaminated foods and drink. A high infective dose of 10^8 bacilli is required to bypass the gastric barrier. The ingested organisms pass through the acid barrier of the stomach and multiply in the alkaline medium of the small intestine. Vibrios become adherent to the epithelium. Once epithelial cell attachment occurs, *V. cholerae* produces **enterotoxin** and the disease. Mechanism of action of enterotoxin has been described earlier.

G. Laboratory Diagnosis

1. Specimens

(i) Watery stool
(ii) Rectal swab

2. Collection and Transport

Freshly collected stool is the specimen of choice. Specimens should be collected preferably prior to start of antibiotics. These should not be collected from bedpans due to risk of contamination. Specimens should be immediately transported to the laboratory for processing. In case of delay, stool samples may be preserved in holding media such as VR fluid or Cary-Blair medium for long periods. If the specimen can reach the laboratory in a few hours, enrichment media such as alkaline peptone water or Monsur's medium may be used as transport media. When transport media are not available, strips of blotting paper may be soaked in watery stool and sent to the laboratory after proper packing in plastic envelopes. If possible, specimens should be plated at bedside and the inoculated plates sent to the laboratory.

3. Direct Microscopy

It is not a reliable method. For rapid diagnosis, the characteristic darting motility of the Vibrio and its inhibition by adding antiserum can be demonstrated under the dark field or phase contrast microscope, using cholera stool.

4. Culture

Stool sample is directly cultured on following media.

(a) Selective media (BSA, TCBS or Monsur's GTTA) and non-selective media (blood agar and MacConkey's agar) are inoculated. These plates are incubated overnight at 37°C.
(b) Enrichment media such as alkaline peptone water or Monsur's liquid media are inoculated. These media are incubated at 37°C for 6–8 hours before subculturing on to selective media.

5. Colony Morphology and Staining

After overnight incubation, culture media are examined for typical colonies of *V. cholerae*. On MacConkey's agar, colonies are pale and on Monsur's medium the colony has a black centre with a turbid halo around the colony. TCBS shows yellow colonies and on BSA, translucent colonies are present.

Gram staining from colony shows typical Gram negative comma shaped bacilli. These show darting motility on hanging drop preparation. Further confirmation is done by biochemical reactions and agglutination test.

String test

A loopful of growth of *Vibrio cholerae* is mixed with a drop of 0.5% sodium deoxycholate on a slide. In case of positive test, the suspension losses its turbidity, becomes mucoid and form a 'string' when the loop is lifted away from the suspension.

6. Biochemical Reactions

V. cholerae ferments glucose, mannitol, sucrose, maltose, mannose with acid production. Lactose is usually not fermented. Catalase and oxidase are positive. The El Tor biotype is usually haemolytic, VP positive, agglutinate chick erythrocytes and is resistant to polymyxin B and group IV cholera phage.

7. Agglutination Test

Colonies are picked up with a straight wire and tested with *V. cholerae* 01 antiserum. If positive, the test is repeated with monospecific *Ogawa* and *Inaba* sera for serotyping.

H. Treatment

1. Oral Rehydration Therapy

The most important is prompt water and electrolyte replacement to correct the severe dehydration and salt depletion. This can be achieved by oral rehydration therapy, either alone or supplemented by intravenous fluids.

2. Antibiotics

It is of secondary importance. Tetracycline is useful in reducing the number of stool and it also shortens the period of excretion of vibrios.

I. Prophylaxis

1. General Measures

(i) Purification of water supplies.
(ii) Better provision for sewage disposal.
(iii) Infected patients should be isolated, their excreta disinfected.
(iv) Contacts and carriers are followed up.

2. Specific Measures

Killed parenteral vaccine

It was widely used for active immunisation. This vaccine is **no longer used** as it provides little protection, causes adverse effects and fail to produce local intestinal mucosal immune response.

Killed oral vaccine

Two types of killed vaccine are available:

1. **Whole-cell (WC) vaccine**: It contains killed whole cells of *Vibrio cholerae O1* (classical and El Tor, Ogawa and Inaba) and O139.
2. **Whole-cell recombinant B subunit cholera vaccine (WC/rBS)**: Composition is same as that of WC vaccine alongwith recombinant cholera toxin B subunit.
   Schedule: Two doses are given orally at interval of 7–14 days for adults and children aged 6 years and above. However three doses are given for children 2-5 years. It is not recommended for children less than 2 years.
   Protection: For the first six months after vaccination, the protection rate is 85–90% for WC/rBS vaccine. For WC vaccine protection rate is 66–67% for at least 2 years.
   This vaccine also conferred significant protection against diarrhoea due to *Esch. coli* (LT–ETEC).

Live oral vaccine

Oral live attenuated vaccine (*Vibrio cholerae* O1) is prepared by using mutant strains that lack the gene encoding for cholera toxin.

III. HALOPHILIC VIBRIOS

Halophilic vibrios cannot grow in media lacking sodium chloride. They grow best in the presence of sodium chloride. Their natural habitat is sea water and marine life. Some halophilic vibrios which cause human diseases are *V. parahaemolyticus, V. alginolyticus* and *V. vulnificus*.

KEY POINTS

1. Vibrios are Gram negative, *oxidase positive*, short, rigid, *curved or comma-shaped rods* that are actively motile by a *polar flagellum*.
2. *Vibrio cholerae* is the causative agent of *cholera*. Two serogroups O1 and O139 are responsible for the disease. Both serogroups produce cholera toxin (CT).
3. Two biotypes of *Vibrio cholerae* include *classical* and *El Tor*.
4. Special media with *alkaline pH* are required for growth of vibrios.
5. *Alkaline bile salt agar* (*BSA*) and *Thiosulphate citrate bile sucrose* (*TCBS*) are two important solid media for growing *V. cholerae*.
6. Vaccines are used for protection against cholera.

STUDY QUESTIONS

1. Discuss the laboratory diagnosis of cholera.
2. Write short notes on:
   (i) El Tor vibrios (ii) Non-agglutinating vibrios.

MULTIPLE CHOICE QUESTIONS (MCQs)

1. Which of the following bacteria has darting motility?
   (a) *Escherichia coli*
   (b) *Vibrio cholerae*
   (c) *Salmonella typhi*
   (d) *Pseudomonas aeruginosa*
2. Which of the following media can be used as transport medium for *Vibrio cholerae*?
   (a) Nutrient broth
   (b) Venkatraman-Ramakrishnan medium
   (c) Selenite F broth
   (d) None of the above
3. Stool specimens from cholera cases can be collected and transported to the laboratory using:
   (a) Venkatraman-Ramakrishnan medium
   (b) Cary-Blair medium
   (c) Strips of thick blotting paper
   (d) All of the above
4. Which of the following vaccines is/are available for prevention of cholera?
   (a) Killed parenteral vaccine
   (b) Killed oral vaccine
   (c) Live oral vaccine
   (d) All of the above
5. All of the following are halophilic vibrios except:
   (a) *Vibrio alginolyticus*
   (b) *V. parahaemolyticus*
   (c) *V. vulnificus*
   (d) *V. cholerae*

ANSWERS (MCQs) ...✓

1. (b) 2. (b) 3. (d) 4. (d) 5. (d)

Pseudomonas

26

The genus *Pseudomonas* belongs to the family *Pseudomonadaceae* which contains over 200 species. The most important among these is *Ps. aeruginosa*.

PSEUDOMONAS AERUGINOSA

A. Morphology

It is slender, Gram negative bacillus, 1.5-3 μm × 0.5 μm, non-capsulated, non-sporing and is actively motile by a **polar flagellum**.

B. Culture

It is a strict aerobe and grows well on ordinary media like nutrient broth and nutrient agar. The optimum temperature for growth is 37°C, but growth occurs at a wide range of temperature 5°C to 42°C.

1. Nutrient Agar

Colonies are smooth, large, translucent, low convex, 2–4 mm in diameter. The organism produces a **sweetish aromatic odour**. There is **greenish blue pigment** which diffuses into the medium (Fig. 26.1).

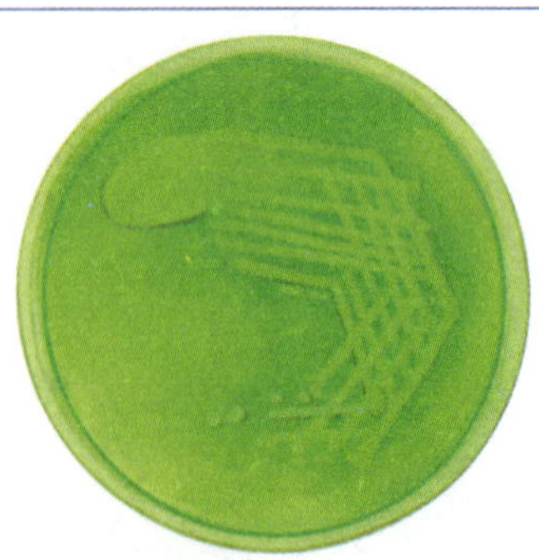

Fig. 26.1 Pseudomonas aeruginosa on nutrient agar

2. Blood Agar

Colony characters are similar to those on nutrient agar. Many strains are haemolytic on blood agar.

3. MacConkey Agar

Colonies are pale or colourless (non lactose fermenters, NLF).

4. Cetrimide Agar

It is a selective medium for *Ps. aeruginosa*.

5. Peptone Water

It forms a turbidity with a surface pellicle. Pseudomonas being a strict aerobe tends to collect at the surface for more oxygen hence forming surface pellicle.

C. Pigment Production

Ps. aeruginosa produces a number of pigments which diffuse into surrounding medium. These pigments are:

1. Pyocyanin

It is a bluish-green pigment. It is not produced by other species of the genus, hence, it is diagnostic of *Ps. aeruginosa*.

2. Fluorescin (Pyoverdin)

It is a greenish yellow pigment. It may be produced by many other Pseudomonas species also.

3. Pyorubin

It is a reddish brown pigment.

D. Biochemical Reactions

Ps. aeruginosa derives energy from carbohydrates by oxidative breakdown rather than a fermentative metabolism. It utilises only glucose oxidatively with acid production. All strains of *Ps. aeruginosa* are oxidase positive and utilise citrate as the sole source of carbon.

E. Resistance

It is killed by heating at 55°C for one hour. It is resistant to the chemical disinfectants and can even grow in certain antiseptics like quaternary ammonium compounds, chloroxylenol and hexachlorophane. It is sensitive to 2% aqueous alkaline solution of glutaraldehyde.

F. Pathogenesis

It causes infections more common in patients with neutropenia, cystic fibrosis, burns and those on ventilators. It is the most important agent causing **healthcare associated (nosocomial) infections**. It is due to its resistance to common antibiotics and antiseptics that it establishes itself widely in hospitals. Equipments such as respirators and endoscopes, articles such as bed pans, and antiseptic or disinfectant solutions may be frequently contaminated. The other common infections caused by it are:

1. Urinary tract infections.
2. Acute purulent meningitis.
3. Post-tracheostomy pulmonary infection.
4. Septicaemia in debilitated patients.
5. Wound and burn infections.
6. Chronic otitis media and otitis externa.
7. Eye infections.
8. Infantile diarrhoea.

G. Laboratory Diagnosis

1. *Specimens*

Pus, wound swab, urine, sputum, blood or CSF

2. *Culture*

Specimens may be inoculated on nutrient agar, blood agar or MacConkey's agar and incubated at 37°C for 18–24 hours. On nutrient agar, there is bluish green pigment diffused in the medium. On MacConkey's agar they grow as pale colonies (NLF). In peptone water, surface pellicle and green pigment can be observed. Selective media such as cetrimide agar may be necessary to isolate *Ps. aeruginosa* from faeces or other samples with mixed flora.

3. *Gram Staining and Motility*

They are Gram negative bacilli and are actively motile.

4. *Biochemical Reactions*

The oxidase test is positive within 30 seconds. They are non-fermenter. They break down glucose oxidatively with acid production only.

5. *Antibiotic Sensitivity Test*

It is useful to select out proper antibiotic as multiple resistance to antibiotics is quite common in *Ps. aeruginosa*.

H. Treatment

It is intrinsically resistant to most of the commonly used antimicrobial agents. Ciprofloxacin, piperacillin, ticarcillin, azlocillin, cefotaxime, ceftazidime, gentamicin and tobramycin are used in treatment of *Ps. aeruginosa* infections.

KEY POINTS

1. The genus *Pseudomonas* comprises of aerobic, Gram negative, *non-fermentative*, non-sporing, *oxidase positive bacilli* which are motile by *polar* flagella.
2. The most important species is *Pseudomonas aeruginosa*. It is a strict aerobe and grows well on ordinary medium like nutrient agar. It produces greenish blue pigment which diffuses into the medium.
3. Different pigments produced by *Ps. aeruginosa* include are *pyocyanin*, *fluorescin* and *pyorubin*.
4. *Ps. aeruginosa* is the most important agent causing *nosocomial infections*. It is due to its resistance to *common antibiotics* and *antiseptics*. The other common infections caused by it are urinary tract infection, acute purulent meningitis, septicaemia, wound and burn infections.

STUDY QUESTION

1. Write briefly about Pseudomonas aeruginosa.

MULTIPLE CHOICE QUESTIONS (MCQs)

1. Which of the following pigment is diagnostic of *Pseudomonas aeruginosa*?
   (a) Pyocyanin
   (b) Fluorescin
   (c) Pyorubin
   (d) Pyomelanin
2. Which of the following infections can be caused by *Pseudomonas aeruginosa*?
   (a) Urinary tract infection
   (b) Wound and burn infections
   (c) Pulmonary infection
   (d) All of the above

ANSWERS (MCQs)

1. (a) 2. (d)

27

Yersinia

The genus Yersinia contains three medically important species — *Y. pestis*, *Y. pseudotuberculosis* and *Y. enterocolitica*.

I. YERSINIA PESTIS

A. Morphology

Y. pestis is a short, ovoid, Gram negative bacillus, about 1.5 μm × 0.7 μm in size, with rounded ends and convex sides, occur singly, in short chains or in small groups. When stained with methylene blue, it shows bipolar staining (***safety pin appearance***) with two ends darkly or densely stained and the central area clear (Fig. 27.1).

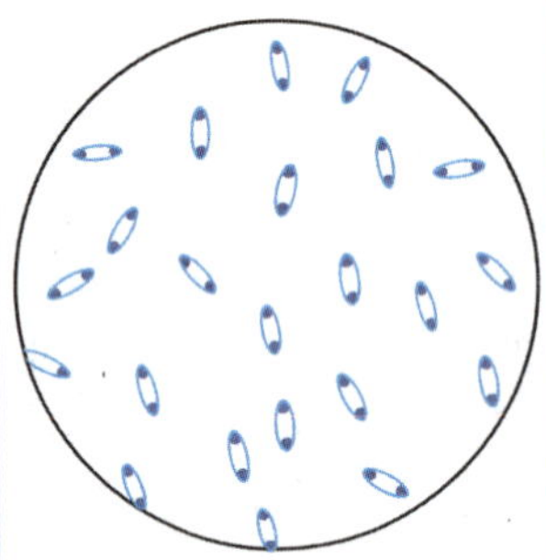

Fig. 27.1. Smear of Y. pestis with bipolar staining

The bacterial body is surrounded by a slime layer (envelope or capsule). It is non-motile, non-sporing and non-acid-fast.

B. Culture

The organism is aerobic and facultatively anaerobic. The optimum temperature for growth (unlike most pathogens) is 27°C. It grows on ordinary media.

1. Nutrient Agar

Colonies are small, delicate, transparent after 24–48 hours of incubation.

2. Blood Agar

Colonies are non-haemolytic and dark brown. Other characters are same as that of the colonies on nutrient agar.

3. MacConkey Agar

Colourless colonies are formed.

C. Biochemical Reactions

Y. pestis ferments glucose, mannitol and maltose with the production of acid but no gas. Lactose and sucrose are not fermented. It is catalase positive, indole negative, urease negative and citrate negative.

D. Pathogenesis

Y. pestis is a natural pathogen of rodents and causes zoonotic disease called ***plague***. Infection is transmitted from one animal to another by the bite of flea.

Plague is a natural disease of rodents and is transmitted to man via the bite of infected rat flea (***Xenopsylla. cheopis***). The incubation period is 2–6 days. In man, plague occurs in three forms: ***bubonic***, ***pneumonic*** and ***septicaemic***.

1. Bubonic Plague

As the plague bacillus usually enters through the bite of infected rat flea on the legs, the inguinal lymph nodes are involved, hence the name bubonic (bubo meaning groin). The inguinal lymph nodes become enlarged and suppurate.

2. Pneumonic Plague

It is highly infectious form of plague involving the lungs producing haemorrhagic pneumonia. It can be transmitted from man to man by droplet infection (**airborne route**) and is virtually always fatal.

3. Septicaemic Plague

The presence of bacteria in blood denotes septicaemic plague. This may occur as primary infection but it usually occurs as the terminal event of bubonic and pneumonic plague. Massive involvement of blood vessels results in haemorrhages in the skin and mucosa. Due to this manifestation, the disease is given the name ***black death***.

E. Laboratory Diagnosis

1. Specimens

(i) Pus or fluid aspirated from bubo in bubonic plague.
(ii) Sputum and blood in pneumonic plague.
(iii) Blood in septicaemic plague.
(iv) Splenic tissue on postmortem.
(v) CSF in meningeal plague.

2. Direct Microscopy

Sputum and aspirate from lymph nodes are stained with Gram's staining and methylene blue. Gram's staining shows characteristic Gram negative coccobacilli. With methylene blue staining, bacilli show typical bipolar staining.

3. *Culture*

Culture is made on blood agar medium and incubated at 27°C. Biochemical tests are performed to confirm the diagnosis.

II. YERSINIA PSEUDOTUBERCULOSIS AND YERSINIA ENTEROCOLITICA

These two organisms resemble *Y. pestis* in that they are small, Gram negative bacilli with bipolar staining and reservoirs of infection are rodents, wild and domestic animals. They differ from *Y. pestis* by their motility at 22°C (and not at 37°C), non-capsulated, urease positive and oxidase negative.

A. Yersinia pseudotuberculosis

It is motile at 22°C and urease positive. Pseudotuberculosis is a zoonosis. Man acquires infection through ingested materials contaminated with animal faeces. Patients develop acute mesenteric lymphadenitis. The term *yersiniosis* denotes infection with yersiniae other than *Y. pestis.*

Laboratory diagnosis includes isolation of the organisms from an excised mesenteric lymph node, or blood and demonstration of antibodies in patient's serum during the acute illness.

B. Yersinia enterocolitica

It is a Gram negative coccobacillus and motile at 22°C. It is aerobic and facultative anaerobe. Optimum temperature for growth is 22°C. On blood agar, smooth translucent, non-haemolytic colonies measuring 2–3 mm in diameter appear after 48 hours incubation at 22°C. On MacConkey agar, it forms pin-point, non-lactose fermenting (NLF) colonies.

Disease occurs via faeco-oral route by contaminated food and water. In man it may cause gastroenteritis, mesentric lymphadenitis and septicaemia.

The laboratory diagnosis consists of isolation of the organism and indirectly by demonstration of antibodies in the patient serum. The organisms can be isolated from faeces, blood or from mesenteric lymph nodes.

KEY POINTS

1. Yersiniae are Gram negative, short bacilli showing bipolar staining (*safety pin appearance*) with methylene blue.
2. The genus yersinia contains three medically important species—*Y. pestis* (the caustive agent of plague), *Y. pseudotuberculosis* (a primary pathogen of rodents) and *Y. entercolitica* (causes human diarrhoeal diseases).
3. Plague is a *zoonotic* disease. It is a natural disease of rodents and is transmitted to man via the bite of infected rat flea (*Xenopsiella cheopis*).
4. In man *Y. enterocolitica* may cause *gastroenteritis*, *mesentric lymphadenitis* and *septicaemia.*

STUDY QUESTION

1. Write short notes on:
   (i) *Yersinia pestis* (ii) *Yersinia enterocolitica.*

MULTIPLE CHOICE QUESTIONS (MCQs)

1. 'Safety pin appearance' on methylene blue staining is a characteristic feature of:
   (a) *Yersinia pestis*
   (b) *Pseudomonas aeruginosa*
   (c) *Burkholderia mallei*
   (d) *B. pseudomallei*
2. What is the causative agent of plague?
   (a) *Yersinia pestis*
   (b) *Y. enterocolitica*
   (c) *Y. pseudotuberculosis*
   (d) *Francisella tularensis*
3. Plague is transmitted to man by bite of infected:
   (a) Sandfly
   (b) Rat flea
   (c) Hard tick
   (d) Mite
4. Pneumonic plague can be transmitted from human to human by:
   (a) Droplet infection
   (b) Ingestion
   (c) Infected sandfly
   (d) All of the above
5. The diseases caused by *Yersinia enterocolitica* in man include:
   (a) Gastroenteritis
   (b) Mesenteric lymphadenitis
   (c) Septicaemia
   (d) All of the above

ANSWERS (MCQs) ...✓

1. (a) 2. (a) 3. (b) 4. (a) 5. (d)

Haemophilus

28

The genus *Haemophilus* contains non-motile, non-sporing, Gram negative bacilli and require one or both of two accessory growth factors (X and V) present in blood.

I. HAEMOPHILUS INFLUENZAE

A. Morphology

It is a small (1.5 µm × 0.3 µm), Gram negative, non-motile bacillus showing considerable pleomorphism. It is non-sporing and non-acid-fast.

B. Culture

H. influenzae has fastidious growth requirements. It grows better in aerobic than in anaerobic conditions. It requires enriched media such as blood agar or chocolate agar because the accessory growth factors known as X ('X' for unknown) and V ('V' for vitamin) present in blood are essential for growth. The optimum temperature for growth is 35–37°C, some strains require 5–10% CO_2. It cannot grow on nutrient agar which lacks the accessory growth factors.

1. X Factor

It is necessary for the synthesis of catalase and other enzymes cytochrome C, cytochrome oxidase, involved in aerobic respiration.

2. V Factor

It is present in red blood cells. Ordinary blood agar is not suitable for the growth of *H. influenzae* where growth is scanty, as the V factor is not freely available, being imprisoned inside the red blood cells. V factor is released from erythrocytes in chocolate agar (heated blood agar at 80-90°C). V factor is also synthesised by Staphylococci. Growth on blood agar can be improved by providing a source of V factor (*Staph. aureus*).

Blood agar with *Staph. aureus* streak and chocolate agar are routinely used for the identification of *H. influenzae*. The colonies are small, translucent and non haemolytic on blood agar.

Satellitism

Although blood agar contains X and V factors, colonies of *H. influenzae* are small due to non-availability of V factor. After inoculating suspected *H. influenzae* on a blood agar plate, *Staph. auerus* is streaked across the same blood agar plate and incubated at 37°C for 18–24 hours. The colonies of *H. influenzae* will be large and well developed alongside the streak of staphylococci while those further away from staphylococcal streak are smaller. This phenomenon is called ***satellitism*** and demonstrates that V factor is available in high concentration near the staphylococcal growth and only in smaller quantities away from it (Fig. 28.1).

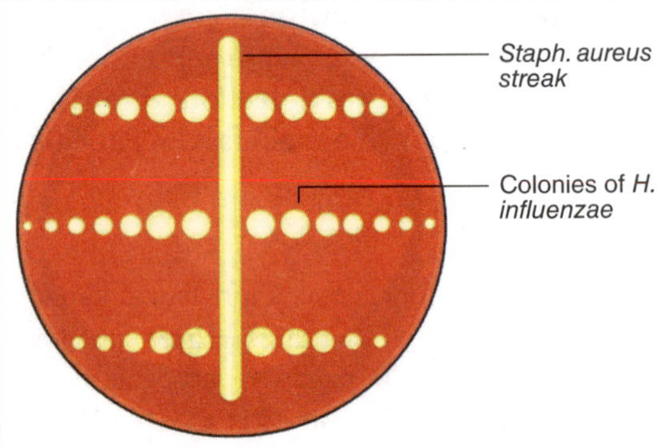

Fig. 28.1 Satellitism

C. Biochemical Reactions

H. influenzae is catalase and oxidase positive, ferments glucose and galactose, reduces nitrate to nitrite. It does not ferment sucrose, lactose and mannitol.

D. Antigenic Structure

The capsulated strains produce a capsule which is polysaccharide in nature. On the basis of capsular material, *Pitman* divided *H. influenzae* into 6 serotypes—a, b, c, d, e, and f. Capsular serotype b strains (Hib) are associated with most invasive infections.

Non-capsulated strains cannot be typed and are called 'non-typable strains'.

E. Pathogenesis

It is an obligate human parasite. The organism enters by respiratory route. The non-capsulated strains of *H. influenzae* are regular commensal in the nasopharynx or oropharynx. Capsulated strains cause invasive infections, type b accounting for most cases. The following infections are caused by *H. influenzae*.

1. Meningitis

This is the most serious disease occurring in children of 2 months to 2 years of age. Majority of the cases are due to type b strains.

2. Acute Epiglottitis

It is the second most common infection caused by *H. influenzae*. This is an acute inflammation of the epiglottis with obstructive laryngeal oedema, seen in children over two years old.

3. Pneumonia

It typically occurs in infants.

4. Bronchitis

H. influenzae is an important pathogen in the acute exacerbations of chronic bronchitis.

5. Suppurative Lesions

Some of the suppurative lesions include septic arthritis, endocarditis, pericarditis and otitis media.

F. Laboratory Diagnosis

1. Specimens

Depending upon the type of lesion, the following specimens may be collected:

(i) Cerebrospinal fluid (CSF)
(ii) Blood
(iii) Throat swab
(iv) Sputum
(v) Pus
(vi) Aspirates from joints, middle ears or sinuses etc.

2. Collection and Transport

Specimens should be collected in sterile containers and under all aseptic conditions. As *H. influenzae* is very sensitive to low temperature, therefore, clinical specimens should never be refrigerated.

3. Direct Microscopy

(i) Gram staining

In meningitis, Gram stained smear of CSF shows pleomorphic Gram negative coccobacilli.

(ii) Quellung reaction

This can be employed for direct demonstration of capsule of *H. influenzae* when a drop of CSF is mixed with specific type b antiserum. Capsular swelling occurs when observed under the microscope.

(iii) Antigen detection

Type b capsular antigen can also be detected in patient's serum, CSF, urine or pus by latex agglutination.

4. Culture

(i) CSF culture

CSF should be plated promptly on blood agar or chocolate agar. A strain of *Staph. aureus* should be streaked across the blood agar plate on which the specimen has already been inoculated. Plates are then incubated at 35–37°C, aerobically with 5–10% CO_2, overnight. The isolate is then identified by its colony morphology, satellitism, Gram staining and serotyping.

(ii) Blood culture

It is usually positive in cases of epiglottitis and pneumonia.

(iii) Sputum culture

Several samples of the sputum are to be cultured to increase the rate of isolation.

5. Colony Morphology and Staining

After overnight incubation, small opaque colonies appear that show satellitism. A smear is made from colony and stained with Gram stain. It shows small Gram negative bacilli or coccobacilli.

II. HAEMOPHILUS DUCREYI

A. Morphology

H. ducreyi is a short, Gram negative coccobacillus, 1–1.5 µm × 0.6 µm in size. They have a tendency to occur in groups or in parallel chains. They frequently take bipolar staining. The microscopic findings have been described as resembling a '***school of fish***' appearance.

B. Culture

It does not grow in ordinary laboratory media. It requires X factor but not V factor for its growth. It can be grown on chocolate agar. It requires 10% CO_2 and high humidity for primary isolation. Optimum temperature for growth is 35°C for 2–8 days.

After 24 hours of incubation, the colonies of *H. ducreyi* are small, pin point to 0.5 mm in diameter, translucent, non-mucoid.

C. Pathogenesis

H. ducreyi causes **chancroid** or **soft sore**, a highly contagious sexually transmitted disease (STD) characterised by tender, non-indurated, irregular ulcers on the genitalia. The infection remains localised, spreading only to the inguinal lymph nodes which are enlarged and painful. Sometimes it leads to inguinal abscess called bubo. Chancroid is also known as ***soft chancre***.

KEY POINTS

1. The genus *Haemophilus* contains non-motile, non-sporing, Gram negative bacilli and require one or both of two accessory growth factors (*X and V*) present in blood.
2. *H. influenzae* and *H. ducreyi* are the major pathogens in the genus *Haemophilus*.
3. *H. influenzae* may cause *meningitis*, pneumonia, epiglottitis, bronchitis, otitis media, septic arthritis and *H. ducreyi* is the causative organism of *chancroid*.
4. *Latex agglutination* is a *rapid test* for *H. influenzae* antigen detection in patient's serum, CSF, or urine.
5. CSF culture is an important test in laboratory diagnosis of meningitis.

STUDY QUESTIONS

1. Discuss the laboratory diagnosis of infections caused by *Haemophilus influenzae*.
2. Write short notes on:
   (i) X and V factors
   (ii) Satellitism
   (iii) *Haemophilus ducreyi*.

MULTIPLE CHOICE QUESTIONS (MCQs)

1. Accessory growth factor/s required by *Haemophilus influenzae* is/are:
   (a) X factor
   (b) V factor
   (c) Both X and V factors
   (d) Neither X nor V factor
2. Which of the following bacteria shows phenomenon of satellitism?
   (a) *Haemophilus influenzae*
   (b) *Listeria monocytogenes*
   (c) *Streptococcus pyogenes*
   (d) All of the above
3. Which of the following infections is/are caused by *Haemophilus influenzae*?
   (a) Meningitis
   (b) Acute epiglottitis
   (c) Both of the above
   (d) None of the above
4. The causative agent of chancroid is:
   (a) *Haemophilus influenzae*
   (b) *H. ducreyi*
   (c) *H. haemolyticus*
   (d) *H. aphrophilus*

ANSWERS (MCQs)

1. (c) 2. (a) 3. (c) 4. (b)

Bordetella

29

I. INTRODUCTION

The genus *Bordetella* contains very small, Gram negative coccobacilli. *B. pertussis* is the most important species.

II. BORDETELLA PERTUSSIS

A. Morphology

B. pertussis is a small, ovoid, 1–1.5 µm × 0.3 µm, Gram negative coccobacillus. It is non-motile, non-sporing and capsulated.

B. Culture

It is aerobic and optimum temperature for growth is 35–36°C. The organism requires a complex medium for its primary isolation. **Bordet - Gengou (glycerol – potato – blood agar)** is a commonly used medium. After incubation for 48–72 hours, colonies on this medium are small, smooth, opaque, greyish white, refractile, resembling ***bisected pearls*** or ***mercury drops***.

C. Biochemical Reactions

B. pertussis is biochemically inactive. It is oxidase positive and usually produces catalase.

D. Pathogenesis

B. pertussis infection is predominantly a childhood disease and is known as **whooping cough**. In human beings, the source of infection is the patient in the early stage. Infection is transmitted by droplets.

E. Laboratory diagnosis

1. Microscopy

Microscopic diagnosis is made by demonstration of the bacilli in respiratory secretions by the fluorescent antibody technique.

2. Culture

For culture, following methods have been used for collection of specimens.

(i) The pernasal swab

A swab is passed along the floor of the nasal cavity and material collected from the pharyngeal wall. The swab is inoculated on Bordet-Gengou medium.

(ii) The cough plate method

A Bordet-Gengou culture plate is held 10–15 cm in front of the patient's mouth during a bout of coughing so that the cough droplets directly inoculate the culture medium.

(iii) The postnasal (peroral) swab

A West's postnasal swab is passed through mouth to collect posterior pharyngeal wall secretions.

The cough plate method and postnasal swabs are no longer recommended.

Medium employed is Bordet and Gengou or charcoal blood agar. Plates are incubated at 35–36°C. Typical pearl like colonies of *B. pertussis* appear in 48-72 hours. These are confirmed by microscopy and slide agglutination.

F. Treatment

Azithromycin or erythromycin is the drug of choice.

G. Prophylaxis

Immunisation of infants and children with killed *B. pertussis* vaccine is very effective. Pertussis vaccine is generally administered in combination with diphtheria toxoid and tetanus toxoid (DPT). Three intramuscular injections at intervals of 4–6 weeks are given before the age of six months, followed by a booster dose at the end of the first year of life.

Under National Immunisation Schedule of India, total five doses are given. Three doses of pentavalent vaccine (containing DPT, hepatitis B vaccine and Haemophilus influenzae type b vaccine) and two booster doses of DPT. Three doses of pentavalent vaccines are given by intramuscular route on anteriolateral side of mid thigh, at 6, 10 and 14 weeks of birth. Booster doses of DPT are given by intramuscular route at 16–24 months and at 5 years.

KEY POINTS

1. The genus *Bordetella* contains very small, Gram negative coccobacilli.
2. *B. pertussis* is the main causative agent of whooping cough.
3. Laboratory diagnosis depends on microscopy and culture.
4. Pertussis vaccine is generally administered in combination with diphtheria toxoid and tetanus toxoid (DPT).

STUDY QUESTION

1. Describe the laboratory diagnosis of whooping cough.

MULTIPLE CHOICE QUESTIONS (MCQs)

1. Which one of the following media is most frequently used for isolation of *Bordetella pertussis*?
   (a) Chocolate agar
   (b) MacConkey agar
   (c) Bordel-Gengou medium
   (d) Tinsdale agar
2. *Bordetella pertussis* infection is transmitted by:
   (a) Droplets
   (b) Inoculation of skin
   (c) Contact
   (d) All of the above

ANSWERS (MCQs)

1. (c) 2. (a)

30

Brucella

BRUCELLA

The genus *Brucella* consists of small, non-motile, aerobic, Gram negative coccobacilli which are strict parasite of animals. Man acquires infection by contact with infected animals or through their products.

A. Morphology

Brucellae are Gram negative, non-motile, coccobacilli or short rods measuring 0.5–0.7 µm × 0.6–1.5 µm. They are arranged singly or in short chains. They are non-sporing and non-capsulated.

B. Culture

Brucellae are strict aerobes. *Br. abortus* is capnophilic, requiring 5–10 per cent CO_2 for its growth. The optimum temperature for growth is 37°C (range 20–40°C) and optimum pH 6.6–7.4.

They may grow on ordinary media, though growth is slow and scanty. The media employed for culture are serum-dextrose agar or trypticase soy agar. The addition of bacitracin, cycloheximide, polymyxin B or vancomycin makes these media selective. On solid media, colonies are small, moist and translucent. In liquid media, growth is uniform.

C. Biochemical Reactions

No carbohydrates are ordinarily fermented but they possess oxidative capacity. They are catalase and oxidase positive. Urease test is very rapidly positive.

D. Pathogenesis

All the three major species of brucellae (*Br. abortus*, *Br. melitensis* and *Br. suis*) are pathogenic to human beings. Brucellosis is a zoonotic disease. Human infection occurs by direct or indirect contact with infected animals. Brucellae are transmitted to humans by:

(i) Drinking contaminated (unpasteurised) raw milk or by ingestion of milk products from infected animals.
(ii) Direct contact with infected animal tissues: butchers, dairy workers, farm workers and veterinarians are particularly at risk.
(iii) Accidental infection may occur in laboratory personnel working with brucellae.

The incubation period varies from 2 to 3 weeks and may extend to 6 months. The onset of symptoms may be acute or insidious. Acute brucellosis is also named as *undulant fever* because of the periodic nocturnal fever that may occur over weeks, months or years especially in untreated cases. When the disease persists for 6 months or more, it is termed as *chronic brucellosis*.

E. Laboratory Diagnosis

1. Specimens

Blood culture is the most definitive method for the diagnosis of acute brucellosis. Brucellae can also be isolated from bone marrow, liver and lymph nodes.

2. Blood Culture

5–10 ml of blood is inoculated into 50–100 ml of serum dextrose broth or trypticase soy broth and incubated at 37°C aerobically in presence of 5–10% CO_2. Subcultures are made on solid media and incubated at 37°C aerobically in presence of 5–10% CO_2.

The need for frequent subcultures can be avoided by use of **Castaneda's method** of blood culture. It contains both liquid (trypticase soy broth) and solid (trypicase soy agar) media in the same bottle (Fig. 30.1). The blood is inoculated into the broth (liquid medium) and the bottle incubated in the upright position. For subculture, the bottle is tilted so that the broth flows over the surface of solid agar slant. It is again incubated in the upright position. In case of positive blood culture, colonies appear on the agar slant. This method reduces the chances of contamination and risk of infection to laboratory workers.

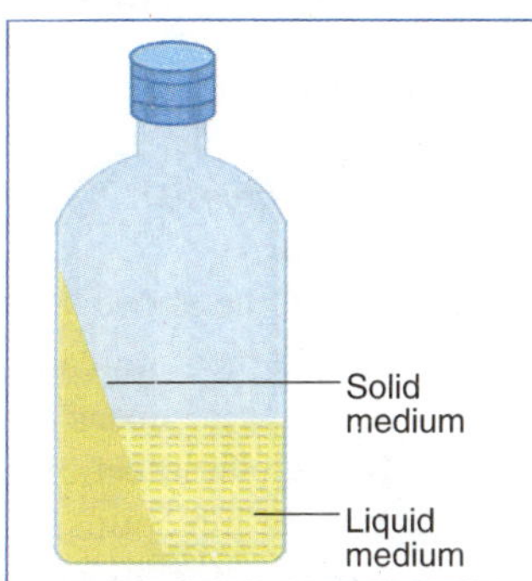

Fig. 30.1 Castaneda's medium

3. Serology

Serological methods are more useful as cultures are negative in high percentage of cases. In chronic brucellosis, only IgG can be demonstrated and IgM may often be absent.

(i) Serum agglutination test (SAT)

Serum agglutination test (SAT) is the most widely used test for diagnosis of brucellosis.

This is a tube agglutination test in which equal volumes of serial two fold dilutions (1 : 20 to 1 : 640) of patient's serum and the standardised antigen (heat killed *Brucella* suspension) are mixed and incubated at 37°C for 24 hours. A single titre of more than 1 : 160 is presumptive evidence of *Brucella* infection. The test can also be done in microplate.

(ii) Castaneda strip test

A loopful of patient's serum is placed on a filter paper strip containing a coloured brucella antigen. Antibody is able to 'fix' the antigen and prevent its movement along the paper.

(iii) Complement fixation test (CFT)

It is more useful in chronic cases as it detects both IgG and IgM.

(iv) ELISA

(v) Indirect immunofluorescent test

4. Hypersensitivity Test (Brucellin test)

It is delayed (type IV) hypersensitivity to *Brucella* antigen (*brucellin*). It is an intradermal test. Positive reaction is indicated by an erythema and induration within 24 hours. This test is not useful for diagnosis of acute infections because test may remain positive for years after acquiring infection. Persistent negative skin test helps to exclude brucellosis.

F. Treatment

Treatment consists of administration of tetracycline (e.g. doxycycline) along with gentamicin.

G. Prophylaxis

1. Persons handling the animals should use protective clothing and gloves.
2. Pasteurisation or boiling of milk should be done.
3. Vaccination of cattle should be done.
4. Unimmunised infected animals should be slaughtered.

KEY POINTS

1. *Brucella melitensis*, *B. abortus* and *B. suis* are the three major species of the genus *Brucella*.
2. Brucellosis is a febrile disease. Man acquires infection by contact with infected animals or through their products.
3. Brucellae are *strict aerobes*. B. *abortus* is *capnophilic*, requiring 5-10 per cent CO_2 for its growth.
4. Laboratory diagnosis depends on culture of brucellae and serology. *Castaneda's method* of blood culture is used. *Standard tube agglutination test* is used for detection of antibodies in patient's serum.

STUDY QUESTIONS

1. Discuss the laboratory diagnosis of brucellosis.
2. Write short notes on:
   (i) Castaneda's medium
   (ii) Serodiagnosis of brucellosis

MULTIPLE CHOICE QUESTIONS (MCQs)

1. The causative agent/s of undulant fever is/are:
   (a) *Brucella abortus*
   (b) *Br. melitensis*
   (c) *Br. suis*
   (d) All of the above
2. Castaneda medium can be used for blood culture in:
   (a) Acute brucellosis
   (b) Bordetella infections
   (c) Yersina infections
   (d) None of the above
3. Brucellae are transmitted to humans by:
   (a) Ingestion of contaminated raw milk
   (b) Direct contact with infected animal tissues
   (c) Accidental mucosal or skin contamination in laboratory personnels
   (d) All of the above

ANSWERS (MCQS)

1. (d) 2. (a) 3. (d)

Mycobacterium

31

Mycobacteria are slender bacilli that are difficult to stain, but once stained, resist decolourisation with dilute mineral acids and are therefore called *acid-fast bacilli* or *AFB*. These organisms are aerobic, non-motile, non-capsulated and non-sporing. Growth is generally slow.

I. MYCOBACTERIUM TUBERCULOSIS

A. Morphology

M. tuberculosis is a slender, straight or slightly curved bacillus with rounded ends, occurring singly, in pairs or in small clumps. It measures 1–4 µm × 0.2 – 0.8 µm (average 3 µm × 0.3 µm) in size. These bacilli are acid-fast, non-sporing, non-capsulated and non-motile. Ziehl-Neelsen staining is useful to study the morphology of these organisms. With this stain, tubercle bacilli are seen bright red (acid-fast), while the tissue cells and other organisms are stained blue (Fig. 31.1). Tubercle bacilli may also be stained with the fluorescent dyes (auramine O, rhodamine) and appear yellow luminous bacilli under the fluorescent microscope. Beaded or barred forms are frequently seen in *M. tuberculosis*. They are Gram positive but are difficult to stain with the Gram stain.

B. Culture

M. tuberculosis is an obligate aerobe. The bacilli grow slowly (generation time 14–15 hours) and colonies appear only in about two weeks and sometimes it may take up to 6–8 weeks.

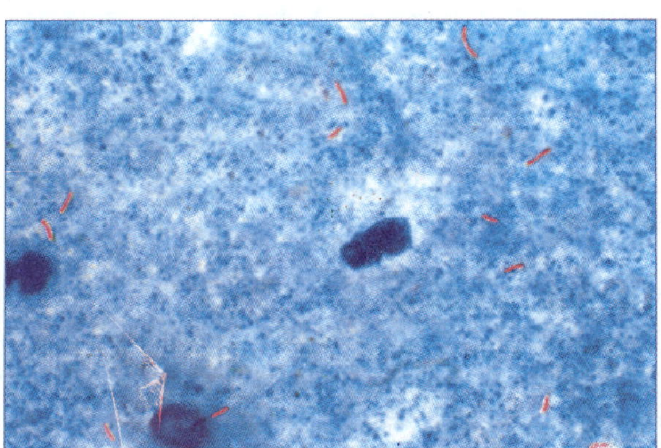

Fig. 31.1 Mycobacterium tuberculosis in Ziehl-Neelsen stained smear

Optimum temperature for growth is 37°C (range 30–40°C). Optimum pH is 6.4 to 7.0. Tubercle bacilli can grow on a wide range of enriched culture media but **Lowenstein–Jensen (LJ) medium** is the most commonly used. This medium consists of beaten eggs, asparagine, mineral salts, malachite green and glycerol or sodium pyruvate. It is solidified by heating (inspissation). Malachite green inhibits the growth of organisms other than mycobacteria and provides a colour to the medium. Colonies of *M. tuberculosis* are dry, rough, buff coloured, raised, with a wrinkled surface (Fig. 31.2). *M. tuberculosis* has a luxuriant growth (*eugonic growth*).

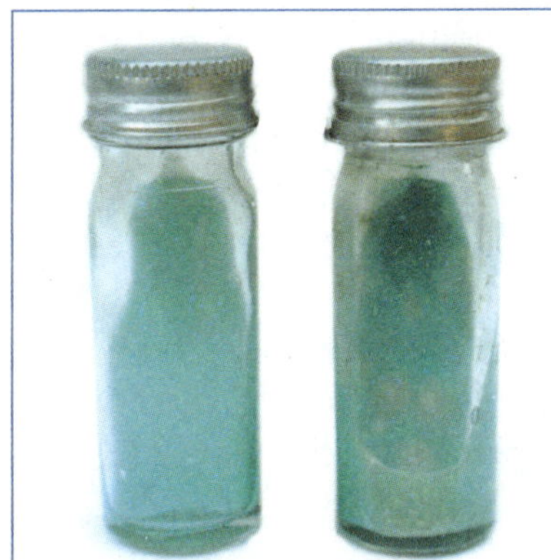

Fig. 31.2 LJ media without growth and with growth

In liquid media, the bacilli grow as surface pellicle. Virulent strains tend to grow as *serpentine cords* in the liquid media, while avirulent strains grow in a more dispersed fashion.

C. Biochemical Reactions

Mycobacterial species can be identified by several biochemical tests. Niacin test and Nitrate reduction test are two important biochemical tests, which are positive in *M. tuberculosis.*

D. Pathogenesis

Tuberculosis may involve lungs (pulmonary) or sites other than lungs (extrapulmonary).The infection is commonly acquired by inhalation of infected droplets coughed or sneezed into the air by a patient with pulmonary tuberculosis. In bovine tuberculosis, infected cows develop lesions in the udder and bacilli are excreted in the milk which can then infect people who drink it raw. In developed countries, pasteurisation of milk has virtually eradicated this organism.

Tubercle bacilli are engulfed by macrophages but they survive and multiply in macrophages. The cell mediated immunity (CMI) plays a major role to interact with these macrophages whereas humoral immunity appears to be irrelevant.

E. Koch's Phenomenon

The response of a tuberculous animal to reinfection was best explained by Robert Koch. When a healthy guinea pig is inoculated subcutaneously with virulent tubercle bacilli, the puncture site heals quickly and there is no immediate visible reaction. After 10–14 days, a nodule appears at the site of injection which ulcerates and the ulcer persists till the animal dies of progressive tuberculosis. The regional lymph nodes are enlarged and caseous. If on the other hand, virulent tubercle bacilli are injected in a guinea pig, which had received a prior injection of tubercle bacilli 4–6 weeks earlier, an indurated lesion appears at the site of injection in a day or two which undergoes necrosis in another day or so to form a shallow ulcer. This ulcer heals rapidly without involvement of the regional lymph nodes or tissues. This is called *Koch's phenomenon.* This phenomenon is a combination of hypersensitivity and immunity.

F. Tuberculin Skin Test

1. Principle

Tuberculin skin test (TST) is delayed or type IV hypersensitivity reaction.

2. Reagents

(i) Old tuberculin (OT)

It was originally described by Robert Koch. This crude product may lead to serious complications in some patients, it is now rarely used.

(ii) Purified protein derivative (PPD)

A purified preparation of the active tuberculoprotein (PPD-S) was prepared by *Seibert* (1941). It was prepared by growing *M. tuberculosis* in a semisynthetic medium. It is called *purified protein derivative* (PPD). The dosage of PPD is expressed in tuberculin unit (TU). Another PPD is PPD RT-23. I TU of PPD RT-23 is equivalent of 5TU of PPD-S.

3. Method

Mantoux test

0.1 ml of PPD containing 5 TU of PPD-S is injected intradermally into flexor aspect of forearm. A PPD-S dose of 1 TU is used when extreme hypersensitivity is suspected. In India 1 TU of PPD RT-23 is recommended and not PPD-S.

4. Result

In the Mantoux test the site of injection is examined after 48–72 hours and interpreted as follows:

Positive test

In a positive reaction, there is induration (local oedema) of 10 mm diameter or more surrounded by erythema at the site of inoculation. Positive test only confirms past infection with tubercle bacilli but does not indicate presence of active state of the disease.

G. Laboratory Diagnosis

Bacteriological diagnosis can be established by microscopy, culture examination, by animal inoculation test or by molecular method.

1. Specimen

Specimen collection depends on the site of involvement. Tuberculosis may involve lungs (pulmonary) or sites other than lungs (extrapulmonary).

(i) Pulmonary tuberculosis

Sputum is the most common specimen. It is collected in a clean wide-mouthed container. A morning specimen may be collected on three consecutive days. If sputum is scanty, a 24 hour specimen may be collected. When sputum is not available, laryngeal swab or bronchial washings are collected. In children, gastric washings may be examined as they tend to swallow sputum.

(ii) Meningitis

Cerebrospinal fluid (CSF) from tuberculous meningitis (TBM) often forms a spider web clot on standing, examination of which may be more useful than of fluid.

(iii) Renal tuberculosis

Three consecutive days morning samples of urine are examined.

(iv) Bone and joints tuberculosis

Aspirated fluid

(v) Tissue

Biopsy of tissue.

2. Direct Microscopy

Smear is made from the specimen and stained by the *Ziehl-Neelsen* technique (refer to chapter 2 for method of Ziehl-Neelsen staining). It is examined under oil immersion lens. The acid-fast bacilli (AFB) appear as bright red bacilli against a blue background. A negative report should not be given till at least 300 fields have been examined. Grading of smears is done according to number of bacilli seen (Table 31.1).

Table 31.1: Grading of Ziehl-Neelsen (ZN) Smear

No. of AFB seen in oil immersion field	Report
0 / 300 fields	AFB not seen
1-2 / 300 fields	Doubtful, repeat the smear
1-9 / 100 fields	1+
1-9 / 10 fields	2+
1-9 / field	3+
10 or more / field	4+

If a large number of smears are to be examined, fluorescent microscopy is more convenient. Smears are stained with fluorescent dyes such as auramine 'O' or auramine rhodamine and examined under ultraviolet light. The bacilli appear as bright bacilli against dark background.

However, grading of smears is done differently under Revised National Tuberculosis Programme (RNTCP) (Table 31.2).

Table 31.2: Grading of Ziehl-Neelsen (ZN) Smear according to NTEP (formerly RNTCP)

No. of AFB seen in oil immersion field•	Number of fields examined	Report
>10 AFB/field	20	Positive 3+
1–10 AFB/field	50	Positive 2+
10–99 AFB/100 fields	100	Positive 1+
1–9 AFB/100 fields	100	Doubtful positive
No AFB/100 fields	100	Negative, repeat

3. Concentration of Specimens

Concentration of a specimen is done to achieve:

(a) homogenisation of the specimen
(b) decontamination, i.e., to kill other bacteria present in the specimen.
(c) concentration, i.e., to concentrate the bacilli in a small volume without inactivation.

Such concentrate is used for culture and animal inoculation tests besides smear preparation.

Several concentration methods are in use:

Petroff's method

It is a simple and widely used technique. Sputum is mixed with equal volume of 4% sodium hydroxide and is incubated at 37°C with frequent shaking for about 30 minutes. It is then centrifuged at 3,000 rpm for 30 minutes. The supernatant fluid is poured off and the deposit is neutralised by adding 8% hydrochloric acid in presence of a drop of phenol red indicator. The deposit is used for smear, culture and animal inoculation.

Other methods

mucolytic agents such as N-acetyl-L-cysteine with sodium hydroxide and pancreatin are used for concentration of specimens. In urine and CSF specimens centrifugation is done to concentrate the specimen. Centrifuged deposit is used for smear and culture examination.

4. Culture

Culture is a very sensitive method for detection of tubercle bacilli. It may detect as few as 10 to 100 bacilli per ml. The concentrated material is inoculated on two bottles of **Lowenstein-Jensen medium**. The tubercle bacilli usually grow in 2 to 8 weeks.

In a positive culture, characteristic colonies appear on culture medium. Smear is prepared from isolated colony and stained with Ziehl-Neelsen technique. When acid-fast bacillus (AFB) is slow growing, non-pigmented and niacin positive, it is regarded as *M. tuberculosis*. Confirmation is done by immunochromatographic test (ICT) for detection of MPT 64 antigen.

In radiometric method such as BACTEC, the growth may be detected in about a week by using ^{14}C labelled substrates. Culture media contains ^{14}C-labelled palmitic acid. Mycobacteria metabolise the ^{14}C-labelled substrates and release radioactively labelled $^{14}CO_2$. The instrument measures $^{14}CO_2$. **This significant method has now been discontinued due to radioactivity**.

5. Serology

Serology includes detection of anti mycobacterial antibodies in patient serum. Diagnostic utility of these antibodies is equivocal. WHO has banned the use of these tests for diagnosis of active tuberculosis.

6. Molecular Methods

Polymerase chain reaction (PCR) is a rapid method in diagnosis of tuberculosis. It is based on DNA amplification and has been used to detect *M. tuberculosis* directly in clinical specimens.

Gene Xpert MTB/RIF

Gene Xpert MTB/RIF is an automated diagnostic test. It detects *M. tuberculosis* and rifampicin resistance by PCR. Results can be obtained from sputum specimen with 2 hours. WHO has endorsed this test for use in tuberculosis endemic countries.

Line probe assay (LPA) is used for identification of *M. tuberculosis* complex as well as detection of mutation in drug resistant genes.

H. Treatment

The antitubercular drugs include bactericidal agents such as rifampicin (R), isoniazid (H), pyrazinamide (Z), streptomycin and bacteriostatic agents include ethambutol (E), thiacetazone, ethionamide, paraaminosalicylic acid (PAS) and cycloserine. Short course regimen of 6 months is used. The new daily TB treatment regimen is used. As resistant strains emerge readily by mutation and selection, combinations of two or more drugs are used.

A serious consequence of unchecked drug resistance has been the emergence of ***multidrug resistance tuberculosis* (MDR-TB)**. The term multidrug resistance refers to resistance to rifampicin and isoniazid, with or without resistance to one or more other drugs. MDR-TB is a global problem especially in HIV infected persons. The directly observed therapy under supervision (DOTS) is being used to prevent deterioration of resistance problem by ensuring the patient's compliance.

Another serious condition ***extensively drug resistant tuberculosis (XDR-TB)*** has emerged recently. XDR-TB is due to *M. tuberculosis* strains which are resistant to any fluoroquinolone and at least one additional Group A drug in addition to isoniazid and rifampicin. Currently the Group A drugs include levofloxacin or moxifloxacin, bedaquiniline and linezolid.

I. Prophylaxis

Protection from tuberculosis may be done by public health measures and BCG vaccination. General measures such as nutrition and health education are also important.

BCG Vaccine

Calmette and Guerin (1921) prepared an attenuated strain of *M. bovis*. The strain was attenuated by repeated subcultures. When the strain became incapable of producing tuberculosis in the susceptible guinea pig, it was named *Bacille Calmette Guerin* (BCG).

(i) Dose and administration

Vaccine is given intradermally in a dose of 0.1 ml. BCG vaccine should be given soon after birth failing which it may be administered at any time during the first year of life.

(ii) Protective efficacy

A number of BCG vaccine trials were undertaken and the results varied from 0 to 80%. The immunity has been reported to last for about 10 years. The general opinion at present is that BCG does protect from tuberculosis. Even if disease occurs, it runs a milder course in vaccinated children.

J. National Tuberculosis Elimination Programme (NTEP)

Under NTEP, presumptive pulmonary tuberculosis is referred to a person who has any of following symptoms or signs such as cough for > 2 weeks, fever > 2 weeks, significant weight loss, haemoptysis. Diagnosis is mainly based on good quality microscopy. Two sputum samples are collected from the patient. One early morning specimen and other is collected on spot when patient visits the chest clinic (Fig. 31.3).

II. NON-TUBERCULOUS MYCOBACTERIA

Mycobacteria other than tubercle bacilli, that may occasionally cause human disease resembling tuberculosis, have been called **atypical mycobacteria**. They are also named as *anonymous* or *unclassified mycobacteria*. They normally exist as saprophytes of soil and water. They occasionally cause opportunistic disease in man and hence are also named *opportunistic mycobacteria* or **non-tuberculous mycobacteria (NTM) or MOTT (mycobacteria other than tubercle bacilli)**.

A. Classification

On the basis of pigment production and rate of growth, *Runyon* (1959) classified non-tuberculous mycobacteria into four groups (Table 31.3). Diseases caused by these non-tuberculous mycobacteria are listed in Table 31.4.

Table 31.3: Classification of Non-Tuberculous Mycobacteria

Runyon group	Name	Species
I	Photochromogens	*M. kansasii,* *M. simiae* *M. marinum*
II	Scotochromogens	*M. scrofulaceum* *M. gordonae* *M. szulgai*
III	Non-photochromogens	*M. avium,* *M. intracellulare* *M. xenopi, M. ulcerans,* *M. malmoense*
IV	Rapid growers	*M. chelonei,* *M. fortuitum*

Table 31.4: Diseases Caused by Non-tuberculous Mycobacteria

Disease	Causative agent
Lymphadenopathy	*M. scrofulaceum,* M. avium-intracellulare, *M. szulgai*
Pulmonary disease	*M. avium-intracellulare,* M. kansasii, M. xenopi, *M. simiae*
Skin lesions	
Buruli ulcer	*M. ulcerans*
Swimming pool granuloma	*M. marinum*
Post-injection abscesses	*M. chelonei* *M. fortuitum*
Disseminated disease	
AIDS related	*M. avium-intracellulare*
Non-AIDS related	*M. avium-intracellulare* *M. chelonei*

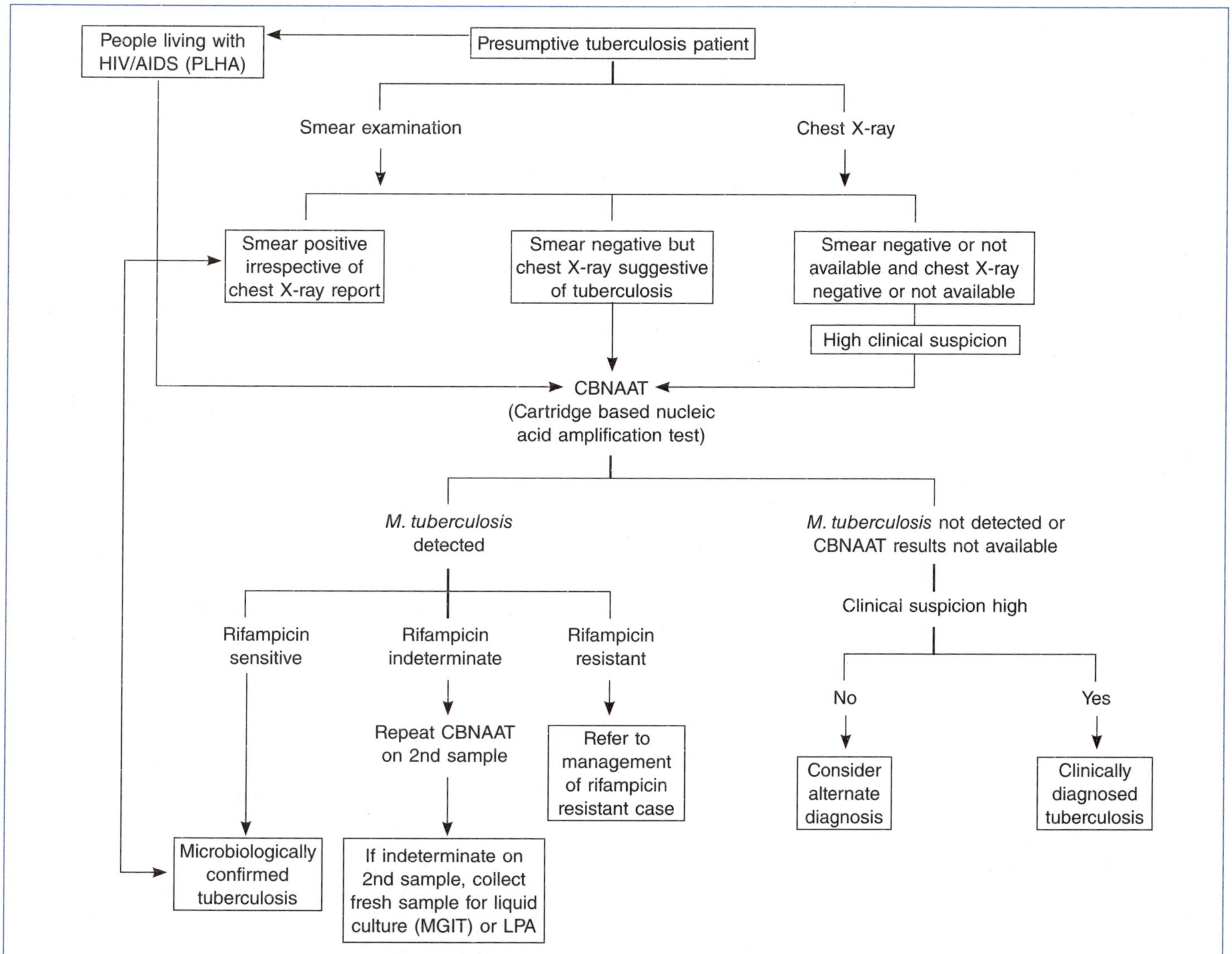

Fig. 31.3 Diagnosis of pulmonary tuberculosis under RNTCP (now NTEP).

B. Culture

Non-tuberculous mycobacteria grow in Lowenstein-Jensen (LJ) medium. Colonies appear within two to three weeks except in case of rapid growers which produce colonies in four or five days. *Photochromogens* form colonies that produce no pigment in the dark, but when colonies are exposed to light, a yellow orange pigment appears. The *scotochromogens* produce pigment in the dark. Non-photochromogens do not form pigment even on exposure to light. Rapid growers may be photo, scoto or non-photochromogens.

III. MYCOBACTERIUM LEPRAE

Leprosy is a chronic mycobacterial disease of ancient world and is still afflicting patients in many parts of world–mainly Asia and Africa. It is caused by *Mycobacterium leprae*.

A. Morphology

M. leprae is a slender, slightly curved or straight bacillus, 1–8 μm × 0.2–0.5 μm. It is acid-fast, but less so than the tubercle bacillus and for which 5% sulphuric acid is used for decolourisation after staining with carbol fuchsin (Fig. 31.4). It is Gram positive and stains more readily.

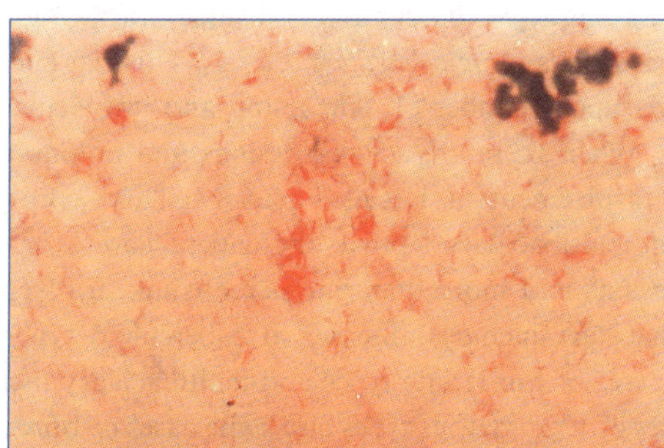

Fig. 31.4 Mycobacterium leprae stained by Ziehl-Neelsen method

The bacilli are seen singly and in groups, intracellularly or lying free outside the cells. Inside the cells they are present as bundles of organisms bound together by a lipid-like substance, the glia. These masses are known as *globi*. The parallel rows of bacilli in the globi give appearance of a *cigar bundle*. In tissue sections, the bacilli are arranged in clumps resembling cigarette ends. The globi are present in Virchow's *lepra cells* or *foamy cells* which are large undifferentiated histiocytes.

B. Cultivation

Lepra bacilli have not yet been grown on artificial culture media or tissue culture.

There have been many attempts to transmit leprosy to different experimental animals. The first breakthrough was achieved by *Shepard* (1960) when he showed that lepra bacilli could multiply in the foot pads of mice.

The nine-banded armadillo (*Dasypus novemcinctus*) is highly susceptible to infection with *M. leprae*.

C. Pathogenesis

Leprosy is a chronic granulomatous disease of humans and the only source of infection is patient. The bacilli localise primarily in the skin, peripheral nerves and nasal mucosa but any tissue or organ may be involved. Due to preference of bacilli for lower temperatures, the superficial and cooler tissues are affected.

Incubation period is very long and variable. Sources of infection are nasal discharge and skin lesions of patients. Prolonged close contact with patients is necessary for transmission of the disease.

D. Ridley and Jopling's Classification

On the basis of clinical, histopathological and immunological findings, *Ridley* and *Jopling* have introduced a scale for classifying the spectrum of leprosy into five groups. These are Tuberculoid (TT), Borderline tuberculoid (BT), Borderline (BB), Borderline lepromatous (BL) and Lepromatous (LL).

According to WHO, leprosy is divided into two groups, *paucibacillary* and *multibacillary* leprosy. This classification depends upon number of skin lesion and involvement of nerves. When there are ≤5 skin lesions and no/one nerve trunk involvement, it is called paucibacillary leprosy. In case of multibacillary leprosy, the patient have 6 or more skin lesions and more than one nerve trunk involvement. Paucibacillary includes all cases of tuberculoid types and some cases of borderline types and multibacillary includes all cases of lepromatous types and some cases of borderline type.

E. Lepromin Test

This reaction was first described by *Mitsuda* in 1919. The original antigen (lepromin) was a boiled, emulsified, lepromatous tissue rich in lepra bacilli. Nowadays, the lepromins used as antigens may be of human origin (lepromin-H) or armadillo derived (lepromin-A).

1. Procedure

The lepromin test is carried out by the intradermal injection of 0.1 ml of lepromin. The response to lepromin is typically biphasic consisting of early reaction of *Fernandez* and late reaction of *Mitsuda*.

(i) ***Early reaction of Fernandez:*** It consists of erythema and induration developing in 24–48 hours and usually remains for 3-5 days.

(ii) ***Late reaction of Mitsuda:*** It appears 1–2 weeks after the injection, reaching a peak in four weeks. The reaction appears in the form of a nodule that may ulcerate.

2. Uses

(i) ***Classification of leprosy:*** The test is positive in tuberculoid leprosy and negative in lepromatous leprosy.

(ii) ***Assessment of prognosis:*** A positive lepromin test indicates a good prognosis and a negative one a bad prognosis.

(iii) ***Assessment of resistance:*** It is done to assess the resistance of an individual to leprosy. Resistance is indicated by positive lepromin test.

F. Laboratory Diagnosis

In lepromatous cases, bacilli are always found in large numbers but in tuberculoid cases, the bacilli are very few and found with great difficulty, or not at all.

1. Specimens

Specimens are collected from the nasal mucosa, skin lesions and ear lobules. The specimens from skin are obtained by **slit and scrape** method. About six different areas should be sampled, including the skin over the buttocks, chin, cheek, forehead and ears. Smears from the nose are made by scraping a little material from the nasal septum.

2. Acid-Fast Staining

Slit-skin smears from skin patches and ear lobes and nasal mucosal scrapings are stained by Ziehl-Neelsen method using 5% sulphuric acid as decolourising agent. Acid-fast bacilli (AFB) arranged in parallel bundles within macrophages (*Lepra-cell*) confirm the diagnosis of lepromatous leprosy. The viable bacilli stain uniformly and the dead bacilli are fragmented, irregular or granular.

The smears are graded, based on the number of bacilli as follows:

1–10 bacilli in 100 fields = 1+
1–10 bacilli in 10 fields = 2+

1–10 bacilli per field = 3+
10–100 bacilli per field = 4+
100–1,000 bacilli per field = 5+
More than 1,000 bacilli, clumps and globi in every field = 6+

(i) Bacteriological index (BI)

It is defined as number of total bacilli in a tissue.

(ii) Morphological index (MI)

It is defined as the percentage of uniformaly stained (viable) bacilli out of the total number of bacilli counted. It provides a method for assessing the progress of patients on chemotherapy.

3. Skin and Nerve Biopsy

These are useful in the diagnosis and accurate classification of leprosy lesion.

G. Treatment

For multibacillary (BB, BL, LL) leprosy, rifampicin 600 mg once a month (supervised), dapsone 100 mg daily (unsupervised), clofazimine 300 mg once a month (supervised), and 50 mg, clofazimine daily (unsupervised) are given for one year. Adult patients with paucibacillary (TT, BT) leprosy are also given the same treatment as that of multibacillary leprosy but for six months.

KEY POINTS

1. Mycobacteria are slender bacilli that are difficult to stain, but once stained, resist decolourisation with dilute mineral acids and are therefore called *acid-fast bacilli* or *AFB*.
2. Ziehl-Neelsen (ZN) staining is useful to study the morphology of these organisms. With this stain, tubercle bacilli are seen bright *red* (acid-fast).
3. Lowenstein-Jensen (LJ) medium is the most commonly used medium to grow *M. tuberculosis*.
4. On LJ medium colonies of *M. tuberculosis* are dry, rough, buff coloured, raised with a wrinkled surface. *M. tuberculosis* has a luxuriant growth (*eugonic growth*). The tubercle bacilli usually grow in 2 to 8 weeks.
5. *M. tuberculosis* may involve lungs (*pulmonary tuberculosis*) or sites other than lungs (*extrapulmonary tuberculosis*).
6. Bacteriological diagnosis of tuberculosis can be established by direct microscopy and culture examination.
7. Drug resistance in *M. tuberculosis* is due to mutation. Emergence of *multidrug resistance tuberculosis* (MDR-TB) is a serious problem.
8. BCG vaccine is used for prophylaxis of tuberculosis. It is given intradermally. It is a live attenuated vaccine.
9. Mycobacteria other than tubercle bacilli, that may occasionally cause human disease resembling tuberculosis, have been called *non-tuberculous mycobacteria* (*NTM*). They are also named as *atypical mycobacteria*, *opportunistic mycobacteria* or *mycobacteria other than tubercle bacilli* (MOTT).
10. They normally exist as saprophytes of soil and water. They occasionally cause opportunistic disease in man.
11. *Mycobacterium leprae* is a slender, slightly curved or straight bacillus. It is acid-fast, but less so than the tubercle bacillus and for which 5% sulphuric acid is used for decolourisation after staining with carbol fuchsin.
12. *M. leprae* has not yet been grown on artificial culture media or tissue culture. However, they can multiply in *foot pads of mice* and *nine-banded armadillos*.
13. *M. leprae* produces leprosy in humans and only source of infection is patient.
14. Laboratory diagnosis depends on demonstration of bacilli in specimens by microscopy. The specimens from skin are obtained by *slit* and *scrape* method.

STUDY QUESTIONS

1. Discuss the laboratory diagnosis of pulmonary tuberculosis.
2. Write briefly about:
   (i) Koch's phenomenon (ii) Tuberculin test (iii) BCG vaccine.
3. Write short note on non-tuberculous mycobacteria.
4. Write short notes on:
   (i) Lepromin test (ii) Laboratory diagnosis of leprosy.

MULTIPLE CHOICE QUESTIONS (MCQs)

1. Eugonic growth on Lowenstein-Jensen medium is a characteristic of:
   (a) *Mycobacterium tuberculosis*
   (b) *M. bovis*
   (c) Both of the above
   (d) None of the above
2. *Myobacterium tuberculosis* infection is commonly acquired by:
   (a) Inhalation
   (b) Ingestion
   (c) Skin contact
   (d) Parenteral
3. A positive tuberculin test is indicated by induration of:
   (a) 10 mm or more in diameter
   (b) 5–9 mm in diameter
   (c) 2–4 mm in diameter
   (d) None of the above
4. Multidrug resistance tuberculosis (MDR-TB) is due to *M. tuberculosis* strain:
   (a) Resistant to rifampicin only
   (b) Resistant to isoniazid only
   (c) Resistant to at least rifampicin and isoniazid
   (d) None of the above
5. BCG vaccine is:
   (a) Live attenuated vaaccine
   (b) Killed vaccine
   (c) Toxoid
   (d) None of the above
6. Which of the following bacteria is photochromogen?
   (a) *Mycobacterium kansasii*
   (b) *M. scrofulaceum*
   (c) *M. gordonae*
   (d) *M. szulgai*
7. Which of the following bacteria is non-photochromogen?
   (a) *Mycobacterium kansasii*
   (b) *M. scrofulaceum*
   (c) *M. gordonae*
   (d) *M. ulcerans*
8. What is the concentration of sulphuric acid used as decolouriser in Ziehl-Neelsen staining method for *Mycobacterium leprae*?
   (a) 20%
   (b) 5%
   (c) 1%
   (d) 0.1%

ANSWERS (MCQs) ...✓

1. (a) 2. (a) 3. (a) 4. (c) 5. (a) 6. (a) 7. (d) 8. (b)

32 Spirochaetes

I. SPIROCHAETES

A. Morphology

The spirochaetes have Gram negative type cell wall composed of an outer membrane, a peptidoglycan layer and a cytoplasmic membrane. They are structurally more complex than other bacteria. They are large, motile, helical bacteria. They are motile because of endoflagella.

B. Diseases

Diseases caused by spirochaetes are shown in Table below.

Genus	Species	Disease
Treponema	*T. pallidum*	Syphilis
	T. pertenue	Yaws
	T. carateum	Pinta
	T. endemicum	Endemic syphilis
Borrelia	*B. recurrentis*	Relapsing fever
	B. vincentii	Vincent's angina
	B. burgdorferi	Lyme disease
Leptospira	*L. interrogans*	Leptospirosis
	L. biflexa	Saprophytes

II. TREPONEMA

A. Treponema Pallidum

Treponema pallidum is the causative agent of syphilis.

1. Morphology

It is a thin, delicate spirochaete with tapering ends, having about ten regular spirals. It is about 10 µm long (range 4–14 µm) and 0.1-0.2 µm wide. It is actively motile, showing rotation round the long axis, backward and forward movements and flexion of the whole body.

It does not take ordinary bacterial stains. Because of thinness of the spirals, *T. pallidum* cannot be seen by light microscope. However, it can be made out by negative staining with India ink. Its morphology and motility can also be seen by dark ground microscopy or phase contrast microscopy. It can be stained with silver impregnation methods. The treponemes reduce silver nitrate to metallic silver that is deposited on the surface enlarging the diameter of the organism.

2. Culture

Pathogenic treponemes cannot be grown in artificial culture media but are maintained by subculture in susceptible animals.

3. Pathogenesis

Natural infection with *T. pallidum* occurs only in human beings. Venereal syphilis is acquired by **sexual contact**. The treponema enters the body through minute abrasions on the skin or mucosa. Clinical disease sets in after an incubation period of about a month (range 10–90 days). There are three clinical stages of the disease in an untreated case—primary, secondary, and tertiary.

(i) Primary syphilis

A papule appears on the genital area that ulcerates forming a classical chancre of primary syphilis, called *hard chancre*. It is a painless, indurated and a circumscribed lesion. The chancre invariably heals within 10–40 days, even without treatment, leaving a thin scar.

(ii) Secondary syphilis

After healing of primary lesion, the patient remains asymptomatic for 2 to 6 months, then secondary syphilis sets in. The secondary lesions are due to widespread multiplication of the treponemes and their dissemination through the blood.

(iii) Congenital syphilis

The treponemes can cross the placental barrier. Infection in foetus usually occurs from primary and secondary infection of the mother.

4. Laboratory Diagnosis

The diagnosis of syphilis consists of *demonstration* of treponemes and detection of antibodies by *serological tests* (Table 32.1). Specimens include collection of exudate from the lesion for direct demonstration of treponemes and serum for serological tests. CSF can be collected for neurosyphilis.

Table 32.1: Diagnostic Methods in Syphilis		
Demonstration of Treponemes	1.	Dark ground microscopy
	2.	Direct fluorescent antibody staining for *T. pallidum* (DFA–TP)
	3.	Treponemes in tissue
		(*i*) Silver impregnation method
		(*ii*) Immunofluorescence staining
Serological tests		
Non-treponemal tests	1.	VDRL
	2.	RPR
Treponemal tests	1.	FTA, FTA-ABS (using killed *T. pallidum*)
	2.	TPHA, (using *T. pallidum* extract)
	3.	TPI test (using live *T. pallidum*)

Demonstration of Treponemes

Demonstration of treponemes by microscopy is applicable in primary and secondary stages and in cases of cogenital syphilis with superficial lesions.

Dark ground microscopy

Treponema pallidum, appears as a slender, spiral organism showing rotational as well as flexion and extension movements (Fig. 32.1).

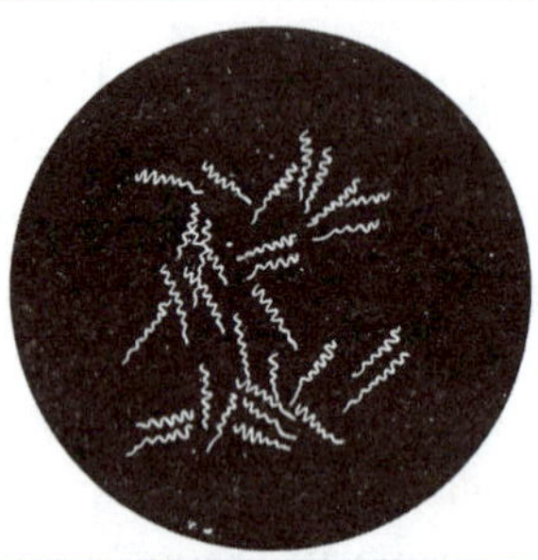

Fig. 32.1 T. pallidum under dark ground microscopy

Serological tests

These tests form the mainstay of laboratory diagnosis. Depending upon the antigen used, serological tests for syphilis are divided into *non-treponemal tests* (cardiolipin or lipoidal antigen is used) and *treponemal tests* (treponemes are used as the antigen).

NON-TREPONEMAL TESTS

In the standard tests for syphilis (STS), reagin antibodies are detected by cardiolipin antigen. Cardiolipin antigen is an alcoholic extract of beef heart tissue to which lecithin and cholesterol are added. The STS includes Venereal Diseases Research Laboratory (VDRL) test, Rapid Plasma Reagin (RPR), Kahn test and Wassermann reaction. The Wassermann reaction is no longer in use. Similarly Kahn test is rarely done.

FLOCCULATION TESTS

Cardiolipin antigen reacts with reagin antibody in syphilitic serum resulting in formation of visible clumps or floccules. Results can be read in a few minutes. *VDRL* and *RPR* tests are equally sensitive.

(a) VDRL (Venereal Disease Research Laboratory) test

It is the most widely used simple and rapid serological test. It is a slide flocculation test.

(b) RPR (Rapid Plasma Reagin) test

It is almost similar to VDRL test. Finely divided carbon particles are added to cardiolipin antigen.

Disadvantages of standard test

The antigen (cardiolipin) is non-specific and hence may react with the sera of patients who may not have syphilis. This accounts for the *biological false positive* (BFP) reactions. These are not caused by technical faults.

Conditions in which BFP reactions occur include:

1. Leprosy (particularly lepromatous leprosy)
2. Malaria
3. Relapsing fever
4. Infectious mononucleosis
5. Tropical eosinophilia
6. Hepatitis
7. Collagen diseases e.g. systemic lupus erythematosus (SLE) and rheumatoid arthritis.

To eliminate these false positive reactions, tests have been developed using treponemal antigens. These treponemal tests are described below.

TREPONEMAL TESTS

Tests using Reiter's Treponemes

Reiter's protein complement fixation (RPCF) test

The principle of the test is same as that of Wassermann reaction, i.e., complement fixation test (CFT).

Tests using T. pallidum (Nichol's Strain)

(i) Using live T. pallidum

Treponema pallidum immobilisation (TPI) test

This test employs live *T. pallidum*. The test serum is mixed with actively motile Nichol's strain of *T. pallidum* and incubated anaerobically. If antibodies are present, the treponemes are immobilised (rendered non-motile), when examined under dark ground illumination.

(ii) Using killed T. pallidum

(a) Treponema pallidum agglutination (TPA) test

A suspension of *T. pallidum*, inactivated by formalin, is mixed with the test serum and examined under dark ground microscopy. The treponemes are found agglutinated in the presence of antibodies.

(b) Treponema pallidum immune adherence (TPIA) test

A suspension of inactivated *T. pallidum* is mixed with the test serum, complement and fresh heparinized whole blood from a normal individual and incubated. The treponemes will be found to adhere to the erythrocytes in the presence of antibodies. Both TPA and TPIA are not used in diagnostic laboratories.

(c) Fluorescent treponemal antibody (FTA) test

It is an indirect immunofluorescence test. Smears of killed *T. pallidum* (Nichol's strain) are prepared on slides and fixed. The patient's serum is allowed to react with the smear. The antibodies that bind to the fixed smear are detected by treating the smear with fluorescein labelled antihuman immunoglobulin (conjugate). The smear is examined under fluorescent microscope. In a positive test, treponemes fluoresce. This test was further modified to fluorescent treponemal antibody absorption (FTA-ABS) test.

(d) Fluorescent treponemal antibody-absorption (FTA-ABS) test

Patient's serum is first absorbed with an extract of non-pathogenic treponemes (Reiter treponemes) to remove reagin and the group-reactive antibody. Method of the test is same as that of FTA test. FTA-ABS test has high specificity and sensitivity. It is the earliest serological test to become positive in syphilis and remains positive for many years even after effective treatment of early syphilis. Another modification, the IgM-FTA-ABS test can detect IgM antibodies in congenital syphilis and helps to differentiate it from seropositivity due to passively transferred maternal antibodies which are IgG in nature.

(iii) Using an extract of T. pallidum

Treponema pallidum haemagglutination assay (TPHA)

Tanned sheep erythrocytes are sensitised with an extract of *T. pallidum*. When these sensitised erythrocytes are mixed with patient's serum containing anti-treponemal antibodies, the erythrocytes clump together.

Table 32.2 shows the reactivity of serological tests in untreated syphilis.

Table 32.2: Reactivity of Serological Tests in Untreated Syphilis

Test	Stage of the disease, % positive		
	Primary	Secondary	Latent
VDRL/RPR	70%	100%	70%
FTA-ABS	80%	100%	65%
TPHA	65%	100%	95%

CHOICE OF SEROLOGICAL TESTS

1. **VDRL** or **RPR** tests are used for **screening** or **for diagnostic** purposes of large number of sera. These tests are also used for quantitative measurement of reagin titre for assessment of clinical activity of syphilis.
2. Treponemal tests **(TPHA or FTA-ABS)** are used to **confirm the diagnosis** with a positive reagin test.

5. Treatment

1. Early syphilis

Primary, secondary and latent infection of two years duration or less are included in early syphilis.

(*i*) Benzathine benzyl penicillin 24 lacs units intramuscularly in a single dose after sensitivity test.

(*ii*) Alternatively, doxycycline 100 mg twice a day, orally for 15 days.

2. Late syphilis

Infection more than two years duration is included in late syphilis.

Benzathine benzyl penicillin 24 lacs units, intramuscularly, once weekly for three weeks.

B. Nonvenereal Treponematoses

Non-venereal treponemal diseases occur in communities with poor standards of hygiene. These include *Yaws*, *pinta* and *endemic syphilis*. Treponemes responsible for these diseases are virtually indistinguishable from *T. pallidum*. Like venereal syphilis, these treponemes also show reactive treponemal and non-treponemal serological tests.

1. Yaws (Framboesia)

It is an endemic disease caused by *T. pallidum* subspecies *pertenue* (still known as *T. pertenue*). *T. pertenue* is morphologically and antigenically indistinguishable from *T. pallidum*.

The primary lesion is an extragenital papule which enlarges and breaks down to from an ulcerating granuloma. Like syphilis, secondary and tertiary manifestations follow. Infection is by direct contact with open ulcers. Flies may act as vectors. Laboratory diagnosis and treatment are similar to that of venereal syphilis.

Yaws has been eradicated from India and WHO declared 'Yaws Free India' on 14th July 2016.

2. Pinta

It is caused by *T. carateum*. The disease is acquired by direct person to person contact. The skin bears the brunt of the disease. Incubation period ranges from 7–21 days. The primary lesion is non-ulcerating extragenital papule which develops into lichenoid or psoriaform patch. Secondary skin lesions are characterised by hyperpigmentation or hypopigmentation. The laboratory diagnosis and treatment are same as those of venereal syphilis.

3. Endemic Syphilis

The disease is caused by *T. pallidum* subspecies *endemicum*. It is transmitted by direct person to person contact and by sharing common contaminated utensils of eating and drinking. Venereal spread is uncommon. Primary chancre is rare but may sometimes be found on nipples of mothers infected by their children. The disease usually manifests with features of secondary syphilis such as mucous patches and skin eruptions. It progresses to tertiary lesions.

The laboratory diagnosis and treatment are same as those of venereal syphilis.

C. Non-Pathogenic Treponemes

Certain commensal treponemes may be found in buccal and genital mucosa and may cause confusion in the diagnosis of syphilis by dark-field microscopy. *T. dentium* is found in the mouth.

T. refringens and *T. gracilis* may be found as commensals in genitalia.

III. BORRELIA

Borreliae differ from other spirochaetes in being larger (8–30 µm × 0.2–0.5 µm) with 3–10 irregular wide and open coils (Fig. 32.2). They are motile, refractile spirochaetes, stain readily with ordinary dyes and are Gram negative. Several species of Borrelia occur as commensals on the buccal and genital mucosa.

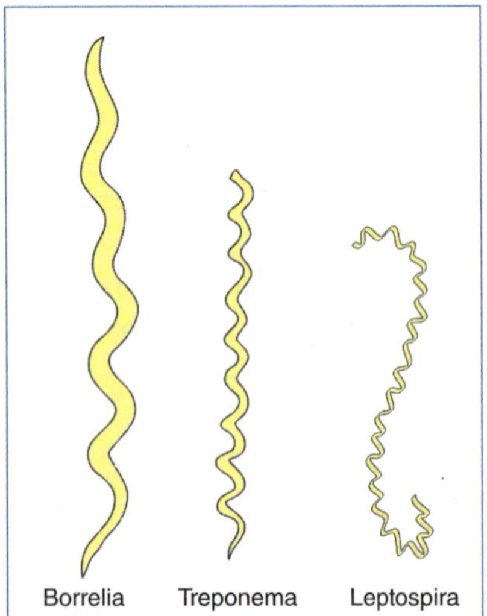

Fig. 32.2 Comparative morphology of different spirochaetes

The important pathogenic borreliae of medical importance include:

1. *B. recurrentis*—causes relapsing fever.
2. *B. vincentii*—causes vincent's angina in association with fusiform bacilli.
3. *B. burgdorferi*—the causative agent of Lyme disease

A. Borrelia recurrentis

Relapsing fever (RF) is an arthropod-borne infection, two types of which are louse-borne and tick-borne.

1. Morphology

Borrelia measure 8–20 µm × 0.2–0.5 µm. They are motile, Gram negative and possess 5–8 irregular spirals. They stain well with Giemsa or Wright stains.

2. Culture

Borreliae are microaerophilic. Optimum temperature for growth is 28–30°C. The organisms can be grown in Noguchi's medium (ascitic fluid containing rabbit kidney), on chorioallantoic membrane (CAM) of chick embryos and in peritoneal cavity of rat or mouse.

3. Pathogenesis

Relapsing fever is transmitted by infected vectors: body louse or tick. Incubation period varies between 2 to 10 days. Disease is characterised by febrile episode of sudden onset. The fever subsides after 3–5 days. There are 3–10 such relapses and then the disease ultimately subsides. Splenomegaly is common.

4. Laboratory Diagnosis

Blood is collected during febrile period and is examined by following methods:

(i) Dark ground microscopy

A wet film of blood is made and examined under the dark ground or phase contrast microscope and borreliae can be detected by their active movements.

(ii) Giemsa or Leishman stain

Blood smears are stained with Giemsa or Leishman stain and examined for borreliae.

(iii) Direct fluorescent antibody test

(iv) Culture

Isolation of *Borrelia* from blood is done by culture.

(v) Segolosy

ELISA is used to detect antibodies in serum.

5. Treatment

Erythromycin is the drug of choice.

B. Borrelia vincentii (Treponema vincentii)

It is a motile spirochaete, about 5–20 µm long and 0.2–0.6 µm wide, with 3–8 coils of variable size. It is easily stained with dilute carbol fuchsin, methyl violet and is Gram negative. It is a normal mouth commensal but a potential pathogen. Under pre-disposing conditions such as malnutrition or viral infections, it gives rise to ulcerative gingivostomatitis or oropharyngitis **(Vincent's angina)**. In these cases, *B. vincentii* is often associated with fusiform bacilli. This symbiotic infection is known as *fusospirochetosis*. Laboratory diagnosis may be made by demonstrating spirochaetes and fusiform bacilli in stained smears of exudates from the lesions. Cultivation is difficult but can be done in enriched media anaerobically. Penicillin and metronidazole are effective in treatment.

C. Borrelia burgdorferi

Borrelia burgdorferi causes Lyme disease.

1. Morphology

It measures 4–30 µm × 0.2–0.25 µm. It is flexible, helical and Gram negative.

2. Culture

It is a microaerophilic spirochaete. It is fastidious bacterium and can be grown in a modified Kelley's (BSK) medium, after incubation for two weeks or more. Optimum temperature for growth is 33–37°C.

3. Pathogenesis

Rodents, deer and other mammals are the natural reservoir hosts. Ixodid ticks are the vectors. The borrelia grows mainly in the midgut of the tick and transmission to humans occurs by regurgitation of the gut contents during biting. *B. burgdorferi* produces Lyme disease and incubation period is about 3–30 days.

4. Laboratory Diagnosis

Laboratory diagnosis can be made by isolation of the organism or by serology. The culture is too slow and difficult for routine use. For the serological diagnosis, ELISA and IF are commonly used.

5. Treatment

Doxycycline or erythromycin is the drug of choice.

IV. LEPTOSPIRA

A. Classification

The genus *Leptospira* is now classified into two species:

1. *L. interrogans*
2. *L. biflexa*

B. Leptospira interrogans

1. Morphology

These are spiral bacteria, 5–20 µm × 0.1 µm with numerous closely set coils and hooked ends (Fig. 32.3). They are actively motile. They stain poorly with aniline dyes but can be observed by fluorescent antibody and silver impregnation techniques. Because of narrow diameter, they are best observed by dark ground, phase-contrast or electron microscopy.

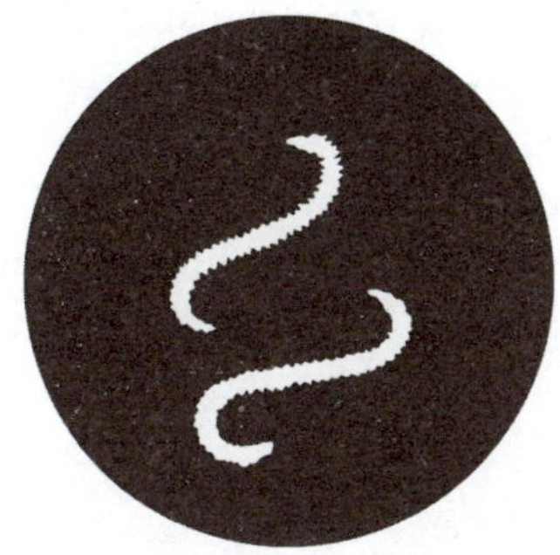

Fig. 32.3 Leptospira—dark ground Illumination

2. Culture

They are aerobic and microaerophilic. Optimum temperature for their growth is 28–32°C and optimum pH 7.2–7.5. They can be grown in media enriched with rabbit serum.

Leptospires may be grown on chorioallantoic membrane (CAM) of chick embryos. They can also be grown in guinea pigs.

3. Pathogenesis

L. interrogans causes a **zoonotic disease** named **leptospirosis** in rodents and sometimes in domestic animals. It is transmitted to humans by **direct or indirect contact with water contaminated by urine of carrier animals**. After an incubation period of 6–8 days, there is onset of febrile illness with leptospires in blood (septicaemic phase) which lasts for 3–7 days. The organisms disappear from the blood but enter into the liver, kidney, spleen and meninges. Leptospirosis is an established cause of aseptic meningitis. They persist in the internal organs, and most abundantly in the kidney and therefore may be demonstrated in the urine in the later stages of the disease. Severe leptospirosis (*Weil's disease*) associated with fever, conjunctivitis, albuminurea, jaundice and haemorrhage is usually caused by *L. icterohaemorrhagiae* serogroup. It is a fatal illness with hepatorenal damage.

4. Laboratory Diagnosis

The diagnosis depends on demonstration of the leptospires microscopically in blood or urine, by isolating them in culture or by animal inoculation or by serological tests.

(i) Demonstration of leptospires in the blood or urine

Leptospires can be observed in the blood by **dark-ground microscopy**. Blood examination is useful in first week as leptospires disappear from blood after 8 days.

Leptospires may be present in the urine in the second week of the disease and intermittently thereafter up to six weeks. Centrifuged deposit of urine may be examined by dark-ground microscopy for leptospires.

(ii) Culture

Specimen of blood during first week and urine in second week (up to six weeks) can be cultured. Centrifuged deposit of urine is cultured. Media are incubated at 28–32°C aerobically and examined by dark ground microscopy.

(iii) Animal inoculation

The blood or urine from the patient is inoculated intraperitoneally into young guinea pigs. From the third day after inoculation, the peritoneal fluid is examined daily for leptospires by dark ground illumination. Heart blood of animal is inoculated into the culture media for isolation of organisms.

(iv) Serological tests

It is very useful method of diagnosis. Two types of serological tests are in use, *screening tests* and the *serotype specific tests*.

(a) *Screening tests*
   Screening tests include complement fixation test, haemagglutination test, enzyme-linked immuno-sorbent assay (ELISA), sensitised erythrocyte lysis (SEL), agglutination test and indirect immunofluorescence. These tests are capable of detecting IgM and IgG leptospiral antibodies. A rapid dip-stick assay has been developed for detection of leptospira-specific IgM antibody.

(b) *Serotype specific tests*
   These serotype specific tests identify the infecting serovar by demonstrating specific antibodies. **Microscopic agglutination test (MAT)** is used for this purpose.

KEY POINTS

1. *Spirochaetes* are large, motile, helical bacteria.
2. The members of genera *Treponema*, *Borrelia* and *Leptospira* are pathogenic to man.
3. *Treponema pallidum* is the causative agent of syphilis. It is a sexually transmitted disease (STD).
4. The laboratory diagnosis of syphilis consists of *demonstration* of *treponemes* and detection of antibodies by *serological* tests.
5. Serological tests form the mainstay of laboratory diagnosis. Two types of antibodies are produced in syphilis, *non-specific* antibody (reagin antibody) and *specific* antitreponemal antibody.
6. In the standard tests for syphilis (STS), reagin antibodies are detected by cardiolipin antigen. The STS includes Venereal Diseases Research Laboratory (VDRL) test and rapid plasma reagin (RPR). These are *flocculation tests*.
7. *Fluorescent treponemal antibody absorption (FTA-ABS) test* and *Treponema pallidum hemagglutination assay (TPHA)* are serological tests for detection of specific antitreponemal antibody. *IgM-FTA-ABS* test, a modification of FTA-ABS, can detect IgM antibodies in *congenital syphilis* and helps to differentiate it from seropositivity due to passively transferred maternal antibodies.

STUDY QUESTIONS

1. Name different spirochaetes and describe the laboratory diagnosis of syphilis.
2. Write short notes on:
   (i) VDRL test
   (ii) TPHA
   (iii) FTA-ABS test
   (iv) *Borrelia vincentii*.

MULTIPLE CHOICE QUESTIONS (MCQs)

1. Which of the following methods can be used to demonstrate *Treponema pallidum*?
   (a) Dark ground microscopy
   (b) Silver impregnation method
   (c) Immunofluorescence staining
   (d) All of the above
2. Which of the following serological test is commonly employed for diagnosis of syphilis?
   (a) Venereal disease research laboratory (VDRL) test
   (b) Kahn test
   (c) Wassermann reaction
   (d) Reiter protein complement fixation (RPCF) test

3. Which of the following serological tests is employed for diagnosis of congenital syphilis?
   (a) FTA-ABS test
   (b) IgM FTA-ABS test
   (c) TPHA test
   (d) Reiter protein complement fixation test
4. The causative agent of lyme disease is:
   (a) *Borrelia recurrentis*
   (b) *B. duttoni*
   (c) *B. vincentii*
   (d) *B. burgdroferi*
5. Which serogroup of *Leptospira interrogans* is responsible for causing Weil's disease?
   (a) *Icterohaemorrhagiae*
   (b) *Hebdomadis*
   (c) *Australis*
   (d) *Canicola*

ANSWERS (MCQs) ...✓

1. (d) 2. (a) 3. (b) 4. (d) 5. (a)

Mycoplasma and Ureaplasma

33

I. MYCOPLASMA

A. Morphology

Mycoplasmas are the smallest free living microorganisms. They can pass through bacterial filters. They are most pleomorphic and may present as small spherical shapes to longer branching filaments. They lack cell wall but have a triple layered cell membrane which is rich in cholesterol and other lipids. They are Gram negative, but are better stained by Giemsa stain.

They are non-sporing and non-flagellated. They are usually non-motile.

B. Culture

Mycoplasmas are generally facultative anaerobes, growth being better aerobically. Optimum temperature for growth is 35–37°C. All mycoplasmas, except *Acholeplasma*, require sterol for growth. They grow on enriched media containing 20% horse or human serum and yeast extract. A medium widely used for the isolation of mycoplasmas is **PPLO broth**. This medium can be made solid by the addition of agar.

Colonies usually appear after incubation for 48–72 hours. Typical tiny ***fried egg* colonies** appear in the medium (Fig. 33.1). Colony size varies from 200–500 μm for 'large colony' mycoplasmas and 15–60 μm for the ureaplasmas.

As the colonies are too small, they cannot be picked with platinum loops. Subcultures are done by cutting out an agar block with colonies and rubbing it on fresh culture plates.

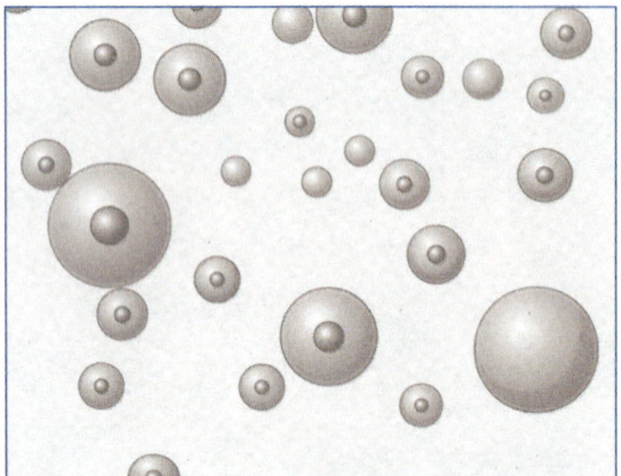

Fig. 33.1 Fried egg colonies

C. Pathogenesis

Mycoplasma causes two types of diseases in man—pneumonia and genital infections.

1. *Mycoplasma pneumoniae*

M. pneumoniae causes **primary atypical pneumonia** (mycoplasmal pneumonia). Transmission is by droplets of nasopharyngeal secretions.

2. *Mycoplasma hominis*

It may be isolated from 20–25% cases with **non-gonococcal urethritis (NGU)**. This has also been incriminated in postpartum sepsis, proctitis, acute salpingitis, pelvic inflammatory disease, cervicitis and vaginitis. It is transmitted by sexual contact.

D. Laboratory diagnosis

Laboratory diagnosis may be carried out by isolation of the organism or by serological tests.

1. Specimen Collection and Transport

The mycoplasmas can be recovered from throat swab, nasopharyngeal swab, respiratory secretions, sputum (*M. pneumoniae*) or urethral secretions, prostatic secretions, cervical swabs, urine (*M. hominis* and *Ureaplasma urealyticum*).

Culture media should be inoculated immediately after collection of specimen. If inoculation is not possible immediately then specimen may be kept at 4°C up to 24 hours. In case of delay more than 24 hours, the specimen should be frozen at –70°C.

2. Culture

PPLO broth medium containing penicillin, polymyxin B, amphotericin B glucose and phenol red (indicator) is inoculated with the specimen and incubated at 37°C. If specimen contains *M. pneumoniae*, growth is detected by turbidity and a colour change (red to yellow) of phenol red indicator, due to fermentation of glucose. Ureaplasma and some other mycloplasmas which do not ferment glucose show only turbidity. It is then subcultured on solid medium containing agar and incubated at 37°C for 5–7 days. Typical ***fried egg* colonies** can be seen. Colonies of *M. pneumoniae* are beta-haemolytic.

3. Serological Tests

(i) Detection of antigen

Antigen can be detected by direct immunofluorescence test, and enzyme immunoassay (EIA).

(ii) Detection of antibody

It can be done by using specific mycoplasmal antigens or by non-specific methods. Among the former are immunofluorescence, enzyme immunoassay (EIA) and latex agglutination test. The non-specific tests are *Streptococcus* MG and *cold agglutination* tests.

(a) *Streptococcus MG agglutination test*: Serial dilution of unheated patient's serum is mixed with heat killed suspension of *Streptococcus* MG and incubated at 37°C for overnight. The agglutination reaction is observed. **It was used in the past.**

(b) *Cold agglutination test*: Cold agglutinins (macroglobulin antibodies) appear in the blood of primary atypical pneumonia. These cold agglutinins have a property to agglutinate human group O erythrocytes at low temperature. Serial dilutions of patient's serum are mixed with washed human O group erythrocytes and kept at 4°C overnight. Clumping is observed. **It is no longer used.**

E. Treatment

Azithromycin is the drug of choice.

II. UREAPLASMA UREALYTICUM

Some strains of mycoplasma form very tiny colonies generally 15–50 µm in size. They are named T strains or T-form mycoplasmas (T for tiny). Now, they are classified as *Ureaplasma urealyticum*. They are peculiar in their ability to hydrolyse urea, which is an essential growth factor in addition to sterol. They are implicated in non-specific urethritis or genital infections. They are transmitted by sexual contact and may cause urethritis, proctitis and Reiter's syndrome in males. In females, they may cause acute salpingitis, pelvic inflammatory disease (PID), cervicitis and vaginitis. Azithromycin is the drug of choice for treatment.

KEY POINTS

1. Mycoplasmas differ from other bacteria in that they *lack a rigid cell wall.*
2. Mycoplasmas are the *smallest* free living microorganisms. They can pass through bacterial filters.
3. *Mycoplasma pneumoniae* causes *primary atypical pneumonia* (*mycoplasmal pneumonia*).
4. *Mycoplasma hominis* causes *non-gonococcal urethritis* (*NGU*).

STUDY QUESTION

Write short notes on:
(i) *Mycoplasma pneumoniae* (ii) Streptococcus MG agglutination test (iii) *Ureaplasma urealyticum.*

MULTIPLE CHOICE QUESTIONS (MCQs)

1. Which of the following bacteria lack cell wall?
   (a) Helicobacter
   (b) Burkholderia
   (c) Mycoplasma
   (d) All of the above
2. Which of the following bacteria may show fried egg colonies on culture medium?
   (a) *Mycoplasma*
   (b) *Helicobacter*
   (c) *Burkholderia*
   (d) *Bordetella*
3. Which is the causative agent of primary atypical pneumonia?
   (a) *Mycoplasma pneumoniae*
   (b) *Streptococcus pneumoniae*
   (c) *Haemophilus influenzae*
   (d) *Influenza virus*
4. Which of the following antibiotics is most suitable for treatment of *Mycoplasma infections*?
   (a) Tetracyclines
   (b) Cephalosporins
   (c) Penicillins
   (d) Norfloxacin

ANSWERS (MCQs)

1. (c) 2. (a) 3. (a) 4. (a)

Actinomycetes

34

The family *Actinomycetes* contains two medically important genera, *Actinomycetes* and *Nocardia*. *Actinomyces* are anaerobic or microaerophilic and non-acid-fast, while *Nocardia* may be acid-fast and aerobic.

I. ACTINOMYCES

A. Morphology

Actinomyces is Gram positive, non-motile, non-sporing, non-acid-fast organism. They often grow in mycelial forms and break up into coccal and bacillary forms. Most of them show true branching.

In tissue, the organisms look different from that of culture. The organisms appear in the pus as ***granules***. When these granules are crushed between two slides and examined by Gram's staining, they consist of a central filamentous Gram positive mycelium surrounded by a peripheral zone of swollen radiating club shaped structures, presenting a ***sun-ray appearance*** (Fig. 34.1).

The sulphur granules are white or yellowish in colour and found only in tissues.

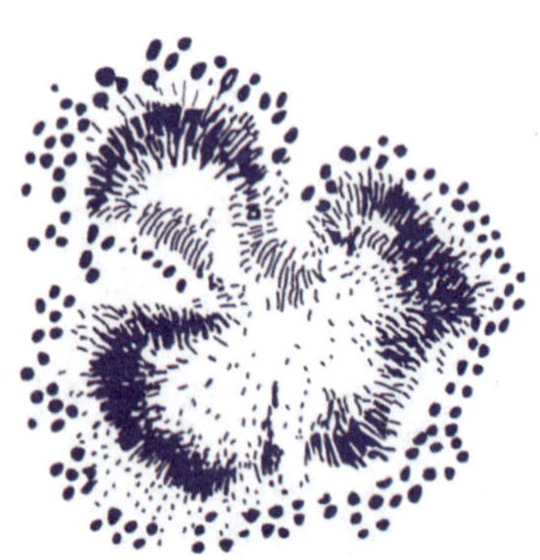

Fig. 34.1 Sun-ray appearance

B. Culture

They grow best under anaerobic or microaerophilic conditions at the optimum temperature of 37°C under 5–10% CO_2. They can be grown on brain heart infusion agar, blood agar or thioglycollate broth.

C. Pathogenesis

The actinomyces causes the disease known as **actinomycosis**. It is a chronic granulomatous disease characterised by multiple abscesses, tissue destruction, fibrosis and formation of multiple sinuses.

Macroscopically, it is a painless indurated swelling with multiple discharging sinuses. The pus contains usually yellow coloured sulphur granules. Actinomycosis may also present as mycetoma.

D. Laboratory Diagnosis

1. *Specimens*

- Pus from lesion or sinuses
- Discharge from fistula
- Sputum in pulmonary disease
- Tissue or biopsy

2. *Microscopy*

Pus is shaken along with some saline in a test tube and the mixture is allowed to settle. The sulphur granules sediment is withdrawn with a capillary pipette. Granules are crushed between two slides and smears are prepared. One smear is stained by Gram stain and other by acid-fast stain (decolourisation with 1% sulphuric acid). Gram staining shows a *sun-ray appearance* (Fig. 34.1). Acid fast staining shows central part as non-acid-fast surrounded by acid-fast 'clubs'.

3. *Culture*

The sulphur granules or pus containing 'Actinomycetes' are washed and inoculated into thioglycollate broth and streaked on brain heart infusion agar (BHI agar) and blood agar. Cultures are incubated anaerobically and aerobically with 5% CO_2 at 37°C for at least 2 weeks. *Actinomyces* produces ***spider colonies*** that resemble molar teeth. The isolate is identified by microscopy, biochemical reactions and fluorescent antibody methods.

E. Treatment

Surgical removal of affected tissue along with penicillin therapy are effective.

II. NOCARDIA

Nocardiae resemble Actinomyces morphologically but are strictly aerobic.

A. Species

The important species include *N. asteroides, N. brasiliensis* and *N. caviae.*

B. Morphology

Nocardiae are Gram positive bacteria and form a mycelium, that fragments into rod shaped and coccoid elements. *Nocardia* resembles *Actinomyces*, but some species are acid-fast, and a few are non-acid-fast.

C. Culture

Nocardiae readily grow in ordinary media. They are strict aerobes. They can be grown on nutrient agar, Sabouraud dextrose agar (SDA) and brain heart infusion agar (BHI agar). Nocardiae form dry, granular, wrinkled colonies with pigmentation (white, yellow, pink or red).

D. Pathogenesis

Nocardiae produce opportunistic pulmonary disease known as *nocardiosis* in immunocompromised individuals including those with AIDS. Man acquires infection by inhalation of the bacteria from environmental sources. It causes systemic nocardiosis which manifests primarily as pulmonary disease, pneumonia, lung abscess or other lesions resembling tuberculosis.

It may also cause mycetoma. It is a chronic granulomatous lesion involving the subcutaneous and deeper tissues mainly localised in the region of foot. It presents as a tumour with multiple sinuses. It came to be known as *Madura foot* or *Madura disease*.

E. Laboratory Diagnosis

1. Specimens

Pus or purulent sputum

2. Microscopy

The smears are stained with Gram staining and Ziehl-Neelsen (ZN) technique using decolourisation with 1% sulphuric acid. Gram positive filamentous bacteria can be seen on Gram staining. Acid-fast bacilli are detected on ZN technique though some species are non-acid-fast.

3. Culture

The specimens are inoculated on nutrient agar, SDA and BHI agar and incubated at 36°C for 3 weeks. Colony morphology is seen and bacteria are identified by staining.

F. Treatment

Cotrimoxazole is the drug of choice.

KEY POINTS >>>

1. Actinomyces is a Gram positive, non-motile organism. Most of them show true branching.
2. In the pus, the organisms appear as *granules*.
3. The *Actinomyces* causes a disease known as actinomycosis.
4. *Nocardiae* resemble actinomyces morphologically but are acid-fast. They produce opportunistic pulmonary disease known as *nocardiosis* in immunocompromised individuals. It may also cause *mycetoma*.

STUDY QUESTION

1. Write short notes on:
   (i) Actinomycosis (ii) Nocardia.

MULTIPLE CHOICE QUESTIONS (MCQs)

1. 'Sun-ray appearance' morphology is characteristic of:
   (a) *Actinomyces*
   (b) *Nocardia*
   (c) *Streptomyces*
   (d) *Actinomadura*

2. Which of the following organs is the most commonly involved in nocardiosis?
   (a) Lung
   (b) Skin
   (c) Spleen
   (d) Bone

ANSWERS (MCQs) ...✓

1. (a) 2. (a)

Miscellaneous Bacteria

35

I. CAMPYLOBACTER

There are ten species in Genus *Campylobacter* but only a few are of medical importance.

A. Morphology

Campylobacters are small, curved, Gram negative bacilli measuring 0.5–5 µm × 0.2–0.5 µm. They are motile by single polar flagellum (monotrichate) or amphitrichate flagella.

B. Culture

Growth of campylobacters occurs under strict microaerophilic conditions. They grow readily on simple media in an atmosphere of a mixture of oxygen (5%), CO_2 (10%) and nitrogen (85%). *C. jejuni, C. coli* and *C. lari* grow optimally at 42°C. However, *C. fetus* and most other campylobacters produce visible growth at 37°C. Campylobacters growing at 42°C are referred to as the thermophilic group.

Colonies are circular and convex but those of thermophilic group, particularly *C. jejuni,* are flat and tend to swarm on moist agar. Well formed colonies are seen only after 48 hours.

C. Biochemical Reactions

All produce oxidase and most species are catalase positive. They are biochemically inactive and do not utilise sugars or produce indole.

D. Pathogenesis

C. jejuni has emerged as the most important human pathogen in diarrhoeal diseases and accounts for 90% of campylobacter infections. The incubation period varies from 3–10 days. All the campylobacters appear to be inhabitants of the gastrointestinal tract of animals. Ingestion of raw milk, contaminated water or partially cooked poultry are common sources of human infections.

E. Laboratory Diagnosis

1. Direct Microscopy

(i) Gram staining

Gram stained smear of faeces may show Gram negative, curved bacilli.

(ii) Dark ground or phase contrast microscopy

Wet preparations examined by dark ground or phase contrast microscopy may reveal the darting or tumbling motility of the spiral rods.

Direct microscopy may be useful for rapid presumptive diagnosis

2. Culture

Faeces or rectal swabs are plated on selective media. The selective media commonly used are Butzler's selective medium, Skirrow's *Campylobacter* selective medium and Campy BAP selective media. Inoculated plates are incubated at 42°C for growth of the thermophilic campylobacters (*C. jejuni, C. coli* and *C. lari*). If the presence of *C. fetus* (non-thermophile) is suspected, additional plates should be incubated at 37°C for its growth. Plates are incubated in an atmosphere of 5% O_2, 10% CO_2 and 85% N_2. After 48 hours incubation, well formed colonies are observed. The growth is identified by Gram staining (Gram negative curved bacilli), motility (darting motility), oxidase test (oxidase positive) and biochemical reactions (catalase positive, nitrate reduction). Only *C. jejuni* hydrolyses hippurate.

II. HELICOBACTER

These are strict microaerophiles with a spiral morphology. They possess sheathed flagella. Three species *H. pylori, H. cinnaedi* and *H. fennelliae* are of medical importance.

Helicobacter pylori

It can be distinguished from campylobacters by its multiple sheathed flagella and strong hydrolysis of urea.

1. Morphology

H. pylori is a short curved, spiral or S shaped Gram negative bacterium measuring 3 µm × 0.5–0.9 µm. It is motile by a tuft of unipolar sheathed flagella (lophotrichate) while campylobacters have a single unsheathed flagella.

2. Culture

It is strict microaerophilic and grows in an atmosphere of 5% O_2, 10% CO_2 and 85% N_2. It does not grow anaerobically.

High humidity and 5–10% CO_2 are required for growth. The optimum temperature for growth is 37°C and not 42°C. It can grow in moist freshly prepared chocolate agar and campylobacter selective media. After incubation at 37°C under microaerophilic atmosphere for 3–5 days, *H. pylori* produces circular, convex and translucent colonies.

3. Biochemical Reactions

H. pylori is biochemically inactive in most conventional tests but produces urease, catalase and oxidase. It produces abundant urease.

4. Pathogenesis

H. pylori is implicated to cause chronic active gastritis, duodenitis and peptic ulcer.

5. Laboratory Diagnosis

(i) Specimens

Biopsy of gastric mucosa

(ii) Direct microscopy

(a) Gram staining
Gram staining of the specimen shows short curved, spiral Gram negative bacteria.

(b) Haematoxylin-Eosin staining
It can be used in histological sections.

(c) Warthin-Starry silver staining
Organisms can be seen most clearly with this method.

(iii) Culture

Specimen is inoculated on chocolate agar and campylobacter selective medium followed by incubation as mentioned above. The organism is identified on the basis of colony morphology, Gram staining and biochemical reactions.

(iv) Biopsy urease test

The biopsy material is placed in urea solution with an indicator and incubated at 37°C. If the tissue contains *H. pylori*, pH changes due to production of ammonia. Urea is broken down to ammonia by action of enzyme urease produced by the organism.

(v) Urea breath test

Urea labelled with an isotope of carbon is given orally to the patient. If the patient's stomach contains *H. pylori,* urea is converted into ammonia and CO_2. This labelled CO_2 appears in the breath where it can be measured.

(vi) Serology

Antibodies to *H. pylori* can be detected in patient serum by ELISA.

III. LEGIONELLA PNEUMOPHILA

A. Morphology

L. pneumophila is a Gram negative bacilli measuring 2–5 µm × 0.3–0.9 µm. It is motile with polar or subpolar flagella. It is non-capsulated, non-sporing and non-acid- fast.

B. Culture

These are fastidious organisms and do not grow on ordinary media. They are strict aerobes and grow best at pH 6.8 to 7.8 and at 35–37°C temperature. They can be grown on buffered charcoal-yeast extract agar (BCYE) and Mueller-Hinton medium supplemented with essential growth factors.

Colonies are circular, 1–2 mm in diameter, grey or grey blue and low convex with a slightly irregular edge.

C. Biochemical Reactions

L. pneumophila is catalase positive and oxidase variable. It hydrolyses hippurate, starch and gelatin.

D. Pathogenesis

The natural habitat of *L. pneumophila* is water. The organisms have been isolated from cooling towers, airconditioning systems, humidifiers, whirlpool baths, showers and respiratory ventilators.

Legionella infection may occur in two main forms which are designated as Legionnaire's disease and Pontaic fever, together known as *legionellosis*.

E. Laboratory Diagnosis

1. Microscopy

Legionellae can be detected in the clinical specimens (sputum, bronchial aspirate, pleural fluid, lung biopsy or autopsy material) by direct immunofluorescence test. Gram-stained smears are of little value as legionellae stain poorly.

2. Culture

Specimen is inoculated on culture media and incubated at 35–37°C up to 10 days. Bacteria from colonies are identified by direct immunofluorescence test.

3. Detection of Legionella Antigen

Legionella antigen can be detected in the urine by enzyme linked immunosorbent assay (ELISA).

4. Serological Test

Antibodies in serum can be detected by indirect fluorescent antibody test (IFAT).

IV. LISTERIA

A. Morphology

The organisms of the genus *Listeria* are small, Gram positive coccobacilli or rod shaped measuring 1–3 µm × 0.5 µm. They are motile at 25°C showing tumbling motility but are non-motile at 37°C. They are non-sporing, non-capsulated and non-acid-fast. They may resemble the morphology of diphtheroids.

B. Culture

Listeriae can grow at wide range of temperature, 4°C–45°C, but the optimum temperature for the growth is 37°C. They are aerobic or microaerophilic but better growth is obtained when cultures are incubated in presence of 5–10% CO_2. They grow on ordinary media but growth is improved by the addition of glucose, blood or liver extract. Colonies are 1–2 mm in diameter, round, smooth, translucent, easily emulsifiable and non-pigmented. On blood agar, colonies are surrounded by a narrow zone of β–haemolysis.

C. Biochemical Reactions

Listeriae produce acid from glucose. They are catalase positive but oxidase, urease and indole negative. H_2S is not produced by these organisms.

D. Pathogenesis

Eight species of Listeria are recognised. All the eight species may cause disease in animals. Only *L. monocytogenes* and very rarely *L. ivanovii* are likely to be associated with human disease. Human infections result from contact with infected animals, inhalation of contaminated dust or ingestion of contaminated milk or food. Hospital-acquired infections have also been reported. Infections caused by *L. monocytogenes* can be divided into following groups:

1. Neonatal Infections

Infection from pregnant woman to foetus is transmitted either transplacentally or intrapartum. It may lead to abortion or stillbirth or neonatal disease. Meningitis or septicaemia may occur in neonates.

2. Adult Infections

Meningitis accounts for the most cases of listeriosis. Other forms of listeriosis include encephalitis, brain abscess, spinal abscess, septicaemia and endocarditis. Butchers, poultry workers and veterinarians may develop cutaneous infections due to the direct contact with infected animals or birds.

E. Laboratory Diagnosis

1. Specimens

(i) Blood
(ii) CSF
(iii) Amniotic fluid
(iv) Pus
(v) Swabs from cervical and vaginal secretions
(vi) Meconium
(vii) Cord blood

2. Direct Microscopy

In Gram stained smears of CSF sediments, the organisms may be seen as Gram positive coccobacilli.

Leucocytes in CSF are raised, of which 40-60% may be lymphocytes. Protein content of CSF is raised and glucose is slightly lowered.

3. Culture

Specimens should be inoculated on
(i) blood agar
(ii) chocolate agar

These specimens may also be added to nutrient broth and incubated at 35–37°C for 5 days followed by subculture on solid media.

Blood agar shows small colonies surrounded by a narrow zone of β-haemolysis. The bacteria are actively motile when grown at 25°C. The isolate is identified by its morphology and biochemical tests.

F. Treatment

Ampicillin or amoxycillin and gentamicin are drugs of choice. Cotrimoxazole may also be used.

KEY POINTS »»

1. Campylobacters are small, curved, Gram negative bacilli. They are *microaerophilic*. *C. jejuni* is the most important species and is reponsible for diarrhoea.
2. Helicobacters are *strict microaerophiles* with a spiral morphology. *Helicobacter pylori* is the most important species. It causes chronic active gastritis, duodenitis and peptic ulcer. It is also recognised as a risk factor for gastric malignancies.
3. *Legionella pneumophila* is a Gram negative bacillus and motile. The natural habitat of *L. pneumophila* is water. The organism have been isolated from cooling towers, airconditioning systems, showers and respiratory ventilators. Legionella infection may occur in two main forms—*Legionnaire's disease* and *Pontaic fever*, together known as *legionellosis*.

4. The organisms of the genus *Listeria* are small, Gram positive coccobacilli or rod shaped. They are motile at 25°C showing *tumbling motility* but are *non-motile* at *37°C*. *Listeria monocytogenes* is the important species for human diseases.

STUDY QUESTIONS

1. Write short notes on:
   (i) *Campylobacter* (ii) *Helicobacter pylori.*
2. Write briefly about:
   (i) *Legionella pneumophila* (ii) *Listeria monocytogenes.*

MULTIPLE CHOICE QUESTION (MCQ)

1. Tumbling motility is characteristic of:
   (a) *Listeria monocytogenes*
   (b) *Proteus vulgaris*
   (c) *Enterobacter cloacae*
   (d) *Hafnia alvei*

ANSWER (MCQ)

1. (a)

Rickettsia, Orientia and Coxiella

36

The family *Rickettsiaceae* contains small coccobacillary organisms which cause typhus fever and related diseases. It consists of two genera, *Rickettsia and Orientia. Coxiella* and *Ehrlichia* are now included in family *Coxiellaceae* and family *Anaplasmataceae*. Previously both these genera belonged to family *Rickettsiaceae* (Table 36.1).

I. RICKETTSIA

A. Morphology

Rickettsiae are pleomorphic, coccobacilli, 0.3–0.6 μm × 0.8–2.0 μm in size, non-motile, non-capsulated and Gram negative, though they do not take the stain well. The organisms stain bluish purple with Giemsa stain.

B. Culture

Rickettsiae are unable to grow in cell free media. They are cultivated in yolk sac of chick embryo. The optimum temperature for growth is 32–35°C. They can also grow on HeLa, HEp 2 and other continuous cell lines.

C. Animal Inoculation

Laboratory animals like mice and guinea pigs are useful for primary isolation of rickettsiae from clinical materials.

D. Pathogenesis

Rickettsiae are generally transmitted to humans by the bite or by the faeces of an infected arthropod vector. Diseases caused by various species of the genus *Rickettsia* include **typhus fevers** and **spotted fevers** (Table 36.1).

1. Typhus Fever Group

This group consists of epidemic typhus and its recrudescent infection (Brill-Zinsser disease) and endemic (murine) typhus.

Neil-Mooser or tunica reaction: When male guinea pigs are injected intraperitoneally with blood from a case of endemic typhus or with a culture of *R. mooseri*, they develop fever and a characteristic scrotal inflammation. The scrotum becomes enlarged and the testes cannot be pushed back into the abdomen because of the adhesions due to inflammation between the layers of tunica vaginalis. This is known as *Neil-Mooser* or *tunica reaction*. This reaction is negative in epidemic typhus (*R. prowazekii*). **It is not in use nowadays.**

2. Spotted Fever Group

The diseases of this group include Rocky Mountain spotted fever (RMSF), boutonneuse fever, Australian tick typhus, Siberian tick typhus and rickettsial pox.

E. Laboratory Diagnosis

Laboratory diagnosis of rickettsial diseases may be carried out by

1. Serology
2. Isolation of rickettsiae
3. Molecular methods

1. Serology

Serological diagnosis may be done by (i) Weil-Felix reaction or by (ii) specific tests using rickettsial antigens.

(i) Weil-Felix reaction

It is a heterophile agglutination test which detects anti-

Table 36.1: Organisms of the Family Rickettsiaceae

Genus	Species	Disease	Insect vector
Rickettsia	*R. prowazekii*	Epidemic typhus, Brill-Zinsser disease	Human body louse
	R. typhi (R. mooseri)	Endemic typus	Rat flea
	R. rickettsii	Rocky-Mountain spotted fever	Ixodid ticks
	R. conori	Boutonneuse fever	Ixodid ticks
	R. australis	Australian tick typhus	Ixodid ticks
	R. siberica	Siberian tick typhus	Ixodid ticks
	R. akari	Rickettsial pox	Mites
Orientia	*O. tsutsugamushi*	Scrub typhus	Trombiculid mites

rickettsial antibodies that cross react with certain non-motile proteus strains OX 19, OX 2 and OX K. The basis of the test is the sharing of an alkali stable carbohydrate antigen of some rickettsiae with non-motile strains of proteus, *P. vulgaris* OX 19, and OX 2 and *P. mirabilis* OX K. The proteus organisms are used as antigens.

Sera from patients with epidemic and endemic typhus strongly agglutinates OX 19 and sometimes OX 2 also. In Brill-Zinsser disease the test is negative or weakly positive. In spotted fevers both OX 19 and OX2 are agglutinated. OXK agglutinins are found only in scrub typhus. The test is of no value in diagnosis of rickettsial pox (Table 36.2).

Table 36.2: Weil-Felix Reaction in Diagnosis of Rickettsial Diseases

Disease	Agglutination with Proteus strain		
	OX19	OX2	OXK
Epidemic typhus	++++	±	–
Brill-Zinsser disease	∓	–	–
Endemic typhus	+++	±	–
Spotted fever group	++	++	–
Scrub typhus	–	–	+++
Rickettsial pox	–	–	–

(ii) Specific tests using rickettsial antigens

Serological methods using rickettsial antigens are specific, which include indirect immunofluorescence antibody (IFA) test, latex agglutination test and enzyme immunoassay.

2. Isolation of Rickettsiae

Blood clot ground in skimmed milk is inoculated intraperitoneally in male guinea pigs or mice. The inoculated animals are to be observed for 3 to 4 weeks. The response of animals to different rickettsial infections vary.

For demonstration of rickettsiae, smears from peritoneum, tunica and spleen of infected animals may be stained by Giemsa or Gimenez methods.

Rickettsiae can also be grown in the yolk sac of chick embryo. Rickettsiae grow well on Vero and Hela cell line cultures.

3. Molecular Methods

Polymerase chain reaction (PCR) is available for detection of specific rickettsial DNA.

F. Treatment

Doxycycline is the drug of choice for treatment of rickettsial infections.

II. ORIENTIA

Scrub typhus is caused by *O. tsutsugamushi*. The disease is transmitted by the larval forms of the mite. Human infection occurs by an infected mite. The incubation period is 7–10 days. The clinical features are similar to those of epidemic typhus. A necrotic lesion (eschar) occurs at the site of bite in the skin.

Laboratory diagnosis is same as that of rickettsial diseases.

III. COXIELLA

Coxiella is named after Cox who first isolated the agent and introduced the technique of yolk sac inoculation for its cultivation. It differs from rickettsiae in being smaller, more resistant to physical and chemical agents and transmissible without arthropod vectors. It belongs to family *Coxiellaceae* (Table 36.3).

Table 36.3: Family Coxiellaceae

Genus	Species	Disease	Insect vector
Coxiella	*C. burnetii*	Q fever	1. Extrahuman-Tick 2. Human-Nil

C. burnetii is an obligate intracellular pathogen. It is pleomorophic, occurring as small bacilli, 0.2–0.4 μm × 0.4–1.0 μm in size. It is Gram negative. It can remain infectious for months in milk, water, soil and on wool. It can survive in dust and aerosols, therefore, can be transmitted as an airborne infection. It can be inactivated by 2% formaldehyde, 5% hydrogen peroxide and 1% lysol.

Q fever is primarily a zoonosis. Wild animals may constitute the primary reservoir. Infection is transmitted among them by ticks. Human infections have been traced to (i) consumption of infected milk (ii) handling of infected wool (iii) contaminated soil and (iv) contaminated clothing. Man to man transmission can occur but is rare. Ticks do not play any significant role in transmission of the disease to man. The incubation period is 2–4 weeks.

Laboratory diagnosis is mainly by serology using indirect immunofluorescene assay (IFA). **IFA is the method of choice**. ELISA kits are commercially available and have sensivities and specificaties similar to those of IFA test. Weil-Felix test is negative in Q fever. Isolation of organisms from clinical specimens is possible, but is not recommended due to the hazard of laboratory infection.

Care in the handling of animals and their products will be helpful in prophylaxis of Q fever.

KEY POINTS

1. Rickettsiae are pleomorphic, coccobacilli, non-motile, non-capsulated and Gram negative, though they do not take the stain well.
2. *R. prowazekii* causes epidemic typhus.
3. Endemic typhus is caused by *R. typhi* (*R. mooseri*).
4. *R. rickettsii* is responsible for Rocky-Mountain spotted fever.
5. *Orientia tsutsugamushi* is the causative agent of *scrub typhus*.
6. Q fever is caused by *Coxiella burnetii.*
7. Laboratory diagnosis of rickettsial diseases may be carried out by *serology* and *isolation of rickettsiae*.
8. *Weil-Felix reaction* is a heterophile agglutination test which detects anti-rickettsial antibodies that cross react with certain non-motile proteus strains OX19, OX2 and OXK.

STUDY QUESTIONS

1. Discuss the laboratory diagnosis of rickettsial diseases.
2. Write short notes on:
   (i) Q fever
   (ii) Neil-Mooser reaction
   (iii) Weil-Felix reaction.

MULTIPLE CHOICE QUESTIONS (MCQs)

1. What is the causative agent of epidemic typhus?
   (a) *Rickettsia prowazekii*
   (b) *R. typhi*
   (c) *R. conori*
   (d) *R. australis*
2. Endemic typhus is caused by:
   (a) *Rickettsia prowazekii*
   (b) *R. typhi*
   (c) *R. conori*
   (d) *R. australis*
3. What is the causative agent of Rocky-Mountain spotted fever?
   (a) *Rickettsia prowazekii*
   (b) *R. typhi*
   (c) *R. rickettsii*
   (d) *R. conori*
4. Insect vector for epidemic typhus is:
   (a) Human body louse
   (b) Rat flea
   (c) Tick
   (d) Mite
5. What is the causative agent of rickettsial pox?
   (a) *Rickettsia prowazekii*
   (b) *R. typhi*
   (c) *R. akari*
   (d) *R. conori*
6. Scrub typhus is caused by:
   (a) *Rickettsia prowazekii*
   (b) *Ehrlichia sennetsu*
   (c) *Coxiella burnetii*
   (d) *Orientia tsutsugamushi*
7. Q fever is caused by:
   (a) *Rickettsia prowazekii*
   (b) *Ehrlichia sennetsu*
   (c) *Coxiella burnetii*
   (d) *Orientia tsutsugamushi*

ANSWERS (MCQs) ...✓

1. (a) 2. (b) 3. (c) 4. (a) 5. (c) 6. (b) 7. (c)

Chlamydia and Chlamydophila

37

Chlamydiae are obligate intracellular parasites which are small, non-motile and Gram negative.

I. CHLAMYDIAE

A. Species

The family *Chlamydiaceae* previously contained a single genus *Chlamydia* having four species, *C. trachomatis, C. psittaci, C. pneumoniae* and *C. pecorum*. According to revised classification, the family *Chlamydiaceae* has been divided into two genera *Chlamydia* and *Chlamydophila*. *Chlamydia psittaci*, *Chlamydia pneumoniae* and *Chlamydia pecorum* are placed into new genus *Chlamydophila*. *C. trachomatis* is classified into two biovars, namely, TRIC (causing trachoma, inclusion conjunctivitis) and LGV (causing lymphogranuloma venereum).

Diseases caused by these species are shown in Table 37.1.

B. Morphology and Development Cycle

Chlamydiae exist in two forms, the elementary body and the reticulate (initial) body.

1. Elementary Body (EB)

It is a spherical particle measuring 200–300 nm in diameter. It is the extracellular infective form.

2. Reticulate (Initial) Body (RB)

Reticulate body is non-infectious in nature. It is the intracellular growing and replicative form.

The infectious particle (EB) enters the host cell by phagocytosis. It enlarges to form reticulate body, 500–1000 nm in size. It divides repeatedly by binary fission to produce a large number of elementary bodies. The newly formed infectious particles (EB) on liberation from host cell, may infect new cells and the cycle is repeated (Fig. 37.1).

C. Culture

Chlamydiae can be isolated by

1. Animal inoculation
2. Yolk sac inoculation
3. Tissue culture.

1. Animal Inoculation

Mice are inoculated by intranasal, intraperitoneal or intracerebral inoculation. The mice die within 10 days and smears from various tissues (lung, peritoneal exudate, spleen or brain) show the elementary bodies.

2. Yolk Sac Inoculation

Yolk sac of chick embryo is inoculated and the organisms can be detected in impression smears.

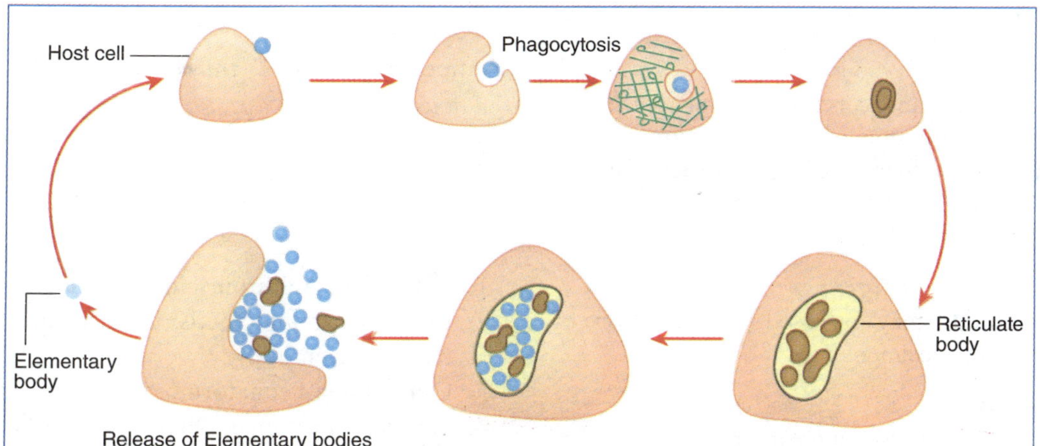

Fig. 37.1 Development cycle of Chlamydiae

Table 37.1: Diseases Caused by Chlamydia and Chlamydophila

Species	Serotype	Disease
C. psittaci	Many serotypes	Psittacosis and ornithosis
C. trachomatis	A, B, Ba, C	Trachoma
C. trachomatis	D, Da, E, F, G, H, I, Ia, J, Ja, K	Inclusion conjunctivitis (neonatal and adult), Non-gonococcal urethritis, salpingitis, cervicitis, pelvic inflammatory disease (PID), epididymitis, proctitis, pneumonia of newborns
C. trachomatis	L1, L2, L2a, L2b, L3	Lymphogranuloma venereum
C. pneumoniae (formerly called TWAR strain)	One serotype	Acute respiratory disease (ARD)

3. Tissue Culture

McCoy cells treated with cycloheximide are the most commonly used cell line. The organisms in the tissue culture can be detected by staining for inclusions or elementary bodies.

D. Pathogenesis

Chlamydial infections in man occur in three forms:

1. Ocular infections
2. Genital infections
3. Respiratory infections.

Different species of *Chlamydia* responsible for these diseases are shown in Table 37.1.

1. Ocular Infections

(i) Trachoma
(ii) Inclusion conjunctivitis
(iii) Ophthalmia neonatorum (Inclusion blennorrhoea)

2. Genital Infections

(i) *Non-gonococcal urethritis*
(ii) *Lymphogranuloma venereum*

3. Respiratory Infections

(i) *Pneumonia*
(ii) *Psittacosis* and *ornithosis*

E. Laboratory Diagnosis

Specimens

Ocular, urethral, vaginal and cervical specimens are best collected by scraping the mucosa. In addition, blood, sputum, respiratory secretions, and other tissues can also be collected. In case of LGV, pus or discharge from bubo should be collected.

1. Direct Detection of Antigens

The following methods may be used for detection of chlamydial antigens in specimens.

(i) Light microscopy

C. trachomatis infections of conjunctiva, urethra and cervix may be diagnosed by demonstrating inclusion bodies in the smears stained with Giemsa method. The inclusion bodies of *C. trachomatis* contain a glycogen matrix, therefore, these may also be stained with iodine solution.

(ii) Direct Immunofluorescence (DIF)

It is a rapid test. Smears are stained with FITC-labelled monoclonal antibodies and fluorescence can be detected in positive smears.

(iii) ELISA

Sensitivity and specificity of ELISA is similar to that of immunofluorescence test.

(iv) Nucleic acid amplification tests (NAATs)

PCR and real time PCR are used. These are the tests of choice for the diagnosis of chlamydial infections.

2. Isolation

Chlamydiae may be isolated by inoculation into mice, yolk sac of chick embryo or in tissue cultures.

The organisms in the tissue culture can be detected by staining for inclusions. Immunofluorescence is a better method to identify these inclusions.

3. Serology for Antibody Detection

(i) Complement fixation test (CFT)

It was used in the past.

(ii) Microimmunofluorescence

Antibodies against *C. trachomatis* and *C. pneumoniae* can be detected.

(iii) ELISA Test

F. Treatment

1. Trachoma: Azithromycin is the drug of choice.
2. Inclusion conjunctivitis: Tetracycline or azithromycin may be given orally.
3. Ophthalmia neonatorum: Azithromycin may be given.
4. Genital infections: Doxycycline or azithromycin are administered.
5. LGV: Doxycycline for 3 weeks is the drug of choice.
6. *C. psittaci* and *C. pneumoniae* infections: Tetracycline and azithromycin can be used.

KEY POINTS

1. Chlamydiae are obligate intracellular parasites which are small, non-motile and Gram negative.
2. *C. trachomatis* causes *trachoma, inclusion conjunctivitis, non-gonococcal urethritis, salpingitis, cervicitis* and *lymphogranuloma venereum* (*LGV*). *C. pneumoniae* is responsible for *acute respiratory disease* (ARD).
3. *C. trachomatis* has serotypes A to K and L1 to L3.
4. Laboratory diagnosis of chlamydial infections depends on direct detection of antigens, isolation of organism and serology for antibody detection.

STUDY QUESTION

1. Write short notes on:
   (i) TRIC agents
   (ii) Laboratory diagnosis of chlamydial infections.

MULTIPLE CHOICE QUESTIONS (MCQs)

1. Which of the following serotypes of *Chlamydia trachomatis* cause hyperendemic trachoma?
   (a) A, B, Ba, C
   (b) D to K
   (c) L1 to L3
   (d) None of the above
2. Which of the following serotypes of *chlamydia trachomatis* cause non-gonococcal urethritis?
   (a) A, B, Ba, C
   (b) D to K
   (c) Both of the above
   (d) None of the above
3. Which of the following serotypes of *Chlamydia trachomatis* cause lymphogranuloma venereum?
   (a) A, B, Ba, C
   (b) D to K
   (c) L1 to L3
   (d) None of the above
4. Which of the following methods can be used for isolation of chlamydiae in specimens?
   (a) Inoculation in mice
   (b) Inoculation in yolk sac of chick embryo
   (c) Inoculation in tissue cultures
   (d) All of the above

ANSWERS (MCQs)

1. (a) 2. (b) 3. (c) 4. (d)

Unit IV

VIROLOGY

38 General Properties of Viruses

Viruses are the smallest obligate intracellular infective agents containing only one type of nucleic acid (DNA or RNA) as their genome. They have no metabolic activity outside the living cells. They do not possess a cellular organisation and lack the enzymes necessary for protein and nucleic acid synthesis. They multiply by a complex process and not by binary fission. They do not grow in inanimate media. They are resistant to antibiotics. The major differences between prokaryotes and viruses are shown in Table 38.1.

Table 38.1: Differentiating Features of Prokaryotes and Viruses

Properties	Bacteria except chlamydiae	Chlamydiae	Viruses
Cell wall	+	+	–
Ribosomes and cellular enzymes	+	+	–
DNA and RNA	Both present	Both present	Only one present
Binary fission	+	+	–
Growth on inanimate media	+	–	–
Sensitivity to antibacterial antibiotics	+	+	–
Sensitivity to interferon	–	+	+

I. MORPHOLOGY OF VIRUSES

A. Size

Viruses are much smaller than other organisms. The extracellular infectious virus particle is called the *virion*. The size of viruses ranges from 20 to 300 nm in diameter. The **largest virus** is the smallpox virus (300 nm) and the **smallest** is the parvovirus (20 nm) (Fig. 38.1).

B. Structure and Symmetry

1. Structure

The virion consists of a nucleic acid core (genome) surrounded by a protein coat, the *capsid*. The capsid together with the enclosed nucleic acid is known as the *nucleocapsid*. The capsid is composed of a large number of protein subunits (polypeptides) which are known as *capsomers*. Certain viruses also contain envelope that surrounds the nucleic acid. It is lipoprotein in nature.

2. Symmetry

Three types of symmetry are determined by the arrangement of capsid around the nucleic acid core.

(i) *Icosahedral (cubical) symmetry*
(ii) *Helical symmetry*
(iii) *Complex symmetry*

C. Shape

The overall shape of virus particles varies in different groups (Fig. 38.1). Pox virus is brick-shaped and rabies virus is bullet-shaped.

II. CHEMICAL PROPERTIES

A. Nucleic Acid

Viruses contain only one kind of nucleic acid, either single or double stranded DNA or RNA.

B. Viral Protein and Lipids

Viruses contain protein which makes up the capsid. In case of enveloped viruses, they contain lipids (present in the envelope).

III. CULTIVATION OF VIRUSES

As viruses multiply only in living cells, they cannot be grown on any of the inanimate culture medium. Three methods are employed for the cultivation of viruses:

A. Animal inoculation
B. Embryonated egg inoculation
C. Cell culture

A. Animal Inoculation

Infant (suckling) mice are used in the isolation of arboviruses and coxsackie viruses, many of which do not grow in any other system. After inoculation, animals are observed for signs of disease or death. Later on, they are sacrificed and tissues are tested for the presence of virus.

Besides mice, other animals such as guinea pigs, rabbits and ferrets are also used in some situations.

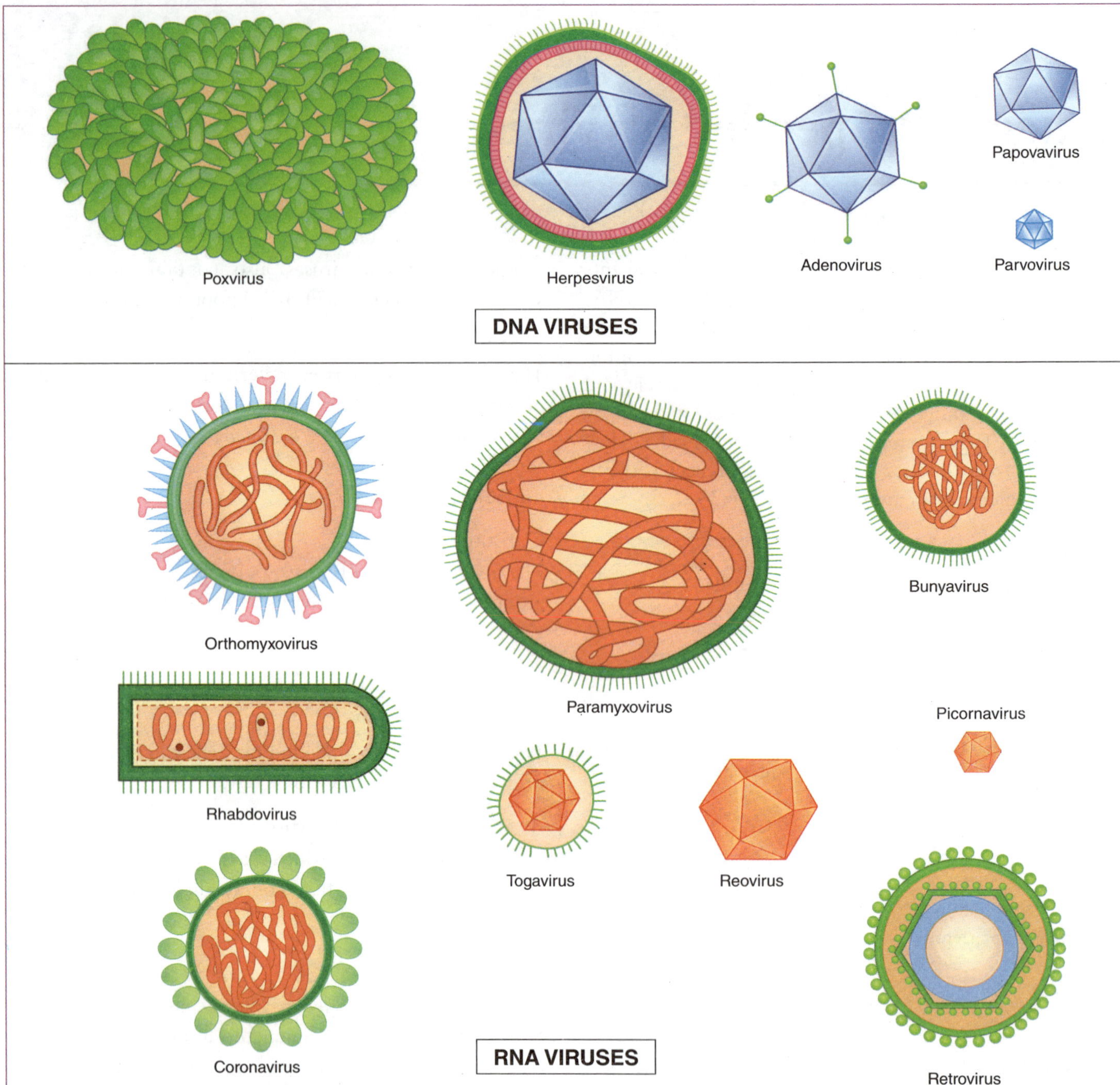

Fig. 38.1 Comparative shapes and sizes of viruses

B. Embryonated Egg Inoculation

Embryonated hen's eggs (7 to 12 days old) are inoculated by one of the several routes (Fig. 38.2) such as chorioallantoic membrane (CAM), allantoic cavity, amniotic sac and yolk sac.

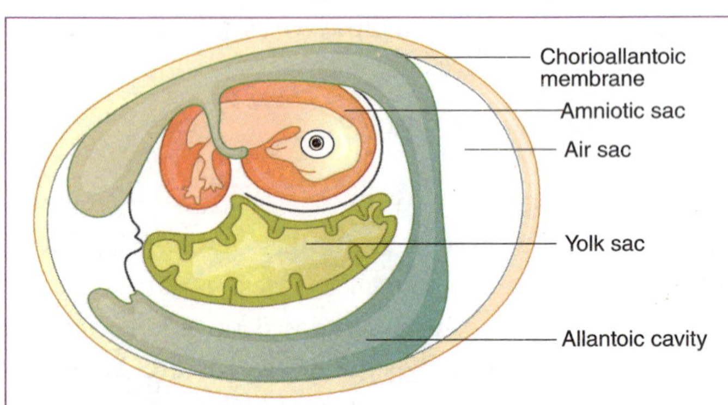

Fig. 38.2 Embryonated egg showing different routes of inoculation.

1. Chorioallantoic Membrane (CAM)

CAM is inoculated mainly for growing poxviruses. It produces visible lesions (**pocks**).

2. Allantoic Cavity

Allantoic inoculation is employed for growing influenza virus for vaccine production.

3. Amniotic Sac

Inoculation into the amniotic sac is mainly used for the primary isolation of the influenza virus.

4. Yolk sac Inoculation

It is inoculated for the cultivation of some viruses and certain bacteria (chlamydia and rickettsiae).

C. Cell Culture/Tissue Culture

This is the type of culture routinely employed for diagnostic virology.

Cell cultures are classified into three different types (Table 38.2).

(i) Primary cell culture
(ii) Diploid cell strains
(iii) Continuous cell lines

Table 38.2: Cell Cultures in Common Use

Type	Name of the cell culture
Primary cell cultures	Rhesus monkey kidney cell culture Chick embryo fibroblast cell culture
Diploid cell strains	WI–38 (Human embryonic lung cell strain) HL–8 (Rhesus embryo cell strain)
Continuous cell lines	HeLa (Human carcinoma of cervix cell line) HEP–2 (Human epithelioma of larynx cell line) Vero (Vervet monkey kidney cell line) McCoy (Human synovial carcinoma cell line)

(i) Primary cell cultures

These are normal cells freshly taken from the organs of animal or human being and cultured. They are capable of very limited growth in culture, perhaps 5-10 divisions at the most.

(ii) Diploid cell strains

They can be subcultured for a limited number. After about 50 serial subcultures they undergo 'senescence' and the cell strain is lost.

(iii) Continuous cell lines

These are cells of a single type that are capable of indefinite growth in vitro. They are usually derived from cancerous tissue. They can be serially cultivated indefinitely, therefore, they are termed *continuous cell lines.*

DETECTION OF VIRUS GROWTH IN CELL CULTURES

Virus growth in cell cultures can be detected by the following methods:

1. *Cytopathic effect*
2. *Haemadsorption*
3. *Transformation*
4. *Immunofluorescence*

IV. LABORATORY DIAGNOSIS OF VIRAL INFECTIONS

In the laboratory, the following methods are commonly employed:

A. Direct demonstration of virus and its components
B. Isolation of virus
C. Detection of the specific antibodies

It is necessary that the appropriate specimens should be collected, preserved and transported to the laboratory in the proper manner.

A. Direct Demonstration of Virus and its Components

1. Electron Microscopy

The detection of virus by electron microscopy (EM) is being used increasingly especially for viruses that are difficult to culture. Clinical applications of electron microscopy include detection of rotavirus and hepatitis A virus in faecal specimens.

2. Fluorescent Microscopy

3. Light Microscopy

Inclusion bodies in tissue sections may be detected by light microscopy. Demonstration of inclusion bodies helps in diagnosis of some viral infections. Negri bodies (inclusion bodies) demonstration in the brain cells of animals is a useful method for presumptive diagnosis of rabies.

4. Viral Antigens

These may be detected by enzyme linked immunosorbent assay (ELISA) and latex agglutination.

5. Polymerase Chain Reaction (PCR)

With a PCR technique, a target DNA sequence can be amplified to the point where it can readily be identified using labelled probes in a hybridisation assay. Thus viral DNA extracted from a very small number of virions or infected cells can be detected. The technique can be used for the diagnosis of infections caused by HIV-1, HIV-2, hepatitis B virus, and Epstein-Barr virus.

B. Isolation of Virus

This is the commonest method used in the diagnosis of virus infections. In general, the viruses can be grown by inoculation into animals, eggs or cell cultures, after the specimen is processed to remove bacterial contaminants. The isolates are identified by neutralisation or other suitable serological techniques. The techniques for the isolation of virus have already been described in detail in this Chapter.

C. Detection of Specific Antibodies

The demonstration of a rise in titre of antiviral antibodies during the course of a disease is strong evidence that it is the aetiological agent. For this, paired sera should be collected from the patient, the *acute* sample collected early in the course of the disease and the *convalescent* sample collected ten to fourteen days later. Examination of a single sample of serum is meaningful when IgM specific antibodies are detected.

V. NOMENCLATURE OF VIRUSES

Viruses are classified on the basis of biological, physical and chemical properties. Viruses are broadly classified into DNA and RNA viruses and then further divided into families, subfamilies, genera and species.

PRIONS

Prions are infectious proteins without any detectable nucleic acid. They are highly resistant to physical and chemical agents. They are resistant to heat (90°C for three minutes), UV rays and nucleases and sensitive to proteases. They produce slow infections with long incubation period (in years). Diseases caused by them include scrapie of sheep and goats, mink encephalopathy, bovine spongiform encephalopathy, Kuru and Creutzfeldt-Jakob disease.

KEY POINTS

1. Viruses are the smallest obligate intracellular infective agents containing only one type of nucleic acid (DNA or RNA) as their genome.
2. Three methods are employed for cultivation of viruses namely *animal inoculation*, *embryonated egg inoculation* and *cell culture*.

STUDY QUESTIONS

1. Discuss the laboratory diagnosis of viral infections.
2. Write short notes on:
   (i) Morphology of viruses (ii) Cultivation of viruses.

MULTIPLE CHOICE QUESTIONS (MCQs)

1. Which of the following characteristics are true for viruses?
   (a) Obligate intracellular infective agents
   (b) Contain either DNA or RNA
   (c) Do not multiply by binary fission
   (d) All of the above
2. Which of the following is the largest virus?
   (a) Smallpox virus
   (b) Parvovirus
   (c) Coronavirus
   (d) Adenovirus
3. Which of the following is the smallest virus?
   (a) Papovavirus
   (b) Parvovirus
   (c) Adenovirus
   (d) Reovirus
4. Which of the following is a diploid cell line?
   (a) Hela
   (b) WI-38
   (c) McCoy
   (d) BHK-21
5. Which of the following routes of inoculating embryonated hen's egg is/are used for cultivation of viruses?
   (a) Chorioallantoic membrane
   (b) Allantoic cavity
   (c) Amniotic cavity
   (d) All of the above

ANSWERS (MCQs) ...✓

1. (d) 2. (a) 3. (b) 4. (b) 5. (d)

DNA Viruses

39

I. POXVIRUSES

Pox viruses belong to the family *Poxviridae* and cause a number of human diseases.

A. Morphology

The Poxviruses are brick-shaped. They are the largest animal viruses measuring 300 × 200 × 100 nm in size and can be seen under the light microscope.

B. Cultivation

They grow in chorioallantoic membrane (CAM) of chick embryo and in tissue culture.

Tissue cultures of monkey kidney, HeLa and chick embryo cells can be used to grow these viruses.

C. Viruses Causing Human Infections

1. Variola

Variola virus causes smallpox. In past, smallpox epidemics appeared in two forms *florid* (fatal disease) occurred in India and *alastrim* (non-fatal disease) seen in Latin America. The name *variola major* was given to the virus causing classical smallpox and *variola minor* to the other virus causing alastrim.

Smallpox has been eradicated and routine vaccination is now stopped. On May 8, 1980, the WHO announced the global eradication of small pox.

2. Vaccinia

Origin of vaccinia virus is not known. It may have evolved from cowpox or smallpox virus. It is an 'artificial virus' and does not occur in nature as such. It causes a localised skin infection. Vaccinia virus is being used as a vector for incorporating genes for protective antigens for several different pathogens.

3. Molluscum Contagiosum

It is a benign epidermal tumour-like lesion, that occurs only in humans. It is a contagious disease. The virus is also transmitted sexually in adults.

D. Prophylaxis

A natural infection of smallpox gives complete protection against reinfection. Vaccination with vaccinia induces protection against smallpox for about five years.

II. HERPESVIRUSES

Herpesviruses are included in the family *Herpesviridae* which has been divided into three subfamilies (Table 39.1).

Morphology

Herpesvirus is 100–200 nm in diameter, contains an icosahedral capsid composed of 162 capsomers, containing linear double stranded DNA genome and is surrounded by a lipid envelope containing peplomers.

Herpes Simplex Virus (HSV)

Man is the only natural host. There are two types of the herpes simplex virus, type 1 and type 2. *Herpes simplex* virus type 1 is usually associated with oral and ocular lesions, while type 2 is responsible for the majority of genital infections.

A. Infections

HSV-1:

1. acute gingivostomatitis
2. herpes labialis
3. keratoconjunctivitis
4. eczema herpeticum
5. encephalitis
6. dendritic keratitis

Table 39.1: Classification of Human Herpesviruses

Subfamily	Scientific name	Common name
Alphaherpesvirinae	Human herpesvirus 1	Herpes simplex virus type 1
	Human herpesvirus 2	Herpes simplex virus type 2
	Human herpesvirus 3	Varicella-zoster virus
Betaherpesvirinae	Human herpesvirus 5	Cytomegalovirus
	Human herpesvirus 6	—
	Human herpesvirus 7	—
Gammaherpesvirinae	Human herpesvirus 4	Epstein-Barr (EB) virus
	Human herpesvirus 8	Kaposi sarcoma associated virus

HSV-2:

1. genital herpes (penis, urethra, cervix, vulva, vagina)
2. neonatal herpes
3. aseptic meningitis

Besides above mentioned primary infections, herpesviruses may present as latent infection, reactivation and recrudescence.

B. Laboratory Diagnosis

1. Specimens

Specimens include vesicle fluid, skin swab, saliva, corneal scrapings, brain biopsy and CSF, according to the site of involvement.

2. Direct Examination

(i) Smears prepared from scrapings from the base of vesicles are stained with toludine blue. Multinucleated giant cells (***Tzanck cells***) are present in a positive smear. ***Cowdry type A* intranuclear inclusion bodies** may be seen in Giemsa stained smears.

(ii) Herpes virions may be demonstrated in specimens by **electron microscopy**.

(iii) Viral antigens can also be demonstrated in the scrapings from the base of the lesions and tissue preparations, stained by **immunofluorescent staining**.

3. Tissue Culture

Virus can be isolated on human fibroblasts, HEp-2 cells, Vero cells and chorioallantoic membrane.

4. Sorology

Primary infection can be diagnosed by detection of virus specific IgM antibody or by a rising titre of IgG antibody.

5. Polymerase Chain Reaction (PCR)

PCR can be used for detection of HSV DNA in CSF.

C. Chemotherapy

HSV infection can be treated with acyclovir (acycloguanosine). It may be used in the form of ointment for the treatment of ocular lesions.

VARICELLA-ZOSTER

Varicella (**chickenpox**) and herpes zoster (**shingles**) are caused by a single virus, for which it is named Varicella-zoster virus (VZV). Chickenpox follows primary infection in a non-immune individual, whereas herpes zoster is a reactivation of the latent virus when immunity falls to ineffective level. VZV is similar to the herpes simplex virus in its morphology.

A. Varicella

Chickenpox is one of the commonest childhood exanthemata. The virus enters through respiratory route. The source of infection is a chickenpox or herpes-zoster patient. It is a highly infectious disease characterised by vesicular rash mostly on the trunk. The rash progresses through macule, papule, vesicle, pustule and scab. The rashes are centripetal in distribution.

B. Herpes zoster

While chickenpox is typically a disease of childhood, herpes zoster is a disease of old age and occurs usually in persons who had chickenpox several years earlier. The virus remains latent in the sensory ganglia. Years after the initial infection, when the immunity has fallen to ineffective levels, the virus may be reactivated. The reactivation is associated with the inflammation of the nerve which leads to neuritic pain that often precedes the skin lesions.

C. Immunity

Although the single virus is responsible for both the clinical entities, one attack of chickenpox confers life long immunity, but antibody fails to eliminate the virus from dorsal root ganglia. Hence, zoster occurs in persons who have immunity to varicella.

D. Laboratory Diagnosis

Diagnosis is usually clinical. Laboratory diagnosis includes:

1. Direct Microscopy

Stained smears from the base of early vesicles show multinucleated giant cells and type A intranuclear inclusions bodies under light microscope. Herpes particles can also be detected by electron microscopy. Direct fluorescent antigen detection using monoclonal antibody is rapid, sensitive and specific method for diagnosis. These methods may be used directly in the vesicle fluid.

2. Virus Isolation

Virus can be isolated in human fibroblast cells, human amnion, HeLa or Vero cells.

3. Polymerase Chain Reaction (PCR)

DNA can be extracted from specimen and amplified by PCR. It is useful for detection of VZV in CSF and other body fluids.

4. Serology

Varicella-zoster specific IgM antibody in patient's serum can be detected by ELISA.

E. Treatment

Acyclovir and vidarabine are effective in the treatment of severe varicella and zoster.

Cytomegalovirus

Cytomegalovirus infections are almost always inapparent, leading to prolonged latency, with occasional reactivation. An individual infected with CMV carries the virus for life. The virus is shed in urine saliva, semen, cervical secretions, tears and breast milk.

A. Pathogenesis

Cytomegalovirus can be transmitted transplacentally from a mother with latent infection to the foetus. Congenital infection may remain inapparent (asymptomatic) at birth or may lead to cytomegalic inclusion disease which is often fatal.

Postnatal infections are usually inapparent. This may be acquired by sexual intercourse, blood transfusion and organ transplantation. Clinical disease in adults resembles infectious mononucleosis. CMV may cause disseminated infection in immunocompromised individuals and can even lead to fatal infections. CMV is an important pathogen in AIDS.

B. Laboratory Diagnosis

1. Specimens

CMV can be isolated from urine, saliva, breast milk, semen, cervical secretions and blood leucocytes.

2. Demonstration of Cytomegalic Cells

Enlarged cells with large intranuclear "**owl's eye**" **appearance** inclusions (**cytomegalic cells**) can be demonstrated in the centrifuged deposits from urine or saliva. It is a simpler but less reliable technique.

3. Isolation of Virus

Virus can be grown in human fibroblast cultures.

4. Serology

CMV-specific IgM can be detected in the serum by ELISA.

5. Polymerase Chain Reaction (PCR)

PCR is the most widely used molecular method for detection of CMV DNA.

C. Treatment

For treatment of severe CMV infections, ganciclovir is the drug of choice.

Epstein-Barr virus (EBV)

EBV has affinity for lymphoid tissue.

A. Clinical Manifestations

Most EBV infections are inapparent. Once infected, the virus is present in the individual for life. The source of infection is usually the saliva of infected persons who shed the virus in oropharyngeal secretions. Intimate oral contact, as in kissing, appears to be the main mode of transmission. EBV has oncogenic properties and may cause Burkitt's lymphoma and nasopharyngeal carcinoma.

The following clinical manifestations may result from EBV infection:

1. Infectious mononucleosis or Glandular fever
2. Infections in immunocompromised hosts
3. EBV-associated malignancies
   (i) *Burkitt's lymphoma*
   (ii) *Nasopharyngeal carcinoma*

B. Laboratory Diagnosis

1. White Blood Cell Count

During the initial phase, patient develops leucopenia due to a drop in the number of polymorphs. Later there is leucocytosis with a predominance of abnormal or **atypical lymphocytes**. These atypical cells are lymphoblasts derived from T cells reactive to the virus infection. These cells are important for diagnosis and constitute about 30-90% of total leucocytes.

2. Paul-Bunnell Test

During infectious mononucleosis, heterophile antibodies appear in the serum of the patient. These are IgM antibodies elicited by EBV infection. These antibodies agglutinate sheep erythrocytes.

(i) Procedure

Inactivated serum (56°C for 30 minutes) in doubling dilutions is mixed with equal volumes of 1% sheep erythrocytes suspension. These tubes are incubated at 37°C for four hours and examined for agglutination. A titre of 100 or above is suggestive of infectious mononucleosis.

(ii) Confirmation

Similar type of antibodies may occur after injections of sera and even sometimes in normal individuals. To confirm these antibodies, absorption of agglutinins with guinea pig kidney and ox red cells is necessary. Forssman antibody induced by injection of horse serum is removed by treatment with guinea pig kidney and ox red cells. Infectious mononucleosis antibody is removed by ox red cells whereas normally occurring agglutinins are removed by guinea pig kidney.

3. EBV–Specific Antibodies

These are specific antibodies against EBV viral capsid antigen (VCA). These can be demonstrated by indirect immunofluorescence or ELISA.

4. Antigen Detection

EBV antigen can be detected by immunofluorescence using monoclonal antibodies.

5. Polymerase Chain Reaction (PCR)

EBV DNA can be detected by PCR.

III. ADENOVIRUSES

Adenoviruses belong to family *adenoviridae*. These are non-enveloped, icosahedral, DNA viruses.

A. Morphology

Adenovirus is 70-75 nm in diameter with an icosahedral capsid containing double stranded DNA.

B. Pathogenesis

Adenoviruses cause infections of the respiratory tract, eye, gastrointestinal tract and urinary tract. Infection occurs through conjunctiva or nasal mucosa. Faeco-oral spread, particularly among children can also occur. Incubation period ranges from 5-7 days.

C. Laboratory Diagnosis

1. Specimens

Throat swab, nasopharyngeal aspirate, bronchial lavage, conjunctival swab, corneal scraping, urine, anal swab, genital secretions and biopsy.

2. Microscopy

Viral particles may be seen directly in stool by electron microscopy. Viral antigens in the cells from respiratory tract, eye, urine and infected cell cultures may be demonstrated by immunofluorescence using monoclonal antibodies.

3. Isolation

Virus may be isolated from the throat, eye, urine or faeces by inoculating the clinical specimen in tissue cultures such as HeLa, Hep-2, and human embryo kidney cells.

IV. PAPOVAVIRUSES

Papova (from *pa*, papilloma; *po*, polyoma; *va*, vacuolating agent) viruses belong to the family *Papovaviridae*. The family contains a group of viruses containing a small icosahedron composed of 72 capsomers and double stranded DNA genome. There are two genera, *Papillomavirus* and *Polyomavirus*.

Papillomaviruses may cause cutaneous warts, genital warts, recurrent respiratory papillomatosis, oral papillomatosis and cervical cancer. These infections are transmitted by indirect or direct contact including sexual contact.

Polyomaviruses produce a variety of malignant tumours in animals hence the name polyoma (poly, many; oma, tumour).

V. PARVOVIRUS

Parvoviruses belong to the family *Parvoviridae* and are very small (about 20 nm), non-enveloped, icosahedral viruses containing a single stranded DNA. They may cause diarrhoea in humans.

VI. HEPATITIS B VIRUS

Due to great importance of Hepatitis B virus (HBV) in nursing care, it has been described in detail in Chapter 41.

KEY POINTS

1. Poxviruses are the *largest* and the most complex of all viruses. They are DNA viruses. *Variola virus* is the causative agent of smallpox. Smallpox has been eradicated and routine vaccination is now stopped.
2. Herpesvirus contains a double stranded DNA genome. Human herpesviruses include human herpesvirus 1 (HHV1) to human herpesvirus 8 (HHV-8). It is simpler but less reliable technique. Epstein-Barr virus (EBV) has affinity for lymphoid tissue.
3. Adenoviruses are non-enveloped, icosahedral, DNA viruses. They cause infections of the respiratory tract, eye, gastrointestinal tract and urinary tract.
4. Papovaviruses (from *pa*, papilloma, *po*, polyoma, *va*, vacuolating agent) are double stranded DNA viruses.
5. Parvoviruses are very small (about 20 nm), non-enveloped, icosahedral viruses containing a single stranded DNA.

STUDY QUESTION

1. Write short notes on:
   (i) Herpes simplex virus
   (ii) Varicella-zoster virus
   (iii) Cytomegalovirus
   (iv) Epstein-Barr virus (EBV).

MULTIPLE CHOICE QUESTIONS (MCQs)

1. Which of the following infections is caused by human herpesvirus 1?
   (a) Acute gingivostomatitis
   (b) Infectious mononucleosis
   (c) Kaposi sarcoma
   (d) None of the above
2. What is the common name for human herpesvirus 4?
   (a) Cytomegalovirus
   (b) Epstein-Barr virus
   (c) Varicella-zoster virus
   (d) Herpesvirus simiae
3. What is the common name for human herpesvirus 5?
   (a) Cytomegalovirus
   (b) Epstein-Barr virus
   (c) Varicella-zoster virus
   (d) Herpesvirus simiae
4. Which of the following diseases can be caused by Epstein-Barr virus?
   (a) Infectious mononucleosis
   (b) Burkitt's lymphoma
   (c) Nasopharyngeal carcinoma
   (d) All of the above
5. Which of the following serological tests is employed for laboratory diagnosis of infectious mononucleosis?
   (a) Paul-Bunnel test
   (b) Widal test
   (c) Weil-Felix reaction
   (d) None of the above

ANSWERS (MCQs) ...✓

1. (a) 2. (b) 3. (a) 4. (d) 5. (a)

40

RNA Viruses

I. PICORNAVIRUSES

Picornaviruses belong to family *Picornaviridae* which consists of six genera.

Picornaviruses of medical importance are shown in Table 40.1.

Table 40.1: Classification of Picornaviruses of Medical Importance

Genus	Species
Enterovirus	Poliovirus Coxsackie virus Coxsackie A Coxsackie B Echovirus Enterovirus
Parechovirus	Parechovirus
Rhinovirus	Rhinovirus
Hepatovirus	Hepatitis A virus

POLIOVIRUSES

Poliovirus is the causative agent of poliomyelitis. The poliovirus strains have been classified into three types: 1, 2 and 3.

A. Morphology

(i) Size: 27-30 nm diameter
(ii) Genome: Single stranded RNA
(iii) Capsid: Arranged in icosahedral symmetry.

B. Pathogenesis

Children are the most susceptible. The virus enters the body by ingestion.

Virus ⟶ Mouth ⟶ Multiplies in lymphatic tissues of oropharynx and intestine
↓
Bloodstream
↓
Spinal cord and brain ⟶ Destroys the anterior horn cells of spinal cord

C. Clinical Features

The earliest manifestations consist of fever, malaise, headache, drowsiness, constipation and sore throat lasting 1–5 days. There are four types of poliovirus infection:

(i) *Inapparent infection* (90-95%)
(ii) *Minor illness* (4–8%)
(iii) *Non-paralytic poliomyelitis* (1-2%)
(iv) *Paralytic poliomyelitis* (0.1-2%)

D. Laboratory Diagnosis

1. Specimens

Virus can be isolated from the faeces (up to 6 weeks), the pharyngeal washings (up to 3 weeks) and autopsy specimen (spinal cord and brain). Virus usually cannot be recovered from CSF.

2. Direct Demonstration of Virus

Virus can be demonstrated in stool by direct electron microscopy or by immune electron microscopy.

3. Isolation of Virus

Specimens are inoculated into tissue culture. Primary monkey kidney cells, HeLa and HEp-2 are usually employed. The virus growth is indicated by typical cytopathic effect seen in cells.

E. Prophylaxis

Two types of vaccines are available, killed polio vaccine (Salk) and live attenuated oral polio vaccine (Sabin).

1. Salk's killed polio vaccine (Inactivated polio vaccine, IPV)

Killed polio vaccine was developed by *Salk* in 1953. It is a formalin inactivated preparation of the three types of the poliovirus. The vaccine is given by intramuscular or intradermal injection.

Under National immunisation programme of India, two doses of IPV are administered by intradermal route at 6 weeks and 14 weeks of age along with oral polio vaccine (OPV). Dose given is fractional dose i.e. 0.1 ml.

It induces serum antibodies (IgM, IgG). It does not induce secretory IgA in the intestine and therefore would not be able to prevent alimentary tract infections.

2. *Live attenuated oral polio vaccine (OPV) (Sabin vaccine)*

Oral polio vaccine was developed by *Sabin* in 1962. It contains live attenuated strains of polio virus types, 1, 2 and 3. It is administered orally and parallels natural infection. It stimulates both local secretory IgA antibodies in the intestine as well as humoral antibodies (IgM and IgG). When the virus is excreted in the faeces, it may spread to close contacts and hence, it protects the individual and the community.

Vaccination schedule

It is administered orally. Three doses are given. In addition to three doses, zero dose is given at birth in institutional deliveries. First dose of OPV is given along with DPT at the age of 6 weeks. The second and third doses are administered at interval of 4–6 weeks. The booster dose is given at the age of 16-24 months. All the doses are generally given along with DPT.

Nowadays, the bivalent vaccine containing type 1 and 3, oral polio vaccine (OPV) is used for immunisation programme. IPV is also introduced along with bivalent OPV and in phased manner. OPV will be phased out.

II. ORTHOMYXOVIRUSES

Orthomyxoviruses are spherical or filamentous, enveloped viruses with single stranded and segmented RNA genome.

INFLUENZA VIRUSES

A. Morphology

Morphology of influenza virus (Fig. 40.1) is as follows:

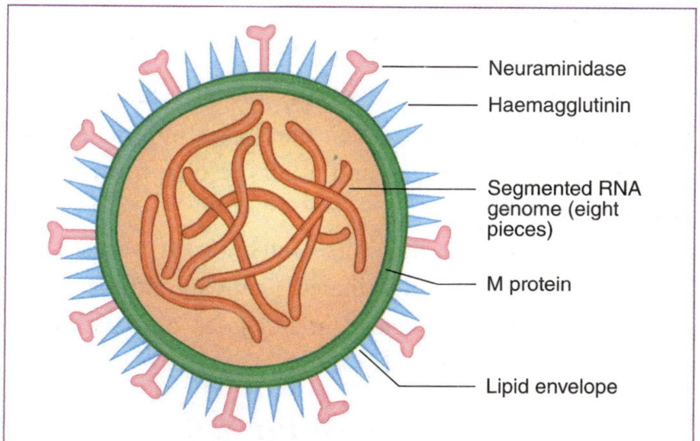

Fig. 40.1 Influenza virus.

(i) Spherical particle

It is typically spherical, 80–120 nm in diameter but pleomorphic and filamentous forms are frequent.

(ii) Helical symmetry

The nucleocapsid has a helical symmetry.

(iii) RNA genome

It contains a single stranded RNA genome which is segmented and exists as eight pieces.

(iv) Envelope

The nucleocapsid is enclosed by an inner protein layer called the matrix or 'M protein' and outer lipid layer.

(v) Peplomers

Attached to the lipid layer of the envelope are two types of glycoprotein peplomers or spikes, the haemagglutinin (HA) and the neuraminidase (NA). Haemagglutinin spikes are triangular in cross section while neuraminidase spikes are mushroom shaped which are less numerous.

B. Antigenic Classification

Based on differences of antigenic structure, influenza viruses are divided into three types: A, B and C. On the basis of antigenic variation of HA and NA antigens, these three types (A, B and C) can be divided into subtypes. Human viruses show 3 HA (H1, H2, H3) and 2 NA (N1, N2) types.

C. Antigenic Variation

Depending on the degree of antigenic change of HA and NA, two distinct forms of antigenic variation are known.

1. *Antigenic Drift*

Antigenic drift refers to the minor antigenic changes in either the haemagglutinin or neuraminidase or both.

2. *Antigenic Shift*

Major antigenic changes in HA (H2 to H3) or NA (N1 to N3) are called antigenic shift, resulting in emergence of a new subtype unrelated antigenically to predecessor strains.

D. Cultivation

1. *Egg Inoculation*

Influenza virus is cultivated in amniotic cavity of 11 to 13 days old chick embryos.

2. *Tissue Culture*

Influenza virus can also be isolated on primary monkey kidney or human embryo kidney cells.

E. Pathogenesis

Influenza virus enters the body by respiratory tract. Incubation period varies from 1–4 days. Subclinical infections are common. Influenza is an acute respiratory disease and clinical features vary from mild coryza to fulminating pneumonia. The uncomplicated disease is usually resolved within 7 days.

F. Laboratory Diagnosis

Laboratory diagnosis depends on demonstration of virus antigens, isolation of the virus and serology.

1. Demonstration of Virus Antigens

Viral antigens in clinical specimens can be detected by **immunofluorescence**. Smears of nasopharyngeal secretions and nasal swab or centrifuged deposit of throat garglings are prepared on slides and treated with fluorescent-tagged influenza antiserum and examined under the fluorescent microscope.

2. Isolation of the Virus

Throat garglings are collected using suitable buffered salt solution. The specimen should be processed immediately. The material is inoculated into:

(i) amniotic cavity of 11 to 13 days chick-embryo or

(ii) monolayers of monkey kidney cell cultures or human embryo kidney cells.

The virus growth can be identified by testing the culture fluid for haemagglutination or by haemadsorption.

3. Molecular Method

It can be used in clinical specimens. Detection of viral RNA by reverse transcriptase polymerase chain reaction (RT-PCR) is highly sensitive method. **Real time RT-PCR** is the **gold standard method** for diagnoses of influenza.

4. Serology

Serological tests are mainly used for seroepidemiology. Various serological tests available are:

(i) ELISA

(ii) Neutralisation test

(iii) haemagglutination inhibition test (HAI test).

III. PARAMYXOVIRUSES

Paramyxoviruses belong to family *Paramyxoviridae*. They possess single-stranded RNA genome as a single piece with helical nucleocapsid. They are enveloped. They are spherical in shape.

Morphology

The paramyxoviruses are spherical enveloped particles 100-300 nm diameter in size. The envelope is covered by projections. These projections are of two types, HN (haemagglutinin, neuraminidase) and F (fusion protein) peplomers. The HN projections of paramyxovirus carry both haemagglutinin and neuraminidase functions. Nucleocapsid is of helical symmetry and contains a single stranded RNA genome as a single piece. Measles virus envelope carries only haemagglutinin but not a neuraminidase.

Viruses of family paramyxoviridae

A. Parainfluenza Viruses

Parainfluenza viruses are acquired by droplets and by contact with respiratory secretions. These viruses are ubiquitous and produce upper respiratory tract infections. In infants and young children, they cause severe respiratory tract disease such as *laryngotracheobronchitis* or *croup*. The patient presents with fever, cough and respiratory obstruction as a result of swelling of larynx and related structures.

B. Mumps Virus

Morphology of the mumps virus is same as described earlier under the heading 'Morphology'.

Mumps or epidemic parotitis is predominantly a disease of childhood and is acquired from direct contact with infected saliva or aerosols from infected patients. Respiratory tract is the portal of entry.

C. Measles Virus

Measles is highly infectious childhood disease spread by respiratory secretions. It is caused by measles virus. The virus resembles paramyxoviruses in morphology.

Measles virus is acquired by inhalation. Measles is characterised by high fever, cough and conjunctivitis. *Koplik's spots* can be seen on the buccal mucosa and are pathognomic of measles. With the decline of acute symptoms in 1-2 days, widespread maculopapular rash appears first on the neck and then spreads to the rest of the body. The rash fades in about a week and the patient recovers uneventfully by 10-14 days.

D. Respiratory Syncytial Virus

It is the most important cause of bronchiolitis and pneumonitis in infants between one to six months of age. Infection in older children and adults results in rhinitis or common cold.

RSV is highly contagious. Infection is transmitted by contact with contaminated hands and surfaces. Nosocomial infections occur in nurseries and paediatric wards. Incubation period is 4–6 days.

IV. RHABDOVIRUSES

Rhabdoviruses are bullet or rod shaped (*rhabdos*, meaning rod) enveloped viruses with single stranded RNA genome. They are included in the family *Rhabdoviridae*.

RABIES VIRUS

A. Morphology

1. Bullet shaped, 75 × 180 nm, with one end round and the other planar or concave.

2. Nucleocapsid shows helical symmetry containing a single stranded, RNA genome.

B. Pathogenesis

Rabies is a natural infection of dogs, foxes, cats, wolves and bats. Man is infected by the bite of rabid dog or other animals. Saliva containing viruses is deposited in the wound. The rabies virus multiplies in muscle or connective tissue at or near the site of introduction before it attaches to nerves.

C. Laboratory Diagnosis

Diagnosis in Humans

(i) Immunofluorescence test

Viral antigens can be detected in hair follicle of the nape of the neck and corneal impression smears by direct immunofluorescence. Diagnosis may be made postmortem using brain as a specimen.

(ii) Demonstration of Negri bodies

This is demonstrated in brain. Negri bodies appear as intracytoplasmic, oval or round, purplish pink (3-27 μm) bodies with characteristic basophilic inner granules.

(iii) Isolation of the virus

The virus can be isolated from specimens like CSF, saliva and urine, by intracerebral inoculation in mice. However, during postmortem, brain tissue is also used. The inoculated mice are examined for signs of illness, and their brains are examined at death or at 28 days after inoculation for Negri bodies. Brains can also be examined by immunofluorescence technique.

D. Prophylaxis

Post-Exposure Prophylaxis

It includes: local treatment; hyperimmune serum; and vaccination

Post exposure prophylaxis is given according to category of exposure (Table 40.2).

Local treatment

The wound should be thoroughly washed with soap and water for 15 minutes. It is very important as soap inactivates the virus by destroying its envelope. After washing, the wound is treated with quaternary ammonium compound (cetavalon) or tincture iodine or alcohol.

Hyperimmune serum

Hyperimmune serum (rabies immunoglobulin) is used along with vaccination in category III exposure. However, in immunocompromised individuals hyperimmune serum treatment along with vaccination is used in both category II and III exposure.

Human antirabies immunoglobulin (20 IU per kg body weight) is reserved for the high risk cases. It is the safest antirabies antiserum. Maximum dose of the antiserum is infiltrated locally in wound and any reminder amount is not needed to be administered intramuscularly at different site.

Vaccination

Vaccines are of two main categories—neural and non-neural. Non-neural vaccines are being used increasingly because neural vaccines are associated with serious risk of neurological complications. Manufacturing and use of neural vaccines have been discontinued in India.

(i) Neural vaccines

The following are some of the infected brain vaccines.

(a) Semple vaccine (sheep brain)

(b) Beta propiolactone (BPL) vaccine

(c) Infant brain vaccine

These infected brain vaccines are encephalogenic and thus are **not in use**.

(ii) Non-neural vaccines

(a) Duck egg vaccine
It is beta propiolactone inactivated vaccine. It has a poor immunogenicity and is therefore **discontinued**.

(b) Duck embryo vaccine
Purified duck embryo vaccine (PDEV) is beta-propiolactone inactivated vaccine. It is also **not in use** for humans.

(c) Cell culture vaccines
The human diploid cell strain vaccine (HDCV) is prepared by growing rabies virus on human diploid cells and is inactivated with beta-propiolactone. This vaccine is highly antigenic and free of side effects. The only disadvantage is its high cost.

Table 40.2: Post-exposure prophylaxis according to categories of exposure

Category	Type and contact	Post-exposure prophylaxis (PEP)
I.	• Touching or feeding of animals • Licks on intact skin	• PEP is not given if reliable case history is available
II.	• Nibbling of uncovered skin • Minor scratches or abrasions without bleeding	• Local wound treatment • Anti-rabies vaccination
III.	• Single or multiple transdermal bites or scratches, licks on the broken skin • Contamination of mucous membrane with saliva (i.e. licks) • Exposure to bat bites	• Local wound treatment • Anti serum (Rabies immunoglobulin) • Anti-rabies vaccine

Other equally effective but more economical cell culture vaccines include 'Purified chick embryo cell culture vaccine' (PCECV) and 'Purified vero cell rabies vaccine' (PVRV).

Commonly used vaccines against rabies are shown in Table 40.3.

Table 40.3: Commonly used Non-neural Antirabies Vaccines

Vaccine	Substrate to grow virus	Type
HDCV	Human diploid cell	Inactivated by BPL
PCECV	Chick embryo cells	Inactivated by BPL
PVRV	Vero cells	Inactivated by BPL

Vaccination schedules

When the biting animal can be observed for ten days and the animal remains healthy, rabies may be excluded and vaccine, if already started, may be discontinued.

Cell culture vaccines

All three cell culture vaccines available in India (HDCV, PCECV, PVRV have the same dose schedule. It is also same for both adults and children. These vaccines can be administered by intradermal (ID) or intramuscular (IM) route.

The dose of 0.1 ml is given for ID route and 0.5 or 1.0 ml (depending on type of vaccine) for IM route. Two types of schedule include injection at two different site at the same time (2-site) and injection at one site (1-site) (Table 40.4).

Postexposure Prophylaxis

Postexposure prophylaxis (PEP) has been summarised in Table 40.4.

Table 40.4 Postexposure Prophylaxis

Regimen	Days				
	0	3	7	14	21
Intradermal (ID), 2-Site regimen	2	2	2	0	0
Intramuscular (IM) regimens					
(i) 1-Site	1	1	1	1*	—
(ii) 2-Site and 1-Site	2	0	1	0	1

* This fourth dose can be given between 14-28 days.
2: Two injections at two different sites.
1: One injection at one site.
0: No injection.

V. ARBOVIRUSES

Arboviruses (arthropod-borne viruses) are RNA viruses that are transmitted by blood-sucking arthropods from one vertebrate host to another.

LABORATORY DIAGNOSIS OF ARBOVIRUSES

Diagnosis may be established by virus isolation or serology.

A. Specimens

Blood, CSF and brain may be used for isolation of virus. As all arboviruses are viraemic, blood is collected during the acute phase of the disease. CSF is useful in encephalitis cases but the best specimen is the brain.

B. Virus Isolation

1. Suckling Mice

Specimens are inoculated intracerebrally into suckling mice. The animal develops fatal encephalitis.

2. Tissue Culture

Some viruses may also be isolated in tissue cultures.

C. Serology

Using ELISA, serotype specific IgM antibody may be detected in patient serum.

Dengue

Dengue is characterised by fever of sudden onset, headache, retrobulbar pain, conjunctival infection, pain in the back and joints (also called break-bone fever), lymphadenopathy and maculopapular rash.

Dengue virus has five serotypes: Dengue virus 1 (DENV 1), dengue virus 2 (DENV 2), dengue virus 3 (DENV 3) and dengue virus 4 (DENV 4) and dengue virus 5 (DENV5). It is transmitted by *Aedes aegypti*.

1. Clinical Features

The disease may occur in two forms: classical dengue fever and dengue in more serious forms with haemorrhagic manifestations.

(i) *Classical dengue fever:* This usually affects older children and adults. It has relatively benign course with fever, headache and pain in muscles and bones. The fever is typically biphasic (saddle back). Incubation period is 5-8 days. The febrile illness lasts for about 10 days after which recovery is generally complete. It is rarely fatal.

(ii) *Other manifestations:* Dengue may also occur in more serious forms, with haemorrhagic manifestations or with shock. These are known as *dengue haemorrhagic fever* (DHF) and *dengue shock syndrome* (DSS).

Initial symptoms are like those of dengue fever but associated with haemorrhagic rash, thrombocytopenia and shock. The mortality rate is 5-10%. All four types of dengue virus are present in India.

2. Laboratory Diagnosis

Isolation of the virus is difficult but serology plays a major role in diagnosis. Demonstration of IgM antibody in serum provides early diagnosis. ELISA is used for detection of IgM antibody. A strip immunochromatographic test for IgM is also available for rapid diagnosis.

Immunochromatographic test (ICT) and ELISA are available for detection of NS1 antigen. NS1 antigen can be detected on the first day of fever before antibody appears. ICT takes about 15 minutes.

Viral RNA can be detected in clinical specimens by reverse transcriptase polymerase chain reaction (RT PCR).

3. Prophylaxis

Control measures include elimination of mosquitoes. No effective vaccine is available.

Rubella Virus

Rubella or German measles is primarily a mild childhood disease. It may be acquired congenitally or postnatally. It is not transmitted by arthropods.

1. Morphology

Rubella virus is a pleomorphic, roughly spherical, 50-70 nm in diameter, enveloped RNA virus. It has single stranded RNA genome.

2. Pathogenesis

(i) Postnatal rubella

Infection is acquired by inhalation. After an incubation period of 2 to 3 weeks, viraemia occurs. The virus is disseminated throughout the body by blood-stream. Patient develops fever, and fine, pink, macular rash, which first appears on the face and then spreads to the trunk and legs. The illness is of short duration and recovery is usually complete.

(ii) Congenital rubella

Rubella virus can cross the placental barrier and can replicate in differentiating cells of the embryo.

3. Laboratory Diagnosis

Routine diagnosis of rubella is not called for but the laboratory diagnosis becomes important in pregnant women suspected to have rubella. Diagnosis can be established by virus isolation or serology.

(i) Virus isolation

Rubella virus can be isolated from adult throat swab. In infants with congenital rubella, the throat swab, urine or CSF can be used for isolation. The virus isolation is not commonly employed for rubella diagnosis because of the difficulties involved.

(ii) Serology

Serological diagnosis is the method of choice in rubella. Antibodies in blood are detected by ELISA. Demonstration of rubella IgM antibody in a single specimen of blood has a diagnostic value. In case of rubella IgG antibody, four-fold rise in titre must be demonstrated between two serum samples collected at 10 days interval. In a newborn baby, rubella specific IgM antibody is diagnostic of congenital rubella as IgM antibodies do not cross the placenta.

4. Prophylaxis

Under National Immunisation Programme of India, MR (Measles, Rubella) vaccine (0.5 ml) is given subcutaneously at 9–12 months of age and second dose at 16–24 months.

VI. ROTAVIRUSES

Rotaviruses are the commonest cause of gastroenteritis in children. Rotavirus (*Rota*, meaning wheel) is a double shelled icosahedral capsid resembling a wheel with short spokes radiating from a wide hub to a clearly defined outer rim. The genome consists of double stranded segmented RNA.

Rotavirus diarrhoea is usually seen in children below the age of five years, but is most frequent between six months and two years of age. Infection is acquired by the faeco-oral route. Incubation period is 2-3 days. The disease is self limiting and recovery occurs within 5-10 days.

Laboratory Diagnosis

1. Demonstration of Virus

During acute stage of the disease, 10^{11} virus particles may be present in the faeces. These can be demonstrated by:

(i) ELISA
(ii) Latex agglutination test
(iii) Electron microscopy
(iv) Immunoelectron microscopy

2. Antibody Detection

Antibodies can be detected in the blood by ELISA. It may be used for seroprevalence.

VII. HEPATITIS VIRUSES

All hapatitis viruses (RNA and DNA) are dealt separately in Chapter 41.

VIII. RETROVIRUSES

Retroviruses especially 'Human immunodeficiency virus (HIV)' has an important role in 'Nursing care', therefore, this RNA virus has been described separately in Chapter 42.

KEY POINTS »»

1. Two types of vaccines are available for immunisation. These are *killed polio vaccine* (*Salk*) and *live attenuated oral polio vaccine* (*Sabin*). Live vaccine (Sabin) is administered orally. Three doses are given.
2. Orthomyxoviruses are spherical or filamentous, enveloped viruses with single stranded and segmented RNA genome. The viruses cause *influenza*, an acute respiratory illness. Laboratory diagnosis depends on *demonstration of virus antigens*, *isolation of the virus* and *serology*.
3. Paramyxoviruses possess single-stranded RNA genome as a single piece with helical nucleocapsid. They are enveloped and spherical in shape. *Parainfluenza virus*, *mumps virus*, *measles virus* and *respiratory syncytial* virus are important paramyxoviruses causing human infections.
4. Rhabdoviruses are *bullet* or rod shaped, enveloped viruses with single stranded RNA genome. Rabies virus is an important rhabdovirus. It causes *rabies*. Man is infected by the bite of rabid dog or other animals. Laboratory diagnosis of rabies in humans depends on *detection of viral antigens*, *demonstration of negri bodies in brain* and *isolation of the virus by tissue culture*. Cell culture vaccines are commonly used antirabies vaccines. These include *human diploid cell strain vaccine* (*HDCV*), *purified chick embryo cell culture vaccine* (*PCECV*), and *purified vero cell rabies vaccine* (*PVRV*). These are *non-neural* vaccines.
5. Arboviruses (arthropod-borne viruses) are RNA viruses that are transmitted by blood-sucking arthropods from one vertebrate host to another. *Dengue* is an important virus causing febrile illness. Dengue virus is transmitted by *Aedes aegypti* mosquito. Laboratory diagnosis of arboviruses may be established by *virus isolation* or *serology*.
6. Rotavirus (*Rota*, meaning wheel) is a double shelled icosahedral capsid resembling a wheel with short spokes radiating from a wide hub to a clearly defined outer rim. The genome consists of double stranded segmented RNA. It is the commonest cause of *diarrhoea in children*. Laboratory diagnosis of rotavirus diarrhoea can be done by *demonstration of virus* in *faeces* by *ELISA*, *latex agglutination test*, *CIEP* and *electron microscopy*.

STUDY QUESTIONS

1. Write short notes on:
   (i) Polio vaccine
   (ii) Morphology of *influenza virus*
   (iii) Parainfluenza viruses
2. Discuss the laboratory diagnosis of rabies.
3. Write short notes on:
   (i) Negri bodies
   (ii) Antirabies vaccines
4. Write short notes on:
   (i) Arboviruses
   (ii) Dengue virus
   (iii) Rubella virus
   (iv) Rotaviruses.

MULTIPLE CHOICE QUESTIONS (MCQs)

1. How many types of poliovirus are there?
   (a) Two
   (b) Three
   (c) Four
   (d) Five
2. How much percentage of poliovirus infections may develop into paralytic poliomyelitis?
   (a) 90–95%
   (b) 4–8%
   (c) 1–2%
   (d) 0.1–2%
3. Which of the following vaccines is killed vaccine?
   (a) Sabin polio vaccine
   (b) Salk polio vaccine
   (c) BCG
   (d) None of the above
4. In which of the following viruses, segmentation of genome is a characteristic feature?
   (a) Influenza virus
   (b) Parainfluenza virus
   (c) Mumps virus
   (d) Measles virus
5. Koplik's spots on the buccal mucosa is a characteristic feature of:
   (a) Mumps
   (b) Measles
   (c) Rubella
   (d) Respiratory syncytial virus
6. Which of the following viruses is bullet shaped?
   (a) Herpes virus
   (b) Variola virus
   (c) Rabies virus
   (d) Parvovirus

7. Negri bodies can be demonstrated in brain of animals who are infected with:
   (a) Street virus
   (b) Fixed virus
   (c) Both of the above
   (d) None of the above
8. Which of the following tests can be used in diagnosis of rabies?
   (a) Direct immunofluorescence test
   (b) Demonstration of negri bodies
   (c) Isolation of virus
   (d) All of the above
9. Which of the following measures can be required for prevention of rabies in humans exposed to bite of rabid animal?
   (a) Local treatment of wound
   (b) Hyperimmune serum administration
   (c) Vaccination
   (d) All of the above
10. How many serotypes of dengue virus are there?
    (a) Three
    (b) Four
    (c) Five
    (d) Eight
11. Which of the following methods can be used for diagnosis of rotavirus infection?
    (a) ELISA
    (b) Latex agglutination test
    (c) Electron microscopy
    (d) All of the above

ANSWERS (MCQs) ...✓

1. (b) 2. (d) 3. (b) 4. (a) 5. (b) 6. (c) 7. (a) 8. (d) 9. (d) 10. (b) 11. (d)

41

Hepatitis Viruses

Viral hepatitis is a systemic disease with primary inflammation in the liver. Till now, there are five hepatitis viruses, i.e., hepatitis A, B, C, D, and E. Hepatitis B is a DNA virus while others (A, C, D, E) contain RNA genome (Table 41.1).

I. HEPATITIS A VIRUS (HAV) (INFECTIOUS HEPATITIS)

The hepatitis A virus enters the body by oral route. The large majority of infections are asymptomatic. Symptoms include fever, malaise, anorexia, nausea, vomiting and liver tenderness. These usually subside with the onset of jaundice. Recovery occurs over a period of 4–6 weeks.

A. Morphology

HAV is 27 nm non-enveloped single stranded RNA virus with an icosahedral symmetry (Fig. 41.1). It belongs to the picornavirus family.

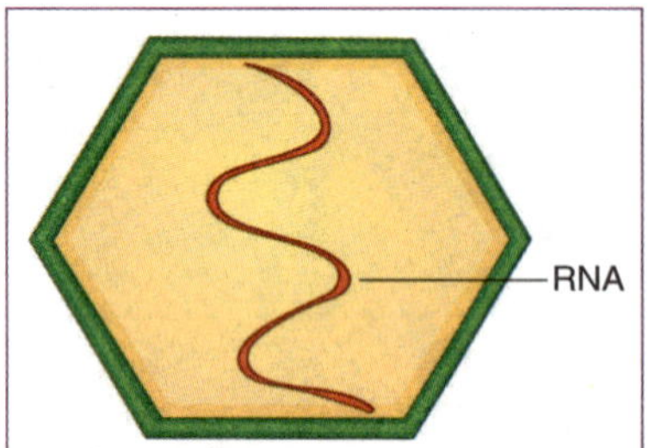

Fig. 41.1 Hepatitis A virus

B. Laboratory Diagnosis

Laboratory diagnosis can be made by

1. Demonstration of virus
2. Detection of antibody

1. *Demonstration of Virus*

The virus may be demonstrated by following methods:

(i) Immunoelectron microscopy (IEM)

The virus can be visualised by IEM in faeces.

(ii) Enzyme-linked immunosorbent assay (ELISA)

HAV antigen can be detected in faeces by ELISA using monoclonal antibodies.

(iii) Isolation

The virus has been grown in human and simian cell cultures but it is not possible to grow them routinely from faeces of patients.

2. *Detection of Antibody*

Because of difficulties of isolation and detection of virus, diagnosis depends on demonstration of specific antibody to HAV in the blood. ELISA kits for detecing IgM and IgG antibodies are available.

C. Prophylaxis

1. As the disease is transmitted by the faeco-oral route, general prophylaxis includes improved sanitation and prevention of faecal contamination of food and water.
2. Passive prophylaxis with normal pooled human immunoglobulin before exposure to the virus or in the early incubation period may prevent or attenuate a clinical illness, while not necessarily prevent virus excretion.
3. A formalin inactivated, alum conjugated vaccine containing HAV grown in human diploid cell culture is available. It is safe and effective. A full

Table 41.1: Characteristic Features of Major Hepatitis Viruses

Feature	HAV	HBV	HCV	HDV	HEV
Genome	RNA	DNA	RNA	RNA	RNA
Nomenclature	*Picornaviridae*	*Hepadnaviridae*	*Flaviviridae*	*Deltavirus*	*Hepeviridae*
Mode of transmission	Enteric	Parenteral, sexual, perinatal	Parenteral, sexual	Parenteral	Enteric
Antigen in blood	HAV	HBsAg, HBeAg	HCV	HDAg	HEV
Antibodies in blood	Anti-HAV	Anti-HBs, Anti-HBe, Anti-HBc	Anti-HCV	Anti-HDV	Anti-HEV
Chronic carrier state	No	Yes	Yes	Yes	No
Hepatic carcinoma	No	Yes	Yes	No	No

course consists of two intramuscular injections of the vaccine. Second dose is administered 6 months after first dose. Protection lasts for 10–20 years.

4. One attack of the disease gives life-long protection against HAV.

II. HEPATITIS B VIRUS (HBV) (SERUM HEPATITIS)

Hepatitis B virus (HBV) belongs to the family *Hepadnaviridae*. It differs from hepatitis A in various aspects (Table 41.2).

A. Morphology

HBV is a complex 42 nm double shelled particle. The outer surface or envelope of virus contains hepatitis B surface antigen (HBs Ag). It encloses an inner icosahedral 27 nm nucleocapsid (core), which contains hepatitis B core antigen (HBc Ag). Inside the core is the genome, a circular double stranded DNA and a DNA polymerase (Fig. 41.2).

Blumberg and coworkers (1965) described a protein antigen in serum of an Australian aborigine, which gave a positive precipitation reaction with sera from two haemophiliacs who had received multiple transfusions. This antigen was named ***Australia antigen***. It was subsequently established to be the surface component of hepatitis B virus (HBsAg). Electron microscopy of sera of hepatitis B patients shows three types of particles (Fig. 41.2). The most abundant form is a spherical particle (22 nm in diameter) and the second type is tubular (22 nm in diameter) particle of varying length. These two types are antigenically identical and are the surface subunits of hepatitis B virus (HBsAg). The third type is a double shelled spherical structure (42 nm in diameter). This particle is the complete hepatitis B virus or ***Dane particle***.

B. Antigenic Structure

1. Hepatitis B surface Antigen (HBsAg)

Surface antigens (envelope protein)

2. Hepatitis B Core Antigen (HBcAg)

It is the core (nucleocapsid) antigen of the virus. It is not detectable in patient's blood.

3. Hepatitis B Precore Antigen (HBeAg)

It is the hidden antigenic component of core.

Table 41.2: Differentiating Features of Hepatitis A and B Viruses

Feature	Hepatitis A	Hepatitis B
1. Virus		
Diameter	27 nm	42 nm
Genome	RNA	DNA
Symmetry	Icosahedral	Icosahedral
Envelope	Non-enveloped	Enveloped
Stability		
60°C for 60 mins	Survives	Survives
100°C for 5 mins	Inactivated	Inactivated
2. Usual mode of infection	Faeco-oral	Parenteral
3. Clinical		
Incubation period	2-6 weeks	2-6 months
Onset	Usually acute	Insidious
Fever less than 38°C	Usual	Rare
Chronicity	Rare	Common
Age incidence	Children and young adults	All ages: commoner in adult
Seasonal distribution	Post monsoon in India Autumn-winter	All the year round
4. Laboratory diagnosis		
HBs Ag	Absent	Present
Raised serum IgM	Common	Rare
Raised serum transaminase	For few days	For many weeks
Virus in faeces	Present early	Absent
5. Mortality	0.1%	1-10%
6. Carrier state		
Blood	Up to 8 months	Up to 5 years
Faeces	Up to 1-3 month	Not known (or negative)

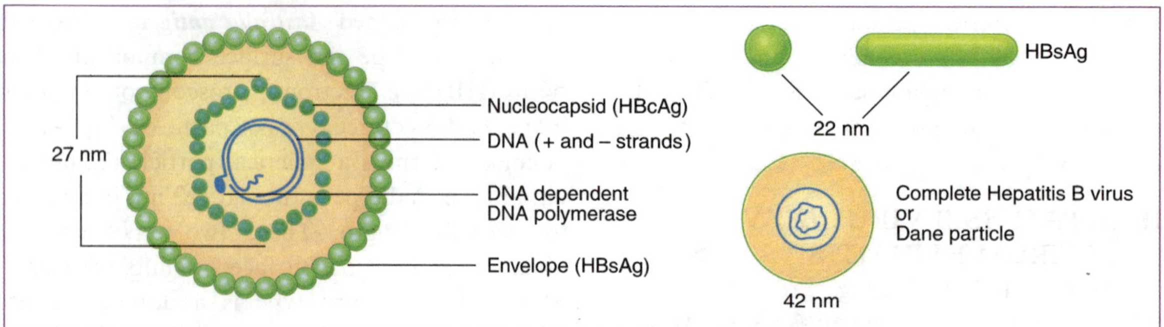

Fig. 41.2 Structure of Hepatitis B virus.

4. Viral Genes and Antigens

The viral genome consists of two linear strands of DNA held in a circular configuration. Associated with one strand of DNA is a viral *DNA polymerase* (Fig. 41.2).

C. Modes of Transmission

There are three important modes of transmission of HBV infection:

1. Parenteral
2. Perinatal
3. Sexual

1. Parenteral Transmission

Transmission of infection may result from accidental inoculation of minute amounts of blood, blood products or fluid containing HBV during medical, surgical or dental procedures.

2. Perinatal Transmission

Transmission probably occurs when carrier mother's blood contaminates the mucous membranes of the newborn during birth.

3. Sexual Transmission

HBV is present in body fluids such as semen and vaginal secretions, hence, it can be transmitted by sexual contact.

D. Clinical Features

Onset is slow, usually insidious but more severe. The incubation period varies from 6 weeks to 6 months. The course of acute HBV infection can be divided into three phases: preicteric, icteric and convalescent.

E. Hepatitis B Carriers

There are two types of hepatitis B carriers: super carriers and simple carriers.

1. ***Super carriers***: They have HBe Ag in blood and are highly infectious. Very minute amount of serum or blood can transmit the infection. These are called super carriers.
2. ***Simple carriers***: They are more common type of carriers who have no HBeAg and a low level of HBs Ag in blood. They transmit the infection only when large volumes of blood or serum are transferred, as in blood transfusion. These are named simple carriers.

F. Laboratory Diagnosis

Laboratory diagnosis of HBV infections can be carried out by detection of **hepatitis B antigens** and **antibodies**. These can be detected by sensitive and specific tests like ELISA and RIA.

1. Detection of Viral Markers

(i) HBsAg

HBsAg is recognised as a **specific marker for HBV infection**. It is the **first marker to appear** in blood after infection. HBsAg disappears with recovery from clinical disease in most patients, however, it persists for years in carriers. Antibody to HBsAg appears within weeks after the disappearance of HBsAg and persists for very long periods. Anti-HBs is the protective antibody.

(ii) HBeAg

Sera containing **HBeAg** are believed to be **highly infectious** and those with anti-HBe of little infectivity. The disappearance of *HBeAg* is followed by appearance of anti-*HBe*.

(iii) HBcAg

It is not detectable in the serum but can be demonstrated in liver cells by immunofluorescence. Anti-HBc antibody usually appears in serum a week or two after the appearance of HBsAg. It remains lifelong and thus serves as a useful indicator of prior infection with HBV, even after all the other markers become undetectable.

2. Viral DNA Polymerase

It appears transiently in serum during pre-icteric phase.

3. Polymerase Chain Reaction (PCR)

HBV DNA level can be detected in serum by PCR. It is a highly sensitive test.

G. Prophylaxis

1. General Preventive Measures

These include health education, improvement of personal hygiene and strict attention to sterility. An important preventive measure is the screening for HBsAg and HBe Ag in blood donors. Use of unsterile needles, syringes and other material must be avoided to prevent hepatitis B infection.

2. Immunisation

(i) Passive immunisation

Passive immunisation may be employed following any accidental exposure to hepatitis B infection. Hepatitis B immunoglobulin (HBIG) is prepared from donors with high titres of anti-HBs. It can be given in a single dose of 0.06 ml/kg (or 10–12 IU/kg) intramuscularly.

(ii) Active immunisation

Recombinant yeast hepatitis B vaccine

It is produced by a recombinant DNA in yeasts in which a plasmid containing the gene of HBsAg has been incorporated. HBsAg particles produced are extracted and purified for use as vaccine. It is safe and free from side effects.

Three doses (1.0 ml each) at 0, 1 and 6 months are administered intramuscularly into deltoid muscle.

III. HEPATITIS C VIRUS (HCV)

Hepatitis C virus (HCV) belongs to the family *Flaviviridae*. It is a 50–60 nm virus with a linear single stranded RNA.

A. Modes of Infection

It is transmitted by needlestick injuries, use of contaminated needles and syringes, transfusion of infected blood and blood products, and sexual intercourse. Maternal-neonatal transmission has also been reported.

B. Clinical Features

Clinical infection with hepatitis C is generally less severe, with milder symptoms, absent or less marked jaundice.

C. Laboratory Diagnosis

It can be established by detection of anti-HCV (antibody) by ELISA. Viral genome (HCV RNA) can be detected by polymerase chain reaction (PCR) PCR is the gold standard method.

D. Prophylaxis

Only general prophylaxis, such as blood or blood products screening, is possible. Avoidance of use of unsterile needles, syringes and other material is another important general prophylactic measure.

IV. HEPATITIS D VIRUS (HDV) (DELTA ANTIGEN)

The HDV is a defective virus as it is dependent on the helper function of HBV for its replication and expression. It belongs to genus *Deltavirus*. It is spherical, 36-38 nm diameter, RNA particle surrounded by HBsAg envelope (Fig. 41.3). The genome is a single stranded small circular molecule of RNA. It encodes its own nucleoprotein, the *delta antigen* or HDAg, but the outer envelope (HBsAg) of HDV is encoded by the genome of HBV coinfecting the same cell. HBV is necessary for the production of HDV virions.

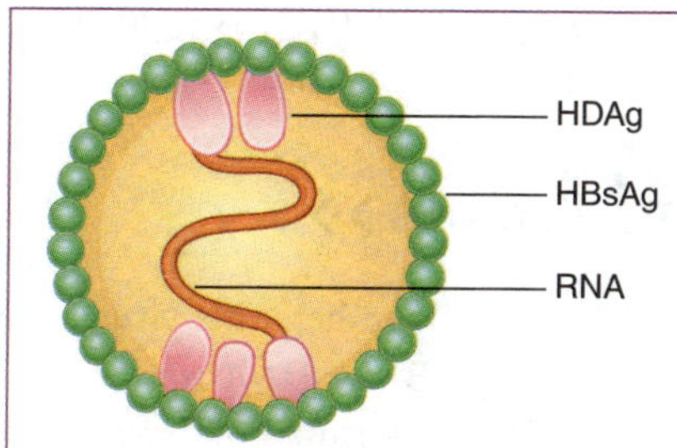

Fig. 41.3 Hepatitis D virus

A. Clinical Features

HDV infection can occur in presence of HBV under two situations:

(i) Simultaneous infection with both HDV and HBV (**coinfection**)

(ii) **Superinfection** of an HBsAg carrier by HDV.

Transmission occurs parenterally.

B. Laboratory Diagnosis

Diagnosis can be made by detecting the **IgM anti-delta antibody** in serum. **ELISA** kits are commercially available for detection of antibodies to HDV. **HDAg** (Delta antigen) is primarily expressed in liver cell nuclei, where it can be detected by **immunofluorescence**. It is occasionally present in serum.

C. Prophylaxis

No specific prophylaxis exists, but immunisation with the hepatitis B vaccine is effective because delta antigen cannot infect persons immune to HBV. Screening of blood donors for HBsAg will also limit blood borne HDV infection.

V. HEPATITIS E VIRUS (HEV)

Hepatitis E virus belongs to family *Hepeviridae* and genus *Hepevirus*. They are spherical, nonenveloped and 27-38 nm in diameter. They possess single stranded RNA genome, which is surrounded by icosahedral capsid.

A. Pathogenesis

It is primarily associated with ingestion of **faecally contaminated drinking water**. Clinically the disease resembles that of hepatitis A. The disease is generally mild and self limited.

B. Laboratory Diagnosis

1. Immunoelectron microscopy

Faeces is examined by electron microscopy of aggregated hepevirus particles using monoclonal antibodies.

2. Serum antibody detection by ELISA test

These are used for detection of IgM and IgG antibodies.

3. Polymerase chain reaction (PCR)

HEV RNA can be detected in faeces or acute phase sera of patients by RT-PCR. It is gold standard test for diagnosis of acute HEV infection.

C. Prophylaxis

Hepatitis E can be prevented by

1. improved standards of sanitation
2. chlorinated water.

VI. NON-A, NON-B (NANB) HEPATITIS

It refers to viral hepatitis resembling type A or type B clinically and epidemiologically but not caused by either of these viruses. Now four types (hepatitis C, D, E, and G) of NANB viruses are known. The diagnosis is possible with serological tests but a few are diagnosed by the process of exclusion.

KEY POINTS »»

1. There are five hepatitis viruses, i.e., hepatitis A, B, C, D, and E.
2. Hepatitis B is a *DNA virus* while others (A, C, D, and E) contain *RNA* genome.
3. Mode of transmission is *enteric* in hepatitis A and hepatitis E viruses while it is *parenteral* and *sexual* in both hepatitis B and hepatitis C viruses.
4. Hepatitis A virus (HAV) can be demonstrated in faeces by *immunoelectron microscopy* (*IEM*) and ELISA. Specific IgM antibody to HAV can also be detected in blood for diagnosis of HAV infection.
5. HBsAg is also named as *Australia antigen*.
6. There are three types of antigen namely *HBsAg* (surface antigen), *HBcAg* (core antigen) and *HBeAg*.
7. *Parenteral*, *perinatal* and *sexual* are three important *modes of transmission* of HBV infection.
8. Laboratory diagnosis of HBV infections can be carried out by detection of hepatitis B antigens and antibodies. These can be detected by ELISA and RIA.
9. HBV infection can be prevented by *general measures* or *immunisation*. General measures include the *screening of HBsAg in blood donors*, *avoidance of use of unsterile needles*, *syringes* and other material.
10. Vaccine is prepared by purifying *HBsAg particles*. Three doses of vaccine at *0*, *1* and *6* months are administered intramuscularly into deltoid muscle.

STUDY QUESTIONS

1. Describe the laboratory diagnosis of infections caused by hepatitis B virus.
2. Write short notes on:
   (i) Hepatitis A virus (HAV)
   (ii) HBsAg
   (iii) Hepatitis B vaccines
   (iv) Hepatitis C virus (HCV)
   (v) Hepatitis E virus (HEV)
   (vi) Non-A, Non-B hepatitis.

MULTIPLE CHOICE QUESTIONS (MCQs)

1. Which of the following hepatitis viruses is DNA virus?
   (a) Hepatitis A virus
   (b) Hepatitis B virus
   (c) Hepatitis C virus
   (d) Hepatitis E virus
2. Which of the following hepatitis viruses can be transmitted by sexual route?
   (a) Hepatitis A virus
   (b) Hepatitis C virus
   (c) Hepatitis E virus
   (d) All of the above
3. Which of the following antigens is present in the envelope of hepatitis B virus?
   (a) HBsAg
   (b) HBcAg
   (c) HBeAg
   (d) None of the above
4. Which of the following viral markers is first to appear in blood after infection with hepatitis B virus?
   (a) HBsAg
   (b) HBcAg
   (c) HBeAg
   (d) Antibody to HBsAg
5. What is the mode of transmission of hepatitis E virus?
   (a) Faecally contaminated drinking water
   (b) Parenteral route
   (c) Sexual route
   (d) None of the above

ANSWERS (MCQs) ...✓

1. (b) 2. (b) 3. (a) 4. (a) 5. (a)

Retroviruses: HIV

42

I. RETROVIRUSES

These are RNA viruses that belong to family *Retroviridae*. Members of this family possess reverse transcriptase (RNA directed DNA polymerase) enzyme which prepares a DNA copy of the RNA genome in host cell. **The presence of enzyme reverse transcriptase is a characteristic feature.**

II. HUMAN IMMUNODEFICIENCY VIRUS (HIV)

HIV occurs in two main types, HIV-1 and HIV-2.

A. Morphology

HIV is a spherical enveloped virus, about 90-120 nm in diameter (Fig. 42.1). It contains two identical copies of single stranded RNA genome. In association with viral RNA is the reverse transcriptase enzyme. The virus core is surrounded by a nucleocapsid composed of protein. The virus contains a lipoprotein envelope. The major virus coded envelope glycoproteins are the projecting spikes on the surface and the anchoring transmembrane pedicles.

B. Modes of Transmission

There are three modes of transmission: sexual contact, parenteral and perinatal.

1. *Sexual contact:* This is the most important mode of transmission. Sexual transmission occurs among both homosexual as well as heterosexual individuals.
2. *Parenteral transmission:* It may occur through blood after receiving infected blood transfusions, blood products, sharing contaminated syringes and needles as in intravenous drug abusers or accidental inoculation.
3. *Perinatal transmission:* Infection may be transmitted from an infected mother to her child either transplacentally or perinatally.

C. Clinical Features

HIV infects all cells expressing at their surface the CD4 antigen, which is the receptor for the virus. It infects primarily the CD4+ lymphocytes. The clinical course of HIV infection can present as follows:

1. *Acute HIV infection*
2. *Asymptomatic infection*
3. *Persistent generalised lymphadenopathy (PGL)*
4. *Symptomatic HIV infection*

When CD4+ cells fall below 200 per mm^3, the titre of virus increases markedly and there is irreversible breakdown of immune defence mechanisms, it is defined as AIDS. Most of the patients with HIV disease die of

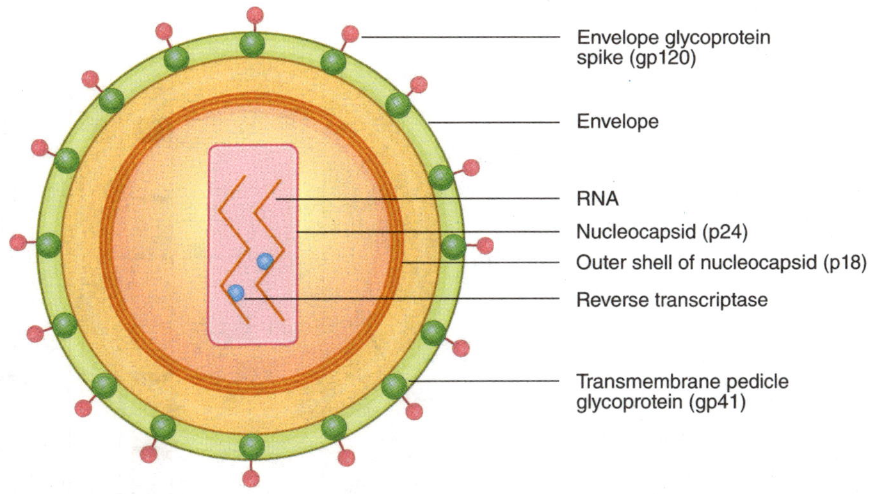

Fig. 42.1 Structure of Human immunodeficiency virus

infections other than HIV e.g. opportunistic infections and malignancies (Table 42.1). AIDS is the end stage of HIV infection.

Table 42.1: Opportunistic Infections and Malignancies Commonly Associated with HIV Infection.

I.	**Bacterial**
	1. Mycobacterial infections—Tuberculosis and non-tuberculous infections
	2. M. avium complex
	3. Salmonellosis
II.	**Viral**
	1. CMV
	2. Herpes simplex
	3. Varicella-zoster
	4. Epstein-Barr (EB) virus
III.	**Mycotic**
	1. *Pneumocystis jiroveci* pneumonia
	2. Candidiasis
	3. Cryptococcosis
	4. Aspergillosis
	5. Histoplasmosis
	6. Coccidioidomycosis
IV.	**Parasitic**
	1. Toxoplasmosis
	2. Cryptosporidiosis
	3. Isosporiasis
	4. Generalised strongyloidiasis
V.	**Malignancies**
	1. Kaposi's sarcoma
	2. B-cell lymphoma or non-Hodgkin's lymphoma

D. Laboratory Diagnosis

1. Specific Tests for HIV Infections

(i) Antigen detection

The p24 antigen is the earliest virus marker to appear in the blood. ELISA can be used for detection of this antigen. Virus isolation is an important test for diagnosis in window period when antibodies are absent in serum of patient.

(ii) Virus isolation

For diagnosis, virus is not routinely isolated. It can be isolated from CD4 lymphocytes of peripheral blood, bone-marrow and serum. Virus isolation is an important test for diagnosis in window period when antibodies are absent in serum of patient.

(iii) Detection of viral nucleic acid

Viral nucleic acid can be detected by polymerase chain reaction (PCR). The test is highly sensitive and specific. It is also useful for diagnosis in window period.

(iv) Antibody detection

Demonstration of antibodies is the simplest and most commonly employed technique for diagnosis. It may take several weeks to months for antibodies to appear after infection. HIV infected persons remain negative for antibodies during *window period*, when initial viral replication takes place for about 2-3 weeks.

There are two types of serological tests—screening and supplemental.

Screening tests

(a) ***ELISA test***: ELISA is the method most commonly used. It is highly sensitive and specific test. It is an extremely good screening test and most laboratories use a commercial ELISA kit that contains both HIV-1 and HIV-2.
Saliva is an acceptable alternative to serum for antibody testing by ELISA.

(b) ***Rapid tests***: These tests take less than 30 minutes and do not require expensive equipment. The rapid tests include dot-blot assay, particle agglutination, HIV spot and comb tests.
Rapid tests are the most commonly used in India.

(c) ***Simple tests***: They take 1–2 hours and do not require expensive equipment.

Supplemental test

Western blot test: In this test, HIV proteins are separated and these proteins are blotted on to strips of nitrocellulose paper. These strips are reacted with test sera. Antibodies to HIV proteins, if present in test serum, combine with different fragments of HIV. The position of the colour band on the strip indicates the fragment of antigen with which antibodies have reacted (Fig. 42.2).

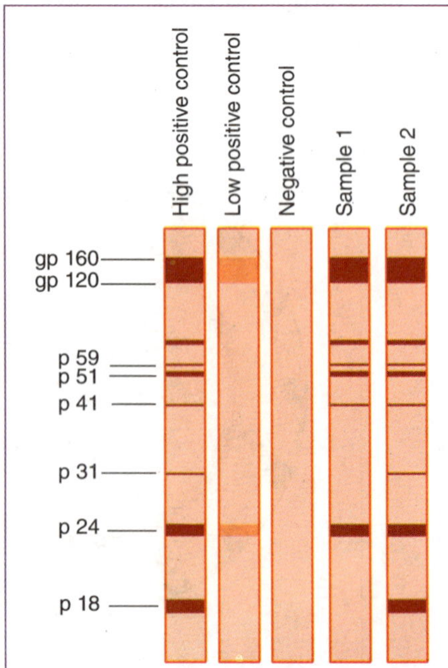

Fig. 42.2 Diagrammatic representation of Western blot test for HIV

A positive result in any one screening test may not be accepted without confirmation. It was the practice to use the Western blot test for confirmation. As the test is cumbersome, costly and not readily available, different strategies are followed for confirmation. The practice now is to perform either two different types of ELISA or an ELISA with any of the rapid tests. A serum positive in both tests is considered positive.

2. *Non-specific Tests*

(i) Total and differential leucocyte count

In AIDS, there is leucopenia with a lymphocyte count less than 400 per mm^3.

(ii) T-lymphocyte subset assays

The normal CD4 : CD8 T-cell ratio of 2 : 1, is reversed to 0.5 : 1 in cases of AIDS. The count of CD4 lymphocytes falls below 200 per mm^3.

E. Prevention

The following preventive measures are recommended.

1. *Sexual contact*: The use of condoms can prevent transmission of the virus.
2. *Sharing needles*: Contaminated syringes or needles should not be shared.
3. *Blood*: All blood and blood products are to be screened for HIV. This also applies to donation of cornea, semen, marrow, kidney and other organs.
4. Isolation of AIDS patient and initiation of treatment.
5. *Control of infection*: Screening of individuals within risk groups helps to identify the HIV infected persons.

F. Prophylaxis

No effective vaccine has yet been found out.

G. Antiretroviral Therapy (ART)

According to NACO guidelines 2018, all patients should be started on ART. This is called **TREAT ALL.**

Specific treatment with antiretroviral drugs is the mainstay in the management of HIV infection. Antiretroviral drugs include both nucleoside and non-nucleoside inhibitors of enzyme reverse transcriptase, viral pretease inhibitors, fusion inhibitor, integrase inhibitor and entry inhibitor (Table 42.2). These drugs have been used in various combinations.

Apart from specific antiretroviral therapy, other measures in the treatment of AIDS include (i) treatment and prophylaxis of opportunistic infections and tumours (ii) general management and (iii) immunorestorative measures.

H. Postexposure Prophylaxis (PEP)

Exposure to blood, body fluid, other potentially infected material or an instrument contaminated with one of these materials may lead to risk of acquiring HIV infection. The risk of infection varies with the type of exposure and other factors. Most exposures do not result in infection. Health workers are normally at very low risk of acquiring infection during management of infected patients. Following exposure, postexposure prophylaxis (PEP) may be required depending upon the category of exposure and HIV status of exposure source. Tenofovir 300 mg + Lamivudine 300 mg + Dolutegravir 50 mg in fixed dose combination (FDC) in one tablet should be given within 2 hours of accidental exposure and then from next day one tablet once a day (OD) for 4 weeks. To be effective these drugs must be started within the first 72 hours and ideally within 2 hours. Both risk of infection and possible side-effects of antiretroviral drugs should be carefully considered when deciding to start PEP. Besides PEP, injured site on the wound should be thoroughly washed with soap and water. Antiseptics may also be used.

Table 42.2 Antiretroviral Drugs

Nucleoside reverse transcriptase inhibitors (NsRTIs)	Non-nucleoside reverse transcriptase inhibitors (NNRTIs)	Protease inhibitors	Fusion inhibitor	Integrase Inhibitors	CCR5 Entry inhibitor
*Zidovudine** *(AZT, ZDV)*	*Nevirapine (NVP)**	*Saquinavir (SQV)*	*Enfuvirtide (T20)*	*Raltegravir* (RGV)*	Maraviroc *(MVC)*
Didanosine (ddI)	*Delaviridine (DLV)*	*Ritonavir (RTV)**		*Elvitegravir (EVG)*	
Zalcitabine (ddc)	*Efavirnez (EFV)**	*Indinavir (IDV)*		*Dolutegravir (DIG)*	
Stavudine (d4T)	*Etravirine (ETR)*	*Nelfinavir (NFV)*			
*Lamivudine (3TC)**	Rilpivirine (RPV)	*Lopinavir (LPV)**			
*Abacavir (ABC)**		*Amprenavir (APV)*			
Emitricitabine (FTC)		*Tipranavir (TPV)*			
		*Atazanavir (ATV)**			
		Fosamprenavir (FPV)			
		*Darunavir (DRV)**			
Nucleotide reverse transcriptase inhibitor (NtRTI) *Tenofovir**					

*Available in National Programme.

KEY POINTS

1. Retroviruses possess *reverse transcriptase* (*RNA directed DNA polymerase*) *enzyme* which prepares a DNA copy of the RNA genome in host cell. The presence of enzyme reverse transcriptase is a characteristic feature.
2. Human immunodeficiency virus (HIV), the causative agent of AIDS, belongs to retroviruses.
3. There are three modes of transmission of HIV infection. These are *sexual contact*, *parenteral* and *perinatal*.
4. HIV infects principally the *CD4 lymphocytes*.
5. Laboratory diagnosis of HIV infection includes specific tests for HIV and non-specific tests. Specific tests include *antigen* (*p24*) *detection*, *virus isolation*, detection of *viral nucleic acid* and *antibody detection*.
6. Demonstration of antibodies is the simplest and most commonly employed technique for diagnosis. *ELISA* is the method *most commonly used method for detection of antibodies*.
7. Specific treatment with *antiretroviral drugs* is the mainstay in the management of HIV infection.
8. *Postexposure prophylaxis* (PEP) may be required when there is exposure to blood, body fluids, other potentially infected material or an instrument contaminated with HIV.

STUDY QUESTIONS

1. Describe the morphology of HIV and laboratory diagnosis of HIV infection.
2. Write briefly about modes of transmission of HIV infection.

MULTIPLE CHOICE QUESTIONS (MCQs)

1. What is the characteristic feature of viruses belonging to family *Retroviridae*?
   (a) Presence of enzyme reverse transcriptase
   (b) Presence of envelope
   (c) Presence of nucleic acid
   (d) Presence of lipid
2. What is the mode of transmission of human immunodeficiency virus?
   (a) Sexual contact
   (b) Parenteral transmission
   (c) Perinatal transmission
   (d) All of the above
3. Which type of cells are most often infected by HIV?
   (a) CD4+T lymphocytes
   (b) CD8+T lymphocytes
   (c) B lymphocytes
   (d) None of the above
4. Which of the following tests is the most commonly employed for diagnosis of HIV infection?
   (a) Virus isolation
   (b) Antibody detection
   (c) Viral nucleic acid detection
   (d) None of the above

ANSWERS (MCQs) ...✓

1. (a) 2. (d) 3. (a) 4. (b)

Unit V

MYCOLOGY

43

Medical Mycology

I. INTRODUCTION

1. Study of fungi is called *Mycology*.
2. All fungi are eukaryotic.
3. Water, soil and decaying organic debris are natural habitat.
4. Fungi are obligate or facultative aerobe.

II. DIFFERENCES OF FUNGI FROM BACTERIA

1. They possess rigid cell walls containing chitin, mannan and other polysaccharides.
2. The cytoplasmic membrane contains sterols.
3. The cytoplasm contains true nuclei with nuclear membrane, mitochondria and endoplasmic reticulum.
4. Fungi may be unicellular or multicellular.
5. They divide asexually, sexually or by both processes.

III. LABORATORY DIAGNOSIS

A. Direct Microscopy

1. Potassium Hydroxide (KOH) Preparation

Specimen is placed in a drop of 10% KOH on a microscopic slide and covered with a coverslip. It is heated gently and examined under microscope. Yeasts cells and hyphae may be observed.

2. Gram Staining

It is done to observe Gram positive yeasts as in case of Candida species.

3. India Ink Preparation

India ink preparation may be used for detection of capsulated yeasts such as *Cryptococcus neoformans* in cerebrospinal fluid (CSF).

B. Culture

1. Sabouraud's dextrose agar (SDA) and SDA medium with antibiotics are inoculated and incubated at 25°C and 37°C for three weeks (Fig. 43.1). Chloramphenicol is added in the culture medium to suppress the growth of contaminating bacteria while cycloheximide (actidione) is incorporated to suppress the contaminating fungi.

   Brain heart infusion (BHI) agar with blood and antibiotics is another medium used for primary isolation of fungi.
2. Microscopy is performed from fungal colony to study the morphology of hyphae, spores and other structures. Teased mounts are prepared in lactophenol cotton blue (LCB) which contains lactic acid, phenol, glycerol and cotton blue.

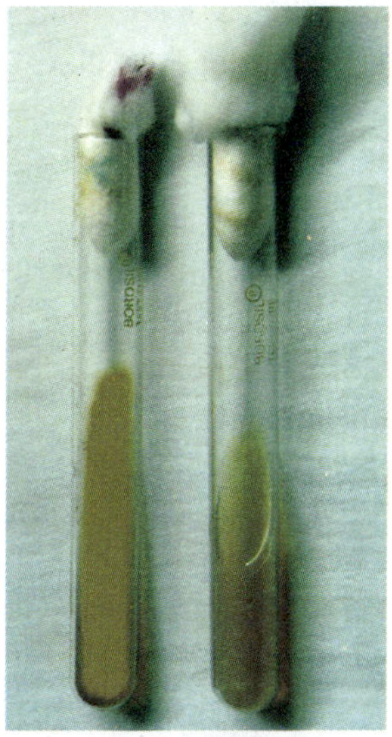

Fig. 43.1 Sabouraud's dextrose agar (SDA) slope with and without antibiotics

IV. FUNGAL DISEASES

A. Superficial Mycoses

Superficial mycoses

- Surface infections, e.g. Tinea versicolor, Tinea nigra, Piedra
- Cutaneous infections, e.g. Dermatophytes

Dermatophytes

(i) Dermatophytes are a group of fungi that infect only superficial keratinised tissue (skin, hair and nails) without involving the living tissue.

(ii) They break down and utilise keratin.
(iii) They are incapable of penetrating subcutaneous tissue.
(iv) They cause *dermatophytoses*, also known as tinea or ringworm.

Classification

Dermatophytes are classified into three genera as follows:

	Genus		Infection of
1.	**Trichophyton**	—	Hair, skin, nail
2.	**Microsporum**	—	Hair, skin
3.	**Epidermophyton**	—	Skin, nail

Laboratory diagnosis

Specimens

Skin scrappings
Hair plucks
Nail clippings

Direct microscopy

- Direct 10% KOH mount may show fungal hyphae.

Culture

- SDA and SDA with antibiotics are used.
- Culture media are incubated at 25–30°C for three weeks.
- Identification of dermatophytes is based on
  - colony morphology
  - pigment production
  - microconidia and macroconidia.
- Colony characters
  - White to creamy, cottony growth
  - Reverse of media is red in *T. rubrum*.
- Microscopy
  - Lactophenol cotton blue preparation from colony reveals microconidia, macroconidia or both.

Treatment of dermatophytoses

Topical antifungal agents are generally used for treatment. Oral griseofulvin is the drug of choice.

B. Subcutaneous Mycoses

1. Mycetoma

(i) Mycetoma is a chronic granulomatous infection of the subcutaneous tissue, usually affects the foot and rarely the other parts of body.
(ii) The disease was first described from Madurai, South India. It is therefore commonly referred to as **Madura foot** or **Maduramycosis**.
(iii) The disease is quite common in Tamil Nadu.

Aetiology

- Mycetoma is caused by a number of actinomycetes and filamentous fungi.

Pathogenesis

- The causative organism is believed to enter the body through minor trauma.
- The disease begins as a **subcutaneous swelling** usually of foot, which enlarges and burrows into the deeper tissues producing characteristic abscess. The abscess bursts with the formation of **chronic multiple sinuses** discharging viscid, seropurulent fluid containing granules.
- The colour and consistency of the granules vary with the different causative agents.

Laboratory diagnosis

- Diagnosis is made from examination of granules.

Treatment

Actinomycotic mycetoma usually respond well to sulphonamides and antibiotics, but mycotic mycetoma may require amputation.

2. Sporotrichosis

(i) Sporotrichosis is a nodular, ulcerating disease of skin and subcutaneous tissue.
(ii) The fungus gains access through thorn pricks or some injuries.

Causative agent

- **Sporothrix schenckii**—a dimorphic fungus

Morphology

- *S. schenckii* occurs in the yeast phase in the tissues and in cultures at 37°C, and in the mycelial phase in cultures at 22°C–25°C (*dimorphic fungus*).
- Yeast phase appears as cigar-shaped cells and mould form contains hyphae carrying flower like clusters of small conidia borne on delicate sterigmata (Fig. 43.2).

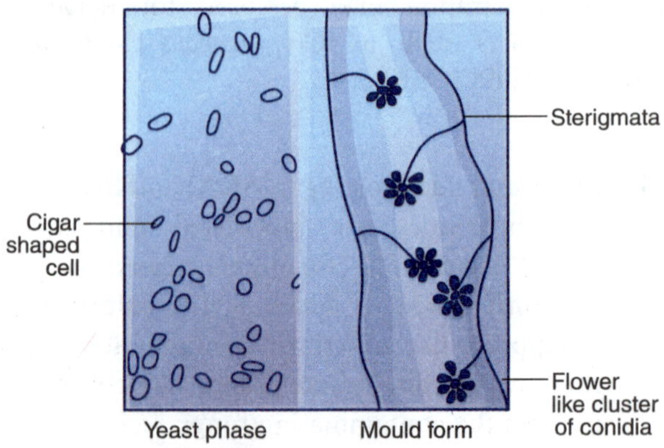

Fig. 43.2 *Sporothrix schenckii*

3. *Rhinosporidiosis*

(i) Rhinosporidiosis is a chronic granulomatous disease characterised by formation of **friable polyps**, usually confined to the **nose**, mouth or eye.
(ii) Causative agent is **Rhinosporidium seeberi.**
(iii) More than 80% cases are reported in India and Sri Lanka.
(iv) The mode of infection is not known but most infections occur in males who have frequent contact with stagnant water or aquatic life.
(v) The fungus has not been cultivated.
(vi) Diagnosis depends on the demonstration of sporangia.

Morphology

- Tissue sections stained with H & E stain show large number of endospores within the sporangia embedded in a stroma of connective tissue and capillaries. The sporangium (10–200 μm) contains thousands of endospores (6-7 μm in diameter) (Fig. 43.3).

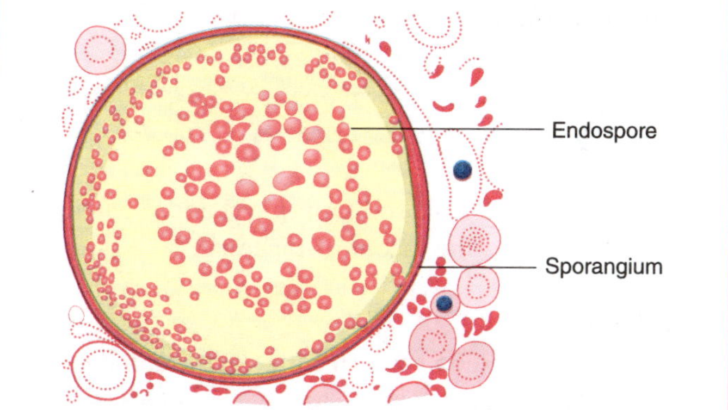

Fig. 43.3 Rhinosporidiosis: sporangium with numerous endospores

C. Systemic Mycoses

1. *Histoplasmosis*

(i) Causative fungus: **Histoplasma capsulatum**, a dimorphic fungus.
(ii) It is primarily a disease of reticulo-endothelial system.
(iii) *H. capsulatum* is an intracellular parasite.

Source of infection

- The fungus is present in the soil enriched with excreta of birds or bats.
- Human infection results from inhalation of spores.

Clinical features

- The large majority of infections are asymptomatic.
- Some individuals develop pulmonary disease which resembles tuberculosis.
- Disseminated histoplasmosis develops only in a minority of infected individuals.
- Involvement of reticuloendothelial system results in lymphadenopathy, hepatosplenomegaly, fever, anaemia and a high rate of fatality.
- Granulomatous and ulcerative lesions may develop on the skin or mucosa.

Morphology

- On microscopy, *H. capsulatum* appears as small oval yeast cell, (2-4 μm in diameter) packed within the cytoplasm of macrophages or monocytes (Fig. 43.4).

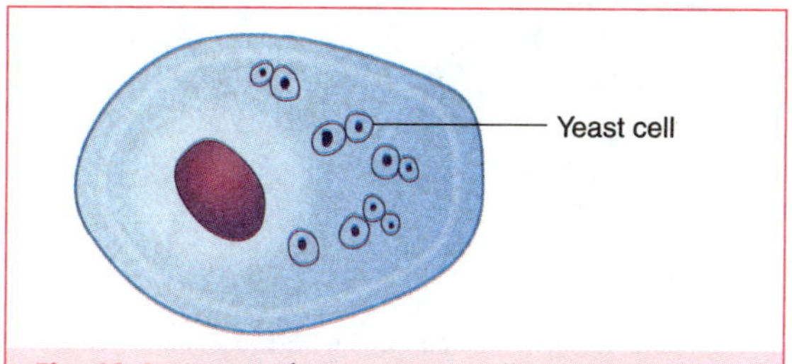

Fig. 43.4 H. capsulatum: yeast cells in macrophage

- The yeast phase is formed in cultures at 37°C. White cottony mycelial growth containing large (8-20 μm) thick walled, spherical spores with tubercles or finger like projections (Fig. 43.5) appears at 25°C.

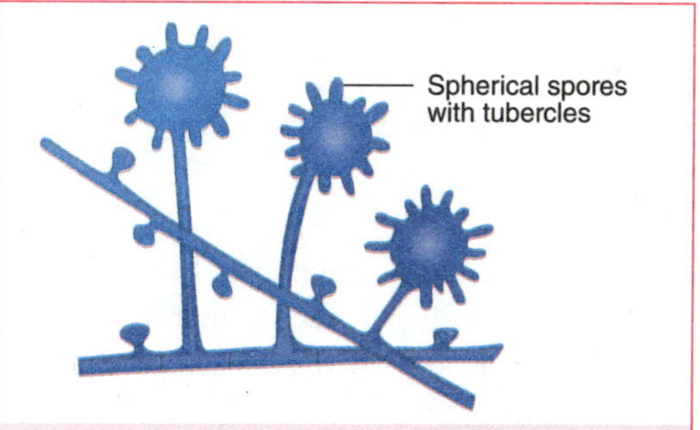

Fig. 43.5 H. capsulatum: mycelial form

2. *Blastomycosis*

(i) Causative fungus: **Blastomyces dermatitidis**, a dimorphic fungus.
(ii) It is a chronic infection of the lungs which may spread to other tissues, particularly skin, bone and genitourinary tract.

Source of infection

- Inhalation of conidia of fungus growing as saprophytes in the soil.

Clinical features

- Asymptomatic
- Mild primary pulmonary disease.
- Disseminated lesions have been found in immunocompromised patients including AIDS.
- Cutaneous blastomycosis.

Morphology

B. dermatitidis is a dimorphic fungus. In tissues and in cultures at 37°C, the fungus appears as spherical or oval budding yeast cells with thick, double contoured walls. Each cell has only a single broad based bud. At 25°C, the culture is filamentous with septate hyphae and many round or oval conidia (Fig. 43.6).

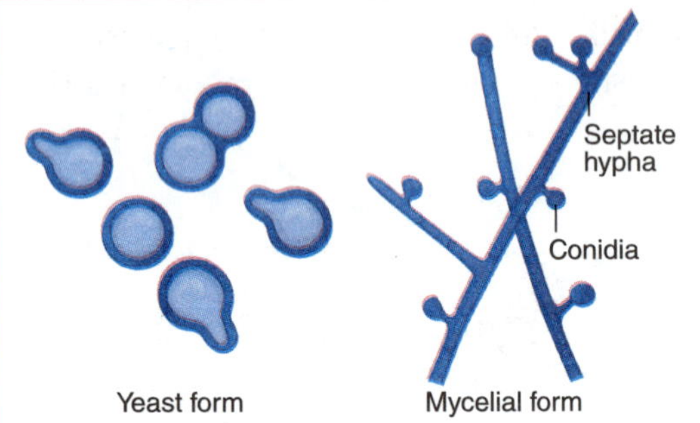

Fig. 43.6 *B.dermatitidis:* yeast and mycelial forms

3. Paracoccidioidomycosis

(i) Causative fungus: **Paracoccidioides brasiliensis**, a dimorphic fungus.
(ii) It is a chronic granulomatous disease involving lungs, mucosa, skin and lymphatic system.

Source of infection

- By inhalation of spores from environmental sources.

Clinical features

- Primary pulmonary infection that spreads by haematogenous route to mucous membranes of mouth, nose, lymph node and adjacent skin, producing chronic granulomatous reaction.
- Ulcerative granulomas of the buccal and nasal mucosa are a prominent feature.

Morphology

- As a dimorphic fungus, it grows as yeast cells with multiple buds in tissues and in cultures at 37°C and in the mycelial phase at 25°C (Fig. 43.7).

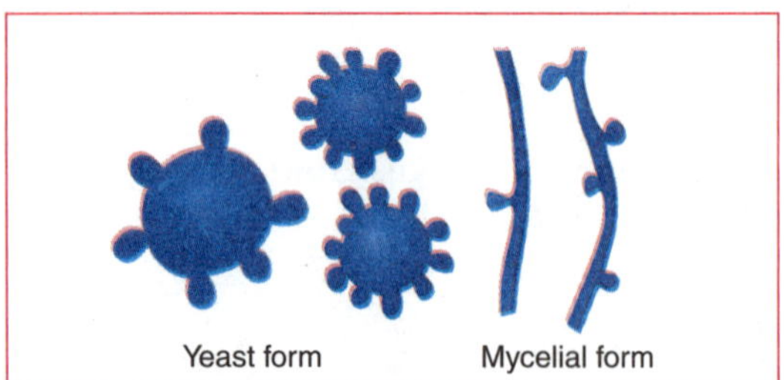

Fig. 43.7 *P. brasiliensis:* yeast and mycelial forms

4. Coccidioidomycosis

Causative fungus: **Coccidioides immitis**, a dimorphic fungus.

Source of infection

- By inhalation of dust containing arthrospores of the fungus.

Clinical features

- Asymptomatic
- Primary pulmonary disease—mild influenza-like fever to severe pneumonia
- Disseminated disease.

Morphology

- Being a dimorphic fungus, it occurs in the tissue as a yeast and in culture (both at 37°C and at 25°C) as the mycelial form.
- The yeast form is a spherule with a thick doubly refractile wall and filled with endospores (Fig. 43.8). Each endospore gives rise to a new spherule.
- The mycelial phase contains pseudo-hyphae which fragment into arthrospores (Fig. 43.8) which are highly infectious.

5. Cryptococcosis

Cryptococcosis is also termed as torulosis.

(i) Causative fungus: *Cryptococcus*, a capsulated yeast.
(ii) *Cryptococcus* has two species *C. neoformans* and *C.gatti*.
(iii) *C. neoformans* is a soil saprophyte and is particularly abundant in the faeces of pigeons.

Morphology

- Spherical budding cell having a prominent polysaccharide capsule (Fig. 43.9).
- It is a true yeast and is Gram positive.
- Capsule may be demonstrated by India-ink or nigrosin staining.

Antigenicity

- On the basis of cryptococcal polysaccharide antigen, *Cryptococcus* has four serotypes (A, B, C and D).

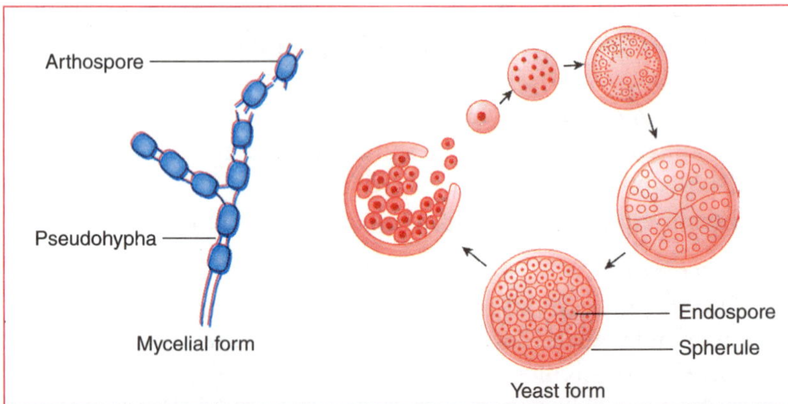

Fig. 43.8 *C. immitis:* arthrospore and spherule stages

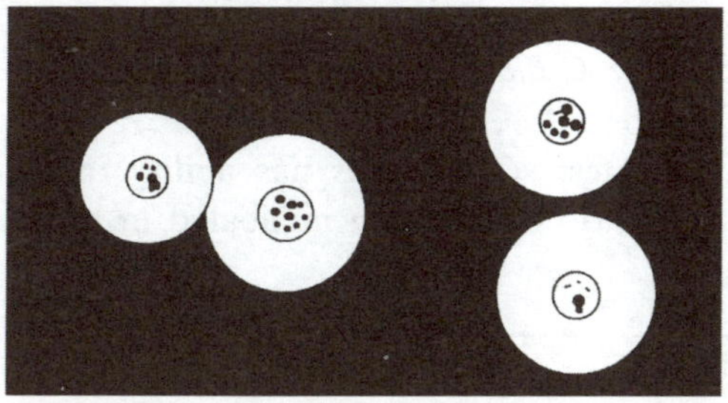

Fig. 43.9 *C. neoformans*

Source of infection

- Infection is usually acquired by inhalation of dust containing yeast cells.

Pathogenesis

- *C. neoformans* is pathogenic in humans and animals.
- The disease is usually seen in immunocompromised host.
- Most infections are asymptomatic.
- Pulmonary cryptococcosis may lead to a mild pneumonitis.
- Cryptococcal meningitis occurs by haematogenous spread. It is often seen in AIDS patients.
- Skin, lymph nodes, bones and other organs may be involved when dissemination of infection occurs. Cutaneous cryptococcosis varies from small ulcers to large granulomas.

Laboratory diagnosis

Specimens

- CSF
- Sputum
- Pus
- Brain tissue

Direct microscopy

- Specimen mixed with a drop of India ink or nigrosin shows round budding yeast cells. In **India ink**, capsule appears as a clear halo around the yeast cells.
- **Gram staining** shows Gram positive yeast cells.

Culture

- Sediment from a centrifuged CSF is inoculated on SDA and incubated at 37°C. Other specimens may also be inoculated on SDA.
- *C. neoformans* grows to form smooth, mucoid, cream coloured colonies.
- Lactophenol cotton blue mount shows budding yeast cells.

Latex agglutination test

- Cryptococcal capsular polysaccharide antigen can be detected in CSF, serum or urine by latex agglutination test.

Animal inoculation test

- Intracerebral or intraperitoneal inoculation into mice leads to a fatal infection in case of *C. neoformans*.

D. Opportunistic Mycoses

Some saprophytic fungi usually do not produce disease but may cause infection under special conditions such as **immunocompromised** individuals and in terminal stages of chronic disease. These are called **opportunistic fungi**.

1. Candidiasis

1. Causative fungus: **Candida albicans** (80–90% of cases)
2. Candidiasis is an infection of skin, mucosa and internal organs, caused by yeast like fungus *Candida albicans*, and occasionally by other candida species.
3. *Candida albicans* is the normal inhabitant of skin, gastrointestinal tract, oral and vaginal cavities.

Morphology

C. albicans is an ovoid or spherical budding yeast cell, 3–5 µm in diameter.

Pathogenesis

(i) Candidiasis is an opportunistic endogenous infection.

(ii) Predisposing factors for candidiasis are diabetes, immunodeficiency, malignancy, prolonged administration of antibiotics, patients on immuno-suppressive drugs and intravenous catheters.

(iii) Lesions caused by candida are as follows:

(a) Mucocutaneous lesions
- Oral thrush
- Vulvovaginitis
- Balanitis
- Conjunctivitis
- Keratitis

(b) Skin and nail infections
- Skin—Infections of axillae, groin, perineum and submammary folds.
- Nails—Infections of finger webs, nail folds and nails may occur. Paronychia and onychia are seen in those persons who frequently immerse their hands in water.
- In infants it may lead to napkin dermatitis.

(c) Systemic candidiasis
- Urinary tract infection
- Intestinal candidiasis: It is a frequent sequel to oral antibiotic therapy and present as diarrhoea.
- Pulmonary candidiasis
- Endocarditis
- Meningitis
- Septicaemia
- Nesocomial candidiasis

Thrush (Pseudomembranous candidiasis): The lesions are soft, white, slightly elevated plaques frequently occurring on the buccal mucosa of tongue, but may also be seen on the gingiva, palate and floor of the mouth. In severe cases, the entire oral cavity may be affected. Thrush is very common in patients with HIV infection or in cancer patients undergoing chemotherapy or radiotherapy. Infection may also be seen in neonates and infants due to incompletely developed immune system. It is also common in debilitated and chronically ill persons.

Laboratory diagnosis

(i) Direct microscopy

Gram stained smears and KOH mounts from lesions of skin, nail or mucous membranes show budding Gram positive yeast cells.

(ii) Culture

(a) Candida species grow well on SDA and ordinary bacteriological culture media e.g. blood agar.
(b) They grow at 25-37°C within 24 hours.
(c) Cream coloured, smooth, pasty colonies appear (Fig. 43.10).

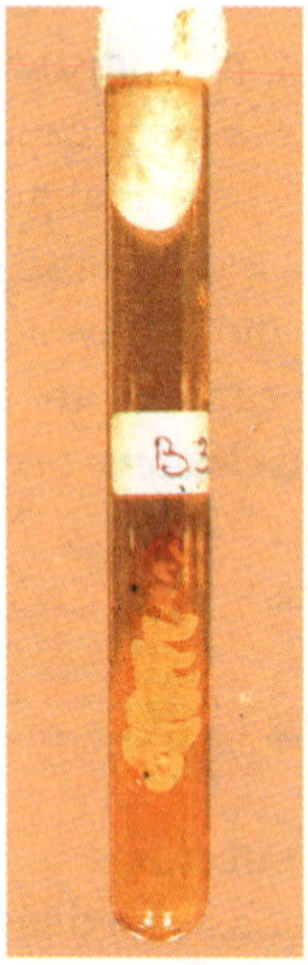

Fig. 43.10 Growth of *Candida albicans* on SDA slope

(d) Gram stained smear from colonies shows Gram positive budding yeast cells (Fig. 43.11).

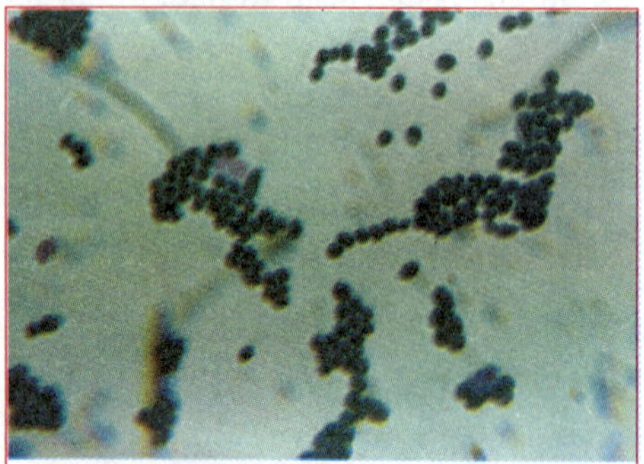

Fig. 43.11 Gram stained smear of *Candida albicans*

(iii) Identification

To differentiate *C. albicans* from other species, the 'Germ tube test' is done.

Germ tube test: *C. albicans* has ability to form germ tubes within two hours when incubated in human serum at 37°C (Fig. 43.12).

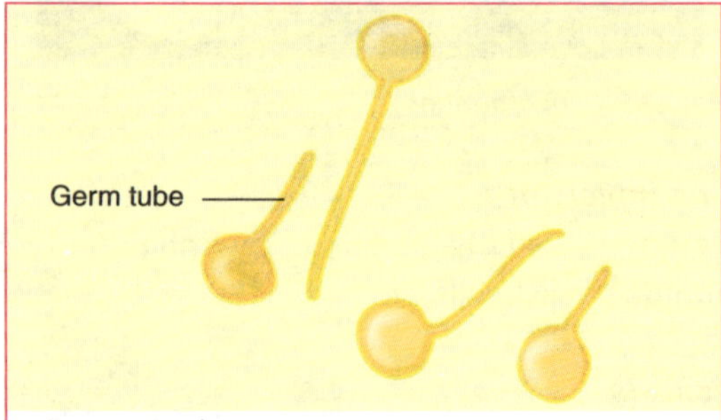

Fig. 43.12 Germ tube formation

2. *Aspergillosis*

1. Aspergilli are ubiquitous in nature.
2. **Aspergillus fumigatus** is the main opportunistic pathogen.
3. Other important species are *A. niger* and *A. flavus.*

Pathogenesis

(i) Aspergillosis is caused by inhalation of *Aspergillus* conidia or mycelial fragments which are present on the decaying matter, soil or air.
(ii) When the host defence is compromised, aspergillosis may develop.
(iii) There are three clinical forms of systemic aspergillosis.
   (a) Respiratory disease
      • Aspergillus asthma
      • Allergic bronchopulmonary aspergillosis (ABPA)
      • Aspergilloma
   (b) Invasive aspergillosis
   (c) Superficial infections
      • Mycotic keratitis
      • Otomycosis

Laboratory diagnosis

(i) Specimens

- Sputum
- Bronchoalveolar lavage
- Biopsy

(ii) Direct microscopy

- KOH preparation of the specimen reveals non-pigmented septate hyphae with characteristic dichotomous branching (at an angle of approximately 45°).
- Biopsy sections can be stained with H & E and PAS staining and examined for the characteristic hyphae.

(iii) Culture

- The clinical specimen is inoculated on SDA without cycloheximide and incubated at 25°C.
- Colonies appear within 1–2 days and show a velvety to powdery surface. Colonies are coloured.
- *A. fumigatus*–green coloured colonies, *A. niger*–black colonies and *A. flavus*—golden-yellow coloured colonies.
- Lactophenol cotton blue preparation from colonies shows branching and septate hyphae. Asexual conidia are arranged in chains, carried on phialides (formerly termed sterigmata), borne on the expanded ends (vesicles) of conidiophores (Fig. 43.13).

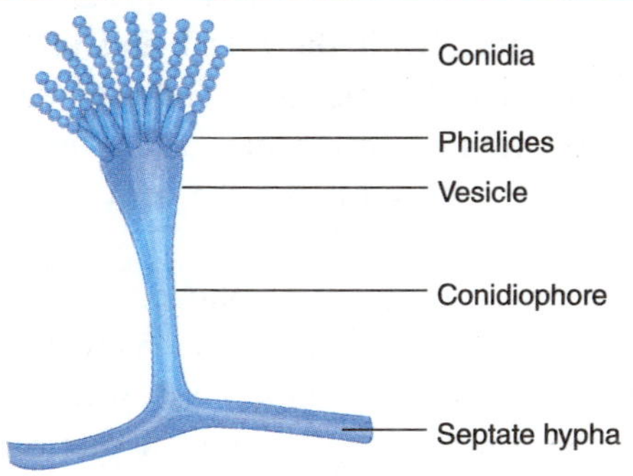

Fig. 43.13 *Aspergillus*

3. Mucormycosis

1. Three main genera *Mucor, Rhizopus* and *Lichtheimia* (formerly *Absidia*) are associated with mucormycosis.
2. These fungi are saprophytes of soil, manure and decaying vegetables.
3. **Mode of infection** is by inhalation of spores.
4. These are normally avirulent and are able to cause disease only when general resistance is extremely low.
5. The **primary infection** is usually in **upper respiratory tract or nose**.
6. Rhinocerebral form of disease **(Rhinocerebral mucormycosis)** is characterised by spreading lesion from nasal mucosa to turbinate bone, paranasal sinuses, orbit and brain. It occurs commonly in patients with diabetic ketoacidosis. It was also isolated from COVID-19 patients.
7. *Mucor* and *Lichtheimia* are most commonly isolated from **mucormycosis**.
8. Rhizopus causes mucormycosis and **otomycosis**.
9. Lichtheimia may also cause **keratitis**.
10. **Pulmonary mucormycosis** is a progressive severe pneumonia. The fungi may spread haematogenously to other areas of the lung and to other organs such as brain.
11. **Gastrointestinal mucormycosis** may occur in malnutrition, uraemia and diarrhoeal diseases.

Laboratory Diagnosis

(i) Specimens

- Scrapings from the lesions
- Pus
- Sputum
- Nasal discharge

(ii) Direct microscopy

- KOH wet mounts of specimens show non-septate hyphae.
- Histological sections stained with H&E stain reveal the presence of hyphae.

(iii) Culture

- Fungi can be readily grown on SDA without cycloheximide at 37°C.
- Lactophenol cotton blue preparation of colonies shows branched sporangiophores arising randomly along aerial mycelium. In the case of mucor rhizoids are absent. Rhizopus has rhizoids, and sporangiospore arise in groups directly above the rhizoids. Lichtheimia has also rhizoids but sporangiophores arise from the aerial mycelium in between the rhizoids (Fig. 43.14).

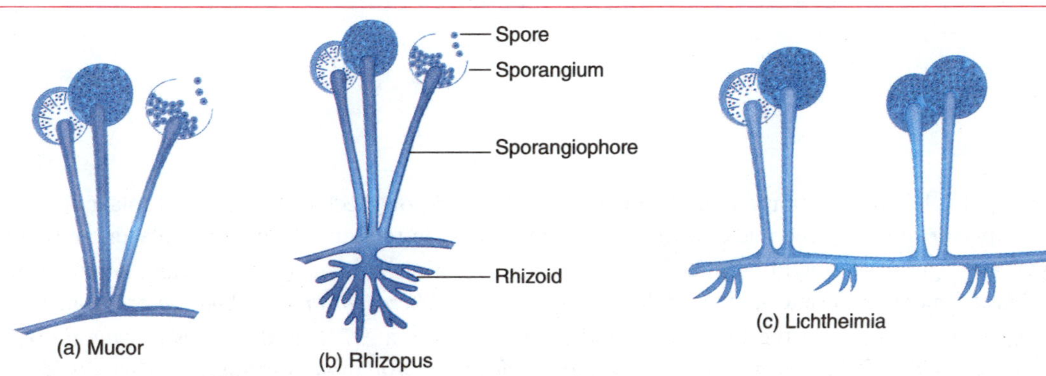

Fig. 43.14 Zygomycetes: (a) Mucor (b) Rhizopus (c) Lichtheimia

Treatment

Amphotericin B is the drug of choice for treatment of mucormycosis.

4. Penicillosis

1. Penicillium species, rarely cause opportunistic human infections.
2. It causes penicillosis, keratitis, otomycosis and rarely deep infections.
3. This saprophytic fungus contains septate hyphae and bears flask-shaped phialides which in turn supports the chains of round conidia. Members of this genus are identified by the brush or broom like arrangement of conidia (Fig. 43.15).

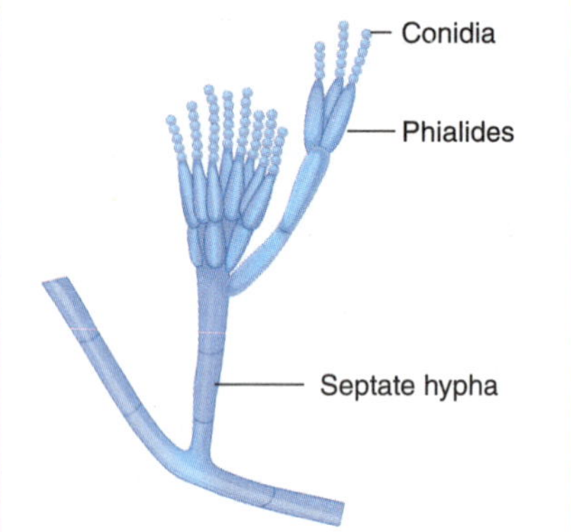

Fig. 43.15 Penicillium

4. The fungus grows rapidly on SDA.
5. The colonies are initially velvety and white but later on become powdery and blue green.
6. *P. marneffei* has been reported as an important opportunist pathogen in the HIV infected individuals.
7. *Useful Penicillium:* Penicillin, an antibiotic was originally obtained from fungus *Penicillium notatum* but the present source is a high yielding mutant of *Penicillium chrysogenum*. Another species *Penicillium comberti* is used in ripening of certain cheese.

PNEUMOCYSTIS JIROVECI

1. *Pneumocystis jiroveci* causes pneumonia in immunocompromised patients. Until recently, it was thought to be a protozoan, but now it has been included in fungi. Molecular studies proved it as a fungus, an ascomycete. Prior to the introduction of chemoprophylaxis, it was a major cause of death among AIDS patients. *P. jiroveci* is a human species and *P. carinii* is found only in rats.
2. *P. jiroveci* has three stages: thin walled trophozoites (1-5 µm), the precyst (5-8 µm) and thick walled spherical cysts (about 8 µm). Cyst contains up to 8 intracystic bodies.
3. Transmission of the organism occurs through the respiratory route, with the cyst being infective stage.
4. Bronchoalveolar lavage, lung biopsy and induced sputum (by administration of a saline mist to induce production of sputum) are the specimens used for diagnosis.
5. Direct demonstration of trophozoites and cysts can be done by Giemsa, toludine blue, methenamine silver and calcofluor white stains. Cyst wall stains black with methenamine silver staining. Cysts often have a punched out "ping-pong ball" appearance. Fluorescent monoclonal antibody staining shows 'honeycomb' appearance of the cyst. The organism can not be cultured.
6. Serological tests can be used for diagnosis in suspected cases. Complement fixation titres of 1:4 or more is indicative of active disease. Latex agglutination test is also used.
7. Polymerase chain reaction (PCR) for amplification of *P. jiroveci* DNA is a rapid method for detection of early infection.
8. Trimethoprim-sulphamethoxazole used in treatment of acute cases of pneumonia.
9. Trimethoprim-sulphamethoxazole or aerosolized pentamidine are used for chemoprophylaxis.

KEY POINTS

1. Fungi possess rigid cell walls containing chitin, mannan and other polysaccharides. The cytoplasmic membrane contains sterols. The cytoplasm contains true nuclei with nuclear membrane, mitochondria and endoplasmic reticulum.
2. Dermatophytes are a group of fungi that infect only superficial keratinised tissue (*skin*, *hair* and *nails*) without involving the living tissue. Three genera of dermatophytes include *Trichophyton*, *Microsporum* and *Epidermophyton*.
3. *Dimorphic fungi* exist as *yeasts* in the host tissue and in the cultures at *37°C* and as *hyphal* (*mycelial*) forms in the soil and in the cultures at *22-25°C*. *Sporothrix schenckii*, *Histoplasma capsulatum*, *Blastomyces dermatitidis*, *Paracoccidioides brasiliensis*, and *Coccidioides immitis* are examples of dimorphic fungi.

4. *Cryptococcosis* is caused by *Cryptococcus*, a *capsulated yeast*. Cryptococcal meningitis is an important manifestation caused by *C. neoformans*. The disease is usually seen in immunocompromised host.
5. Some saprophytic fungi usually do not produce disease but may cause infection under special conditions such as immunocompromised individuals and in terminal stages of chronic disease. These are called *opportunistic fungi. Candida albicans, Aspergillus sp.*, and *Penicillium sp.* are some examples of opportunistic fungi.
6. *Candida albicans* is an ovoid or spherical budding *yeast* cell. It causes *oral thrush, vulvovaginitis, keratitis, paronychia, onychia, napkin dermatitis in infants, urinary tract infection, intestinal candidiasis, pulmonary candidiasis, meningitis* and *septicaemia. C. albicans* has ability to form *germ tube*.
7. Laboratory diagnosis of fungal infections consists of *direct microscopy, and culture* on *Sabouraud's dextrose agar (SDA)*.

STUDY QUESTION

1. Write short notes on:
   (i) Rhinosporidiosis
   (ii) Mycetoma
   (iii) Dermatophytes
   (iv) Histoplasmosis
   (v) Dimorphic fungi
   (vi) Cryptococcosis
   (vii) Opportunistic mycoses
   (viii) Candidiasis
   (ix) *Penicillium species*
   (x) *Pneumocystis jiroveci*

MULTIPLE CHOICE QUESTIONS (MCQs)

1. Which of the following dermatophytes can infect hair, skin and nail?
   (a) Trichophyton
   (b) Microsporum
   (c) Epidermophyton
   (d) All of the above
2. Which of the following fungi has not been cultured?
   (a) *Sporothrix*
   (b) *Rhinosporidium*
   (c) *Acremonium*
   (d) *Blastomyces*
3. Which of the following fungi is a capsulated?
   (a) *Candida albicans*
   (b) *Cryptococcus neoformans*
   (c) *Aspergillus fumigatus*
   (d) None of the above
4. Which animal is used for pathogenicity test in *Cryptococcus neoformans*?
   (a) Mice
   (b) Rabbit
   (c) Guinea pig
   (d) None of the above
5. Which of the following species of *Candida* is responsible for most of the cases in human infections?
   (a) *Candida albicans*
   (b) *C. krusei*
   (c) *C. glabrata*
   (d) *C. stellatoidea*
6. Which of the following infections may occur by *candida albicans*?
   (a) Oral thrush
   (b) Vulvovaginitis
   (c) Poronychia
   (d) All of the above
7. Which of the following *Aspergillus* species produce green coloured colonies on Sabouraud's dextrose agar?
   (a) *Aspergillus fumigatus*
   (b) *A. niger*
   (c) *A. flavus*
   (d) None of the above
8. Which of the following fungi are important opportunistic pathogens in immunocompromised patients?
   (a) *Pneumocystis jiroveci*
   (b) *Penicillium marneffei*
   (c) *Candida albicans*
   (d) All of the above

ANSWERS (MCQs) ...✓

1. (a) 2. (b) 3. (b) 4. (a) 5. (a) 6. (d) 7. (a) 8. (d)

Unit VI

PARASITOLOGY

Medical Parasitology

44

Medical parasitology deals with parasites which infect and produce disease in human beings.

Parasite: A parasite is a living organism which depends on a living host for its survival and derives nutrition from the host, without giving any benefit to the host.

Host: It is defined as an organism which harbours the parasite. Different types of host are as follows:

1. *Definitive host:* It is the host that harbours the adult stage of the parasite or where the parasite replicates sexually.
2. *Intermediate host:* It is the host that harbours the larval stages of the parasite or where the parasite replicates asexually.
3. *Reservoir host:* It is the host that harbours the parasite and acts as an important source of infection.

Classification of Parasites

Parasites are classified into protozoa and helminths. A classification of parasites of medical importance is given in Table 44.1.

Table 44.1: Classification of Parasites

Group	Examples
I. Protozoa (Unicellular)	
1. Amoebae	*Entamoeba histolytica* *E. gingivalis*
2. Flagellates	*Giardia lamblia* *Trichomonas vaginalis* *Leishmania sp.*
3. Sporozoa	*Plasmodium vivax* *P. falciparum* *Toxoplasma gondii*
4. Ciliates	*Balantidium coli*
II. Helminths (Multicellular)	
1. Trematodes	*Fasciola sp.* *Schistosoma sp.*
2. Cestodes	*Taenia sp.* *Echinococcus sp.*
3. Nematodes	Roundworm Hookworm Threadworm

I. PROTOZOA

A. Entamoeba histolytica

Entamoeba histolytica is worldwide in distribution but more common in tropical and subtropical countries. Trophozoites of *E.histolytica* lives in mucosa and submucosa of large intestine of man.

1. Morphology

The parasite exists in three forms: trophozoite, pre-cystic stage and cyst (Fig. 44.1).

(i) ***Trophozoite:*** It measures 18-40 µm (average 20-30 µm) in diameter. The cytoplasm of the trophozoite is divided into two portions—a clear outer *ectoplasm* and a granular *endoplasm*. Trophozoites are motile by pseudopodia. Pseudopodia are long finger-like projections of ectoplasm into which endoplasm flows. Nucleus of trophozoite is spherical in shape and varies in size from 4 to 6 µm. In stained preparation, it shows a small dot like structure, *karyosome*, which is central in position and surrounded by a clear halo. Nuclear membrane is delicate and lined with a layer of chromatin granules. The space between the karyosome and the nuclear membrane is traversed by linin network which has a spoke-like radial arrangement.

(ii) ***Pre-cystic stage:*** It is smaller in size and varies from 10 to 20 µm in diameter. It is round or oval with a blunt pseudopodium. Nucleus has similar characters as that of trophozoite.

(iii) ***Cyst:*** It is round, 10-15 µm in diameter and is surrounded by a highly refractile membrane, called the *cyst wall*. Nuclear structure is similar to that of trophozoite. A mature cyst is a quadrinucleate spherical body. It starts as a uninucleate body but soon divides by binary fission to form two and then four nuclei. Uninucleate and binucleate bodies also possess a glycogen mass and 1-4 chromidial or chromatoid bars. Glycogen mass stains brown with iodine. Chromatoid bars do not stain with iodine but appear as refractile bars with rounded ends in preparations with normal

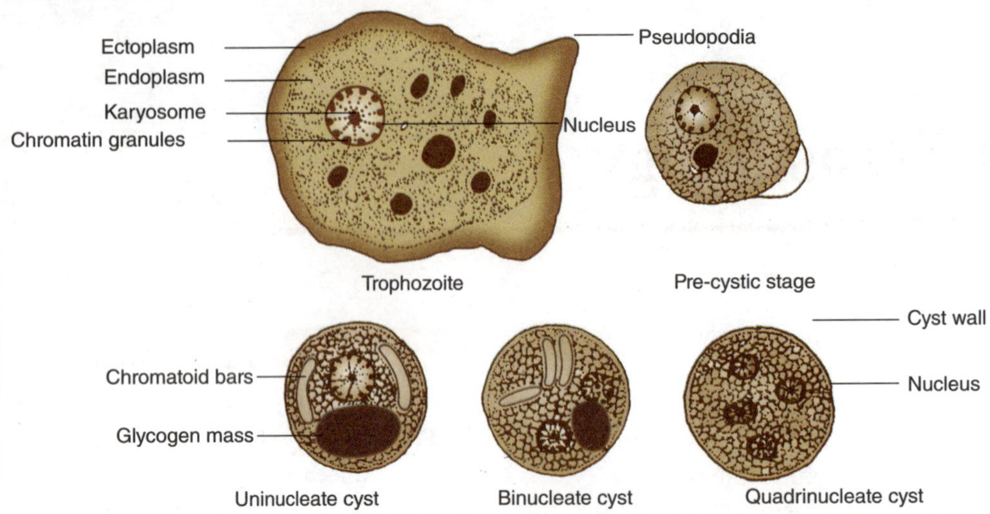

Fig. 44.1 Different morphological forms of *Entamoeba histolytica*

saline. These bars stain black with iron-haematoxylin stain. In a mature cyst (quadrinucleate), both the glycogen mass and chromatoid bars disappear.

2. *Life Cycle*

E. histolytica passes its life cycle in only one host (Fig. 44.2). The mature quadrinucleate cysts are the infective forms. Man acquires the infection by ingestion of water and food containing these cysts. When the cyst reaches the caecum or the lower part of the ileum, the *excystation* occurs. During this process, each mature cyst liberates a single amoeba with four nuclei, a *tetranucleate amoeba* which eventually produces eight *metacystic trophozoites* by the division of nuclei by binary fission. These metacystic trophozoites ultimately lodge in the submucous tissue of the large intestine, their normal habitat. Here they grow and multiply by binary fission.

During growth, *E. histolytica* secretes a proteolytic enzyme which brings about destruction and necrosis of tissues leading to flask-shaped ulcers. A large number of trophozoites are excreted along with blood and mucus in the faeces. This condition is called amoebic dysentery. Sometimes the trophozoites enter into deeper layers and may gain entry into the radicals of portal vein to be carried

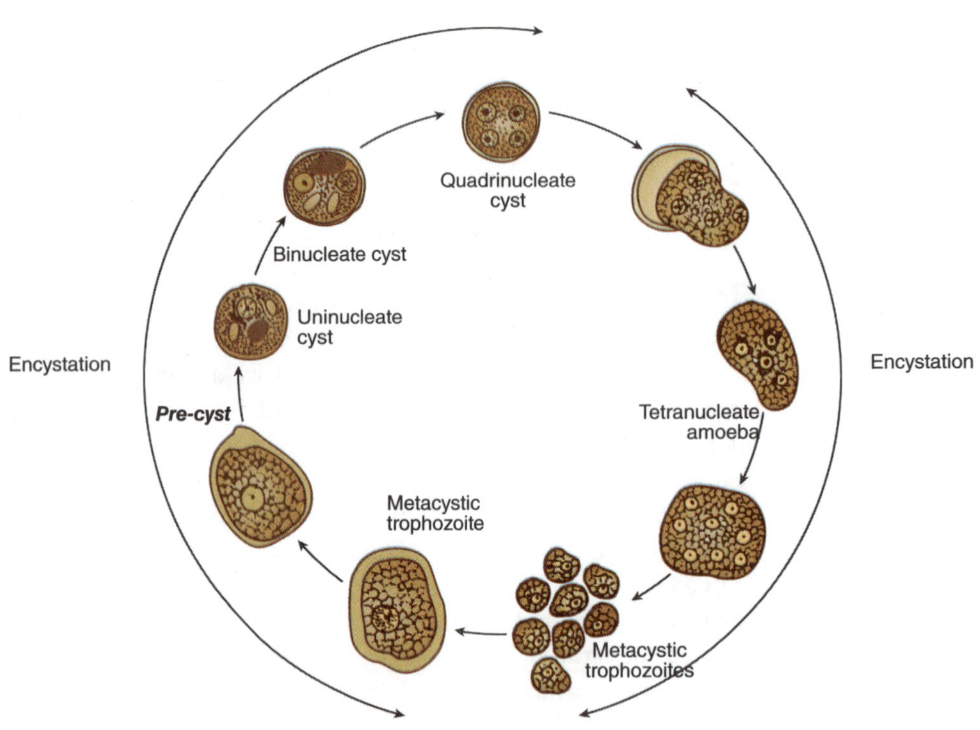

Fig. 44.2 Life cycle of *Entamoeba histolytica*

away to the liver. In the liver, they multiply and produce amoebic hepatitis and amoebic liver abscess.

After some time, when the effect of the parasite on the host is toned down and there is increase in the tolerance of the host, the lesion starts healing. The trophozoites, in the lumen of the large intestine, transform into precysts and then into mature quadrinucleate cysts. This process is known as *encystation*. Cyst formation occurs only within the intestinal tract and not outside the human body.

3. Pathogenesis and Clinical Features

E. histolytica causes amoebic dysentery (intestinal amoebiasis) and extraintestinal amoebiasis.

(i) ***Intestinal amoebiasis:*** Incubation period is 1-4 weeks. The amoebae produce characteristic ulcerative lesions and a profuse bloody diarrhoea. This is called amoebic dysentery. The ulcers may be generalised or may be localised to the ileo-caecal or sigmoido-rectal region.

(ii) ***Extraintestinal amoebiasis:*** Some individuals with intestinal amoebiasis develop hepatic amoebiasis. Amoebic liver abscess is formed. It may occur in any part of the liver but it is generally confined to **posteriosuperior surface of the right lobe of liver.** The pus, of liver abscess, has a characteristic **red-brown anchovy sauce appearance**. The pus may yield trophozoites of the parasite. From the liver, trophozoites may enter into the systemic circulation involving other organs such as lungs, brain, spleen, skin etc.

4. Laboratory Diagnosis

Laboratory diagnosis depends on the demonstration of *E. histolytica* in the material obtained from any particular lesion, such as stool, 'pus' from hepatic abscess cases and sputum.

(i) Intestinal amoebiasis

(a) *Stool examination:* In acute amoebic dysentery, stool or colonic scrapings from ulcers are examined by naked eye and microscopic examination. Normal saline preparation is useful for the demonstration of actively motile trophozoites, while iodine preparation is required for the study of cysts or dead trophozoites. Excretion of cysts in the stool is often intermittent, therefore, at least three consecutive specimens should be examined. *Charcot-Leyden crystals* may appear in saline preparation. These are diamond-shaped crystals, clear and refractile. Amoebic dysentery must be differentiated from bacillary dysentery (Table 44.2).

(b) *Stool antigen detection:* Enzyme-linked immunosorbent assay (ELISA) is used to detect antigens of *E.histolytica* in faeces.

(c) *Serological tests:* In early cases it is always negative. Antibody can be detected in later stages of invasive intestinal amoebiasis. Serological tests used are indirect haemagglutination assay (IHA) and enzyme-linked immunosorbent assay (ELISA).

(d) *DNA probes:* DNA probes have been used to detect *E. histolytica* in stool specimens.

Table 44.2: Distinguishing Features of Amoebic Dysentery and Bacillary Dysentery

Feature	Amoebic dysentery	Bacillary dysentery
Macroscopic		
Number	6-8 motions per day	> 10 motions per day
Amount	Copious	Small
Odour	Offensive	Odourless
Colour	Dark red	Bright red
Reaction	Acidic	Alkaline
Nature	Blood and mucus mixed with faeces	Blood and mucus but no faeces
Consistency	Not adherent to container	Adherent to container
Microscopic		
RBCs	In clumps	Discrete or in rouleaux formation
Pus cells	Scanty	Numerous
Eosinophils	Present	Scarce
Macrophages	Very few	Numerous; many of them contain RBCs; hence mistaken for *E. histolytica*
Ghost cells	Absent	Numerous
Pyknotic bodies	Present	Absent
Charcot-Leyden crystals	Present	Absent
Parasite	Trophozoites of *E. histolytica* present	Absent
Bacteria	Many motile bacteria	Absent

(e) *Polymerase chain reaction (PCR):* *E.histolytica* can be identified in faeces by PCR.

(ii) Hepatic amoebiasis

(a) *Diagnostic aspiration:* Trophozoites of *E. histolytica* may be demonstrated by microscopy of pus aspirated from hepatic abscess.

(b) *Liver biopsy:* Trophozoites may also be demonstrated in the liver biopsy from cases of amoebic hepatitis.

(c) *Stool examination:* In about 15% cases of hepatic abscess, cysts of *E. histolytica* may be demonstrated in the stool. It indicates persistent intestinal infection.

(d) *Serological tests:* Antibody detection is of great value in the diagnosis of hepatic amoebiasis. IHA and ELISA are some serological tests used for diagnosis.

(e) *Antigen detecion:* *E. histolytica* antigen can also be detected in serum by ELISA or coagglutination test. Antigen detection indicates recent and active infection. The antigen disappears when the patient is cured of active disease.

(f) *Polymerase chain reaction (PCR):* It has been employed to detect amoebic DNA in the aspirated pus from amoebic liver abscess.

(g) *Radiological methods:* X-ray, ultrasonography, CT scan and MRI are used for diagnosis of amoebic liver abscess. None of these methods are absolutely specific. These methods cannot differentiate amoebic liver abcess from pyogenic liver abscess.

B. Entamoeba coli

It is world-wide in distribution. It lives in the lumen of large intestine. It is non pathogenic. Life cycle of *E. coli* is similar to that of *E. histolytica*. *Entamoeba coli* also exists in three stages, i.e., trophozoite, pre-cystic stage and cyst. Differences between *E. histolytica* and *E. coli* are shown in Table 44.3.

Table 44.3: Differences between E. histolytica and E. coli

	E. histolytica	*E. coli*
Trophozoite		
Size	20-30 μm	20-40 μm
Motility	Actively motile	Sluggish
Cytoplasm	Clearly demarcated into ectoplasm and endoplasm	Not demarcated
Cytoplasmic inclusions	RBCs, leucocytes and tissue debris but no bacteria	Bacteria and other materials but never RBCs
Nucleus	Not visible in unstained preparation	Visible in unstained preparation
Karyosome	Central	Eccentric
Nuclear membrane	Delicate nuclear membrane lined by fine chromatin granules	Thick nuclear membrane lined by coarse chromatin granules
Cyst		
Size	6-15 μm in diameter	15-20 μm in diameter
Nucleus	1 to 4, central karyosome	1 to 8, eccentric karyosome
Chromatoid bars	Rounded	Filamentous

C. Giardia lamblia

These flagellates inhabit the intestine and are therefore named intestinal flagellates. They are present in **duodenum** and the **upper part of jejunum** of man.

1. Morphology

G. lamblia exists in two phases—trophozoite and cyst (Fig. 44.3). The shape of trophozoite is like that of a tennis or badminton racket. The dorsal surface is convex while ventral surface is concave having a suckling disc. The size of trophozoite is 14 μm long and 7 μm broad. The anterior end is rounded and broad while the posterior end is pointed. It is bilaterally symmetrical, i.e., all the organs of body are paired and hence there are two axostyles, two nuclei and four pairs of flagella.

The cyst is oval in shape and it is 12 μm long and 7 μm broad. There are four nuclei. The axostyles lie diagonally, forming a dividing line within the cyst-wall. The remnants of the flagella and the suckling disc may be seen inside the cytoplasm.

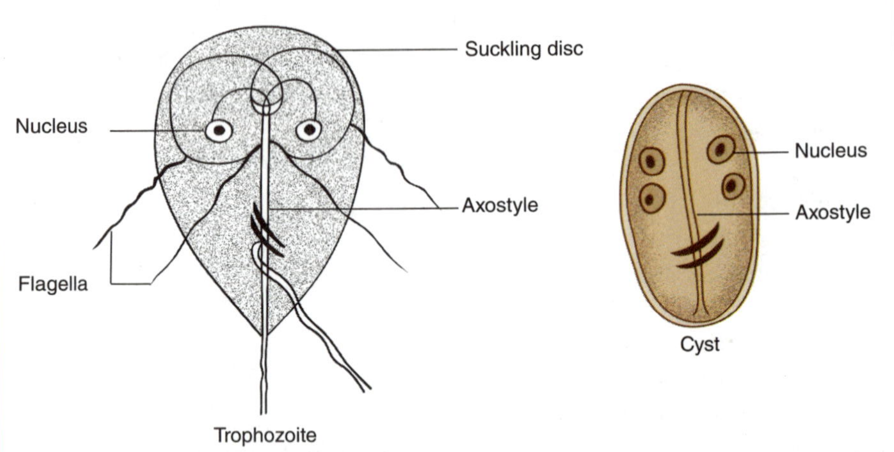

Fig. 44.3 Trophozoite and cyst of *Giardia lamblia*

2. Life Cycle

The trophozoites of the parasite multiply in the intestine of man by binary fission. During unfavourable conditions in the duodenum, encystment occurs, usually in the large intestine. Infection of man occurs by ingestion of cysts. After ingestion, the cyst hatches out two trophozoites which then multiply and colonise in the duodenum. Due to high acidity of duodenum Giardia often localises in the biliary tract.

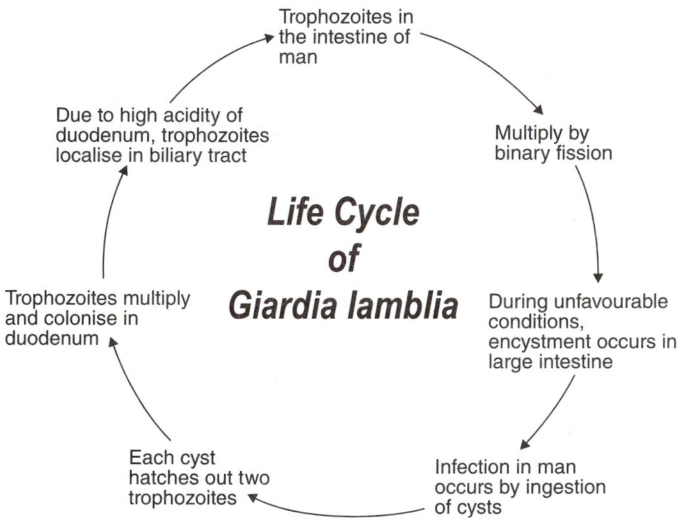

3. Pathogenesis

It may cause a disturbance of intestinal function, leading to malabsorption of fat. The patient may complain of persistent looseness of bowels, and mild steatorrhoea. The patient may present as silent case without any symptom, as chronic enteritis and acute enterocolitis, or as chronic cholecystopathy. Sometimes only general features such as fever, anaemia and allergic manifestations are present.

4. Laboratory Diagnosis

Microscopic examination

Demonstration of Giardia trophozoites and cysts in freshly passed stool by wet preparation (saline and iodine) is useful for diagnosis. Trophozoites may also be recovered in the bile.

5. Treatment

Metronidazole is the drug of choice.

D. Trichomonas

The Trichomonads are flagellate protozoa with 3 to 5 anterior flagella. The genus Trichomonas has been classified into three species according to their habitats:

(i) *Trichomonas vaginalis*—inhabiting the female genital tract; also found in the urinary tract of males and females.

(ii) *Trichomonas tenax*—inhabiting the oral cavity.

(iii) *Trichomonas hominis*—inhabiting the ileocaecal region.

1. Morphology (Fig. 44.4)

These flagellates exist only in the trophozoite phase and there is no cystic phase. They are pear shaped and measure 10-12 μm in length. The anterior end is round. The single ovoid nucleus is present at the anterior end. There are 3 to 5 anterior flagella which are free. A thicker flagellum passes backwards along the side of the body and forms the undulating membrane which comes out free at the posterior end. The undulating membrane is supported at the base by a rod like structure named 'costa'. The axostyle runs down the middle of the body and ends in the pointed tail like extremity.

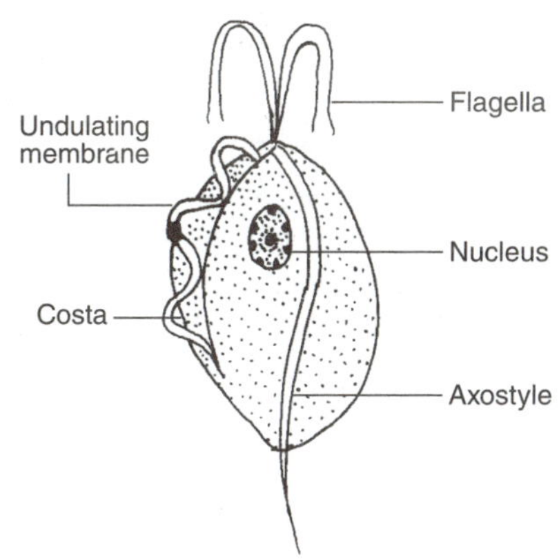

Fig. 44.4 Trophozoites of Trichomonas vaginalis

2. Pathogenesis

T. vaginalis is the causative agent of trichomoniasis in females. In case of males, it causes sexually transmitted disease (STD) causing urethritis. The other two trichomonads (*T. tenax*, *T. hominis*) are non-pathogenic.

3. Laboratory Diagnosis

Microscopic examination

Vaginal or urethral discharge is examined microscopically in a drop of saline for characteristic motile trophozoites.

E. Leishmania donovani

This parasite causes *visceral leishmaniasis* or *kala-azar*. It is endemic in many places in India. It is a parasite of reticuloendothelial system.

1. Morphology

The parasite exists in two forms:

Amastigote : Occurs in man.
Promastigote : Occurs in gut of sandfly and artificial culture.

(i) *Amastigote stage* (Fig. 44.5): It is aflagellar stage and is present in the cells of reticuloendothelial system of vertebrate hosts (man, dog etc.). It is a round or oval body (2 to 4 μm). Nucleus is oval or round and is usually situated in the middle of the cells. Kinetoplast lies at right angle of the nucleus. Axoneme extends from the kinetoplast to the margin of the body. It represents the root of the flagellum.

(ii) *Promastigote stage* (Fig. 44.5): It is a flagellar stage and is present in insect vectors (sandflies) and in cultures. It is long, slender, spindle-shaped body (15-20 μm × 1-2 μm). Nucleus is situated centrally. Kinetoplast lies near the anterior end. Flagellum may be of the same length as the body or even longer.

2. *Life Cycle*

L. donovani passes its life cycle in two hosts, man and also dog in some areas (vertebrate hosts) and female sandfly of the genus *Phlebotomus* (invertebrate host). Indian kala-azar is a non-zoonotic infection with man as the sole reservoir.

The parasite has two stages in its life cycle, i.e., amastigote form and promastigote form. The amastigote form multiplies in the cells of the reticuloendothelium system till the host cell becomes packed with the parasites. The host cell enlarges and eventually ruptures. The parasites are liberated into the circulation. The blood-sucking insect (sandfly) draws these free amastigote forms during its blood-meal.

These amastigote forms develop into promastigote forms which again multiply by binary fission producing a large number of promastigotes. A sandfly species named *Phlebotomus argentipes* acts as Indian vector. Infection occurs by bite of infected sandfly. Incubation period varies from 3 to 6 months.

3. *Clinical Features*

Leishmania donovani produces the disease *kala-azar* or *visceral leishmaniasis*. It is characterised by pyrexia, splenomegaly, hepatomegaly, lymphadenopathy and general features of anaemia.

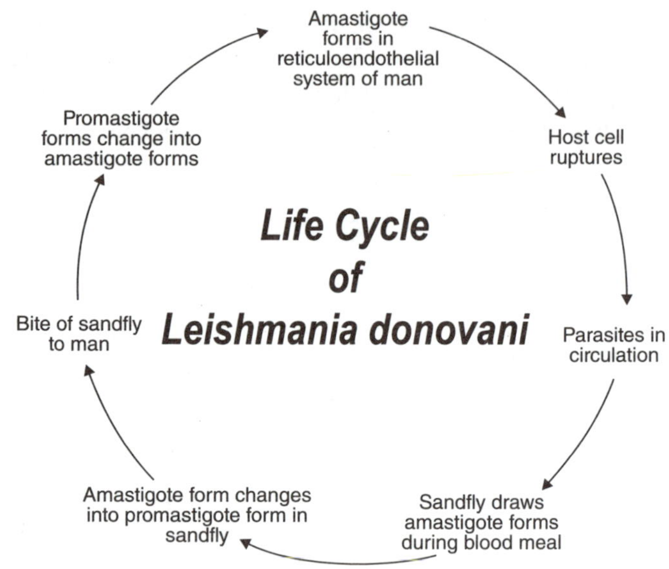

4. *Laboratory Diagnosis*

Laboratory diagnosis of kala-azar depends upon direct evidences and indirect evidences. Direct evidences demonstrate *L. donovani* in specimen.

(i) Direct evidences

(a) *Peripheral blood smear:* Thick blood film is examined for demonstration of amastigote forms. Amastigote forms [Leishman-Donovan (LD) bodies] may be present inside circulating monocytes and less often in neutrophils, in the stained peripheral blood film (Fig. 44.6). Smears are stained by Leishman or Giemsa stain.

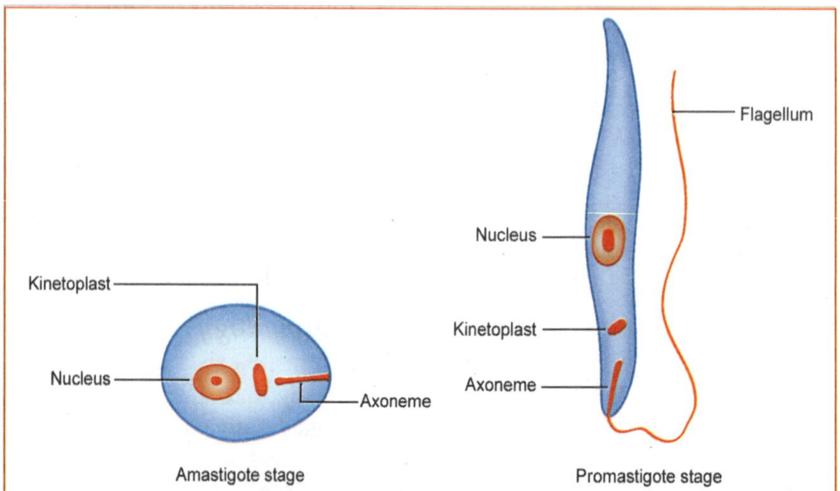

Fig. 44.5 Amastigote and promastigote forms of *Leishmania donovani*

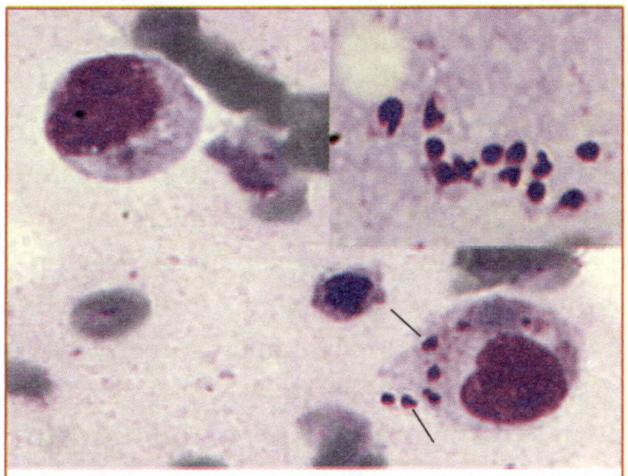

Fig. 44.6 Leishman-Donovan (LD) bodies

(b) *Blood culture:* Blood culture can be done in N.N.N. (Novy, MacNeal, Nicolle) medium and incubated at 22°-24°C. Promastigote forms can be demonstrated.

(c) *Bone marrow aspiration:* Bone-marrow aspiration is a useful method for diagnosis. Amastigote forms can be demonstrated in a stained film. The promastigote forms can be demonstrated when this material is cultured in N.N.N. medium.

(d) *Splenic puncture:* It is one of the most valuable methods for diagnosis. The amastigotes are found in stained films and promastigotes in culture.
The only risk of splenic puncture is that bleeding may continue from the puncture wound resulting in death.

(e) *Antigen detection:* ELISA using species specific monoclonal antibodies and DNA probes are very useful in the direct detection of *Leishmania* antigen.

(ii) Indirect evidences

(a) *Blood count:* There is progressive leucopenia. The proportion of leucocytes to erythrocytes is greatly altered.

(b) *Haemoglobin estimation:* It reveals anaemia.

(c) *Non-specific serological tests*
Napier's Aldehyde test: This test indicates increased serum gamma globulins and thus is non-specific. It is positive only when the disease is of at least three months duration.
Chopra's Antimony test: This test also depends upon increased serum gamma globulin. It is less reliable than aldehyde test.
Complement fixation test with W.K.K. antigen: It detects antibodies in sera of Kala-azar patients. The antigen used was prepared from human tubercle bacillus by Witebsky, Klingenstein and Kuhn, hence named as W.K.K. antigen. The test is considered non-specific since the antigen is not prepared from *L. donovani*.

(d) *Specific tests:* Indirect haemagglutination assay (IHA), indirect fluorescent antibody test (IFAT) and enzyme linked immunosorbent assay (ELISA) are more specific tests.

(e) *Rapid immunochromatographic strip test:* It has been developed for detection of antibodies against rk39 antigen of *L.donovani*. It indicates active kala-azar.

F. Plasmodium

There are four species of Genus *Plasmodium*: *P. vivax*, *P. falciparum*, *P. malariae* and *P. ovale*. They are protozoa, causing malaria in man. In India, *P. vivax* and *P. falciparum* are very common but *P. ovale* does not occur.

1. Life Cycle

The malarial parasites pass their life cycle in two hosts, i.e., **man** (*intermediate host*) and female anopheles **mosquito** (*definitive host*). Asexual development of parasite occurs in man and sexual development in mosquito.

HUMAN CYCLE

The sporozoite is the infective form of the malarial parasite. These sporozoites are present in the salivary gland of female anopheles mosquitoes. Man gets infection by the bite of infected mosquito and sporozoites are introduced directly into the blood circulation. Thus, human cycle starts and it comprises of following stages:

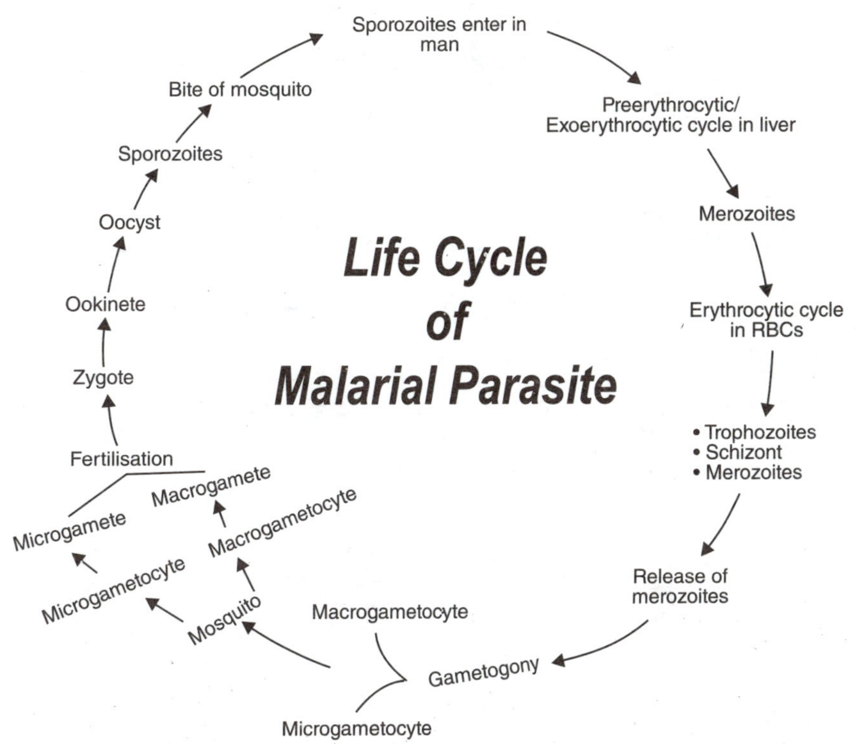

Pre-erythrocytic schizogony
Erythrocytic schizogony
Gametogony
Exo-erythrocytic schizogony

(i) ***Pre-erythrocytic schizogony:*** Before starting erythrocytic schizogony in blood, sporozoites undergo a developmental phase inside the liver cells. This phase of development is known as pre-erythrocytic schizogony. The sporozoites (elongated and spindle-shaped) become rounded inside the liver parenchymal cells. They undergo multiple nuclear division and develop into schizont. The size of schizont varies in different species and it contains 20,000–50,000 merozoites. The pre-erythrocytic cycle lasts for 8 days in *P. vivax*, 6 days in *P. falciparum*, 13-16 days in *P. malariae* and 9 days in *P. ovale*. After completion of this cycle, the liver cells rupture and release merozoites into the blood stream.

(ii) ***Erythrocytic schizogony:*** The merozoites released from pre-erythrocytic schizogony penetrate red blood cells. They pass through the stages of trophozoite, schizont and merozoite (Fig. 44.7). Depending on the species of malarial parasite, there may be 6-24 merozoites in red blood cell. The red blood cells rupture to release the merozoites which attack new red blood cells and continue their erythrocytic schizogony repeating the cycle. In *P. falciparum* infection, erythrocytic schizonts aggregate in the capillaries of the brain and other internal organs, so that only ring forms are found in the peripheral blood. Differential features of various plasmodia are shown in Table 44.4.

(iii) ***Gametogony*** (Fig. 44.8)***:*** Some merozoites of erythrocytic schizogony develop into male and female gametocytes known as **microgametocytes** and **macrogametocytes** respectively. They develop in the red blood cells. These are sexual forms and are found in the peripheral blood. The microgametocytes of all the four species are smaller in size, cytoplasm stains light blue and the nucleus is large and diffuse. In contrast, the macrogametocytes are larger, the cytoplasm stains deep blue and the nucleus is small and compact.

(iv) ***Exoerythrocytic schizogony:*** The exoerythrocytic cycle resembles the pre-erythrocytic cycle. Some sporozoites, on entering into liver cells, do not undergo asexual multiplication but enter into a resting (dormant) phase. The resting stage of the parasite is known as ***hypnozoite***. After some period (usually up to 2 years), hypnozoites reactivate to become schizonts and release merozoites. These merozoites attack red blood cells and are responsible for **relapse** of malaria. Exo-erythrocytic schizogony is absent in *P. falciparum*, therefore, relapses do not occur in malaria caused by *P. falciparum*.

Mosquito cycle

The sexual cycle of malarial parasite actually starts in the human host by the formation of gametocytes which are

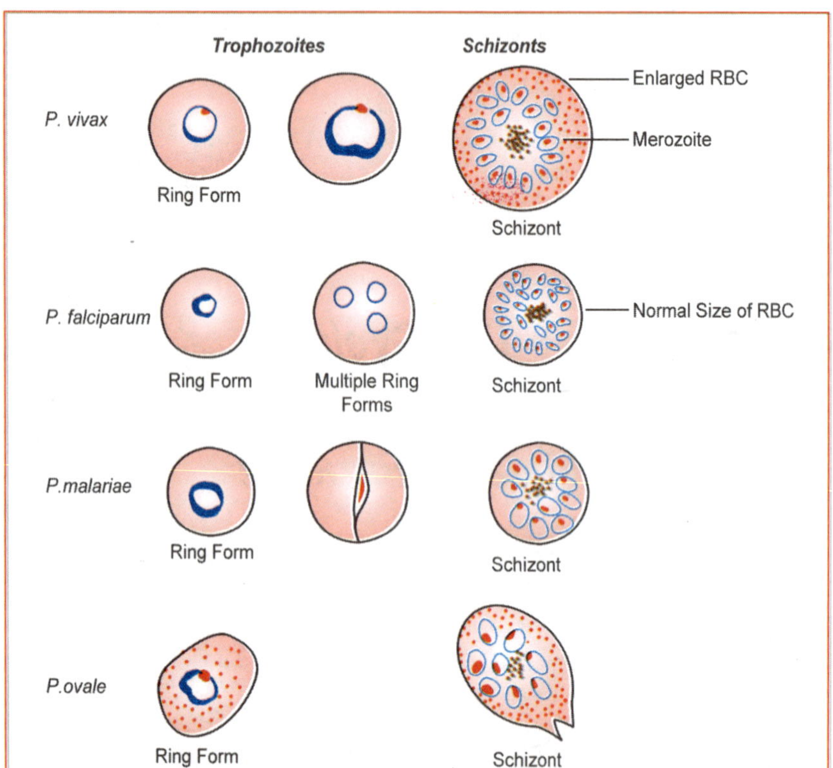

Fig. 44.7 Erythrocytic stages of different species of *Plasmodium*

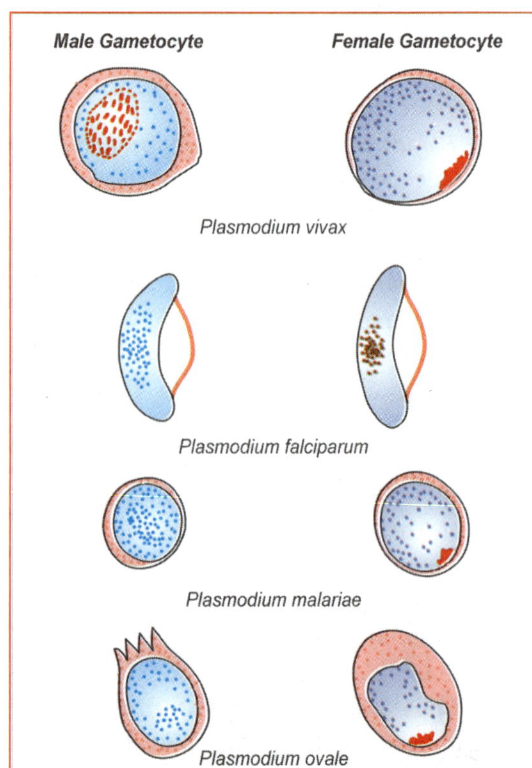

Fig. 44.8 Gametocytes of *Plasmodium species*

Table 44.4: Differential Features of Different Plasmodia of Man

Feature	*P. vivax*	*P. falciparum*	*P. malariae*	*P. ovale*
1. Forms in peripheral blood	Trophozoites, schizonts and gametocytes	Ring forms and gametocytes (crescent shaped)	Trophozoites, schizonts and gametocytes	Trophozoites, schizonts and gametocytes
2. Early trophozoite or ring form	2.5 µm in diameter, cytoplasm opposite the nucleus is thicker	1.25-1.5 µm in diameter, multiple rings in one red blood cell, form *accole*	Similar to that of *P. vivax*	Similar to that of *P. vivax*
3. Trophozoite	Irregular, amoeboid, vacuole present	Compact form, rarely amoeboid, pigments collect into a single mass	Band shaped, slightly amoeboid, vacuole inconspicuous	Compact, not amoeboid, vacuole inconspicuous
4. Schizont	9 to 10 µm in diameter, almost completely fills an enlarged erythrocyte	4.5 to 5.0 µm in diameter, fills two thirds of a normal size erythrocyte	6.5 to 7.0 µm in diameter, almost fills a normal size erythrocyte	6.2 µm in diameter, fills about three quarters of slightly enlarged erythrocyte
5. Merozoites	12-24 in number	18 to 24 in number	6-12 in number	6-12 in number
6. Gametocyte	Spherical, much larger than a red blood cell	Crescentric (sickle-shaped), larger than a red blood cell	Round, size of a red blood cell	Round, size of a red blood cell
(i) Female gametocyte (Macro-gametocyte)	Spherical, larger than male gametocyte, cytoplasm stains deep blue, nucleus is small and compact.	Sickle-shaped, longer, more slender, cytoplasm stains deep blue, nucleus is compact	Similar to that of *P. vivax* but smaller	Similar to that of *P. vivax* but smaller
(ii) Male gametocyte (Micro-gametocyte)	Spherical, smaller than female gametocyte, cytoplasm stains light blue or pale blue, nucleus is large and diffuse	Sickle-shaped, broader, shorter, cytoplasm stains light blue, nucleus is diffuse	Similar to that of *P. vivax* but smaller	Similar to that of *P. vivax* but smaller
7. Malarial pigments	Yellowish-brown	Dark-brown	Dark-brown	Dark yellowish-brown
8. Infected erythrocyte	Enlarged, pale, Schuffner's dots present	Size unaltered, Maurer's dots present	Normal size & no dots, Ziemann's dots on prolonged staining	Slightly enlarged, oval shaped and James's dots present
9. Age of the erythrocytes infected	Young	All ages (young and old)	Old	Young
10. Duration of erythrocytic schizogony	48 hours	≥ 48 hours	72 hours	48 hours

then transferred to mosquito for further development. A female anopheles during its blood meal from the patient, ingests both the asexual and sexual forms of parasite. Only the mature sexual forms are capable of further development in the mosquito and rest die immediately.

In the midgut of the mosquito, one microgametocyte develop into 4 to 8 thread like filamentous structures named ***microgametes***. From one macrogametocyte only one macrogamete is formed. Fertilisation occurs when a **microgamete** penetrates into a **macrogamete**. The fertilised macrogamete is known as ***zygote***. The zygote lengthens and matures into an ***ookinete***. The ookinete develops into an ***oocyst***. As oocyst matures, it increases in size and a large number of sporozoites (a few hundreds to thousands) develop inside it. The number of oocysts in the stomach wall varies from a few to more than hundred. The oocyst ruptures and releases sporozoites in the body cavity of the mosquito. The sporozoites are distributed into various organs and tissues of the mosquito. However, they have a special predilection for salivary glands.

The mosquito is now capable of transmitting the infection to man.

2. Pathogenesis and Clinical Features

Infection with the Plasmodium causes intermittent fever which is named as malaria. Incubation period is 10-14 days in *P. vivax*, *P. falciparum* and *P. ovale* but it is 28-30 days in *P. malariae*. The typical clinical features consist of febrile paroxysm, followed by anaemia and splenomegaly.

P. falciparum is the most pathogenic of the plasmodium species infecting man. There are no relapses in *P. falciparum* infection but relapses occur in *P. vivax* infection.

Pernicious malaria

Pernicious malaria is life threatening complication that sometimes occur in acute falciparum malaria. It is due to heavy parasitization. Various manifestations of pernicious malaria are grouped as cerebral malaria, algid malaria and septicaemic malaria

1. *Cerebral malaria:* It is characterised by hyperpyrexia, coma and paralysis and frequently leads to death even when appropriate therapy has been given. Brain is congested.
2. *Algid malaria:* It is characterised by cold clammy skin leading to peripheral circulatory failure.

Black water fever

It is a manifestation of infection with *P. falciparum* occurring in those persons who have been previously infected and have had inadequate dose of quinine. It is characterised by intravascular haemolysis, fever and haemoglobinuria.

3. Immunity

Immunity is species-specific, stage-specific and strain-specific and lasts only till malarial parasite infection remains active. This type of immunity is known as *premunition immunity*.

4. Laboratory Diagnosis

(i) ***Microscopic examination:*** Microscopic examination of a peripheral blood smear is the most important diagnostic procedure in malaria. Thick and thin smears of the blood are prepared on the same slide or two different slides. Blood for smear should be collected a few hours after the height of febrile paroxysm because the parasites are most abundant during this period. Blood is taken by pricking a finger prior to start of antimalarial therapy. For thick smear, take a drop of the blood on the slide and spread it in an area of 1 cm square. For thin smear, take a drop of the blood at one corner of the slide and spread it with another slide so that tail formation occurs at another end. Both thick and thin peripheral blood smears are stained with Leishman stain. These smears are examined under oil immersion lens.

Malarial parasites may be quickly detected in the thick smear but species identification is difficult. Thin smear is examined for identifying the species of plasmodium.

All asexual erythrocytic stages (ring forms, trophozoites, schizonts), as well as gametocytes can be found in peripheral blood smear in infection with *P. vivax*, *P. malariae* and *P. ovale*, but in *P. falciparum* infection, only the ring forms and gametocytes (crescent shaped) can be seen. Multiple rings in an individual red blood cell with accole forms is diagnostic of *P. falciparum*.

Red blood cells are enlarged in *P. vivax* but there is no enlargement of RBC in *P. falciparum* infection.

(ii) ***Quantitative buffy coat (QBC) test:*** It is a new method for identification of malarial parasite in the peripheral blood. Blood is collected in QBC tube coated with fluorescent dye and is subjected to centrifugation. After centrifugation, the buffy coat in the tube is examined directly under a fluorescent microscope. Acridine orange-stained malarial parasites appear brilliant green. QBC is more sensitive method than the thick blood smear. It can detect 3–4 parasites/μl of blood. However, the species of plasmodium can not be identified. It is costly and needs expensive equipment.

(iii) ***Rapid diagnostic tests:*** Rapid diagnostic tests (RDTs) are based on the detection of antigens using immuno-chromatographic methods. In these tests, a dipstick or teststrip, containing monoclonal antibodies directed against the parasitic antigens, is used. Several commercial kits are available. These tests take about 15 minutes and thus are rapid. Kits available detect histidine-rich protein (HRP-II) of *P. falciparum*. The test is commercially available as the 'Parasite F' test. Parasite lactate dehydrogenase (pLDH) of all four Plasmodium species that infect humans can also be detected using rapid tests. A dipstic test for detecting species specific lactate dehydrogenase is also available. It detects only live parasites therefore it can also be used to confirm cure after treatment.

(iv) ***Serological tests:*** Indirect immunofluorescence test, indirect haemagglutination assay (IHA) and enzyme linked immunosorbent assay (ELISA) are the serological tests used for the diagnosis of malaria.

5. Treatment

Chloroquine along with primaquine is used for treatment of vivax malaria. Artemisinin and its derivatives are the newer drugs used for treatment of foliciparum malaria.

II. TREMATODES

These are leaf-shaped unsegmented worms, called flukes. Each individual worm is hermaphrodite except the Schistosomes which are unisexual. Body cavity is absent. The worm is oviparous (eggs are liberated). Eggs are all operculated (except those of *Schistosomes*) and develop only in water.

Different Trematodes

1. Intestinal trematodes e.g. *Fasciola buski*
2. Hepatic trematodes e.g. *Fasciola hepatica*
3. Lung trematodes e.g. *Paragonimus westermani*
4. Blood trematodes e.g. *Schistosoma haematobium, S. mansoni, S. japonicum*

Mode of Infection

1. By ingestion of encysted cercariae in vegetables (e.g. *F. hepatica, F. buski*), fish or flesh of crab (e.g. *P. westermani*).
2. Free cercariae penetration through the skin e.g. *S. haematobium, S. mansoni.*

III. CESTODES

A. Taenia saginata

Common names for *Taenia saginata* are "The beef tapeworm" and "The unarmed tapeworm". It is worldwide in distribution. The infection occurs by eating raw or insufficiently cooked beef. In India, it is particularly prevalent amongst Muslims but is not found amongst Hindus who do not eat beef.

1. Morphology

(i) ***Adult worm*** (Fig. 44.9): It measures 5 to 10 metres in length but may be up to 24 metres. It is white and semitransparent. It consists of three parts: scolex, neck and proglottids. The scolex or 'head' is quadrate in shape and has four circular suckers which may be pigmented. It measures 1 to 2 mm in diameter. The 'head' does not contain any rostellum or hooklets. The neck is long and narrow, about 0.5 mm in width. Proglottids or segments are 1000 to 2000 in number. The length of a gravid segment is 3 to 4 times its breadth.

(ii) ***Eggs*** (Fig. 44.9): The eggs are liberated by the rupture of ripe proglottids. The characteristic features of the egg are:

(a) Spherical and bile-stained.
(b) 31 to 43 μm in diameter.
(c) The inner embryophore is thick-walled, radially striated and brown in colour.
(d) It contains an oncosphere (measuring 14 to 20 μm in diameter) containing 3 pairs of hooklets.
(e) Does not float in a saturated solution of common salt.
(f) It is infective only to cattle.

B. Taenia solium

Common names for *Taenia solium* are "The pork tapeworm" and "The armed tapeworm". It is also worldwide in distribution. The infection occurs by eating raw or insufficiently cooked pork. It is uncommon in Muslims who are not generally pork-eaters.

1. Morphology

(i) ***Adult worm*** (Fig. 44.9): It measures 2 to 3 metres in length. It also consists of three parts: scolex, neck and proglottids. The scolex or 'head' is globular in shape and has four circular suckers. The 'head' contains a rostellum armed with a double row of hooklets. The neck is short and measures 5 to 10 mm in length. Proglottids or segments are 800 to 900 (less than a thousand) in number (Table 44.5). The gravid segment measures about 12 mm by 6 mm.

(ii) ***Eggs*** (Fig. 44.9): The characteristic features are the same as those described in *T. saginata*. The eggs are infective to both pig and man.

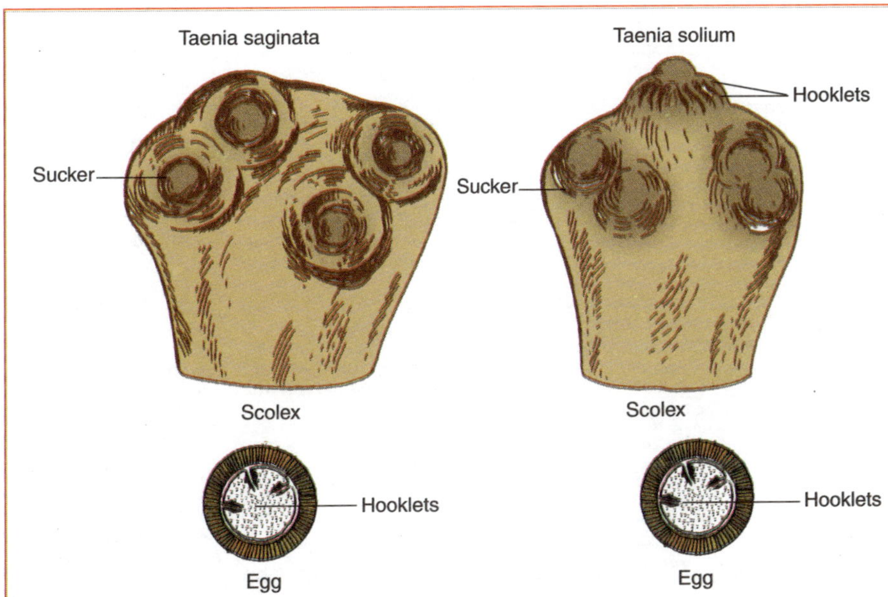

Fig. 44.9 Adult worms and eggs of *Taenia saginata* and *Taenia solium*

Table 44.5: Differentiating Features of Taenia solium and Taenia saginata

Feature	*T. solium*	*T. saginata*
1. Length	2 to 3 metres	5 to 10 metres
2. Head	Small, globular; with rostellum and a double row of hooks. Four suckers present, which are not pigmented	Large, quadrate; without rostellum and hooks. Four suckers present, which may be pigmented
3. Neck	Short	Long
4. Segments (Proglottids)		
(i) Number	< 1000	1000-2000
(ii) Expulsion	Expelled in chains of 5 or 6	Expelled singly
(iii) Uterus	Lateral branches 5 to 10 on each side	Lateral branches 15 to 30 on each side
(iv) Vaginal sphincter	Absent	Present
(v) Ovaries	Two in number with an accessory lobe	Two in number without any accessory lobe
(vi) Testes	150-200 follicles	300-400 follicles
(vii) Larva	Cysticercus cellulosae, present in pig (intermediate) host and may also develop in man (definitive host)	Cysticercus bovis, present in cow (intermediate host) but not in man (definitive host)

2. *Life Cycle*

The worm passes its life cycle in two hosts: the definitive host and the intermediate host. Man is the definitive host (which harbours the adult worm) and pig is the intermediate host (which harbours the larval stage).

The adult worm lives in the small intestine of man and the eggs or gravid proglottids are passed out with the faeces. The animals become infected by swallowing these eggs. After ingestion, oncosphere hatches out and penetrates the gut wall. It is carried in the systemic circulation. The naked oncospheres are filtered out from the circulating blood into the muscular tissue. They are transformed into cysticercus stage in the muscle when these are known as *cysticercus cellulosae*. Human beings are infected by eating uncooked or partially cooked pork containing cysticercus cellulosae. Inside the alimentary canal of man, the scolex of the cysticercus evaginates and attaches to the gut wall by its suckers and then develops into an adult worm.

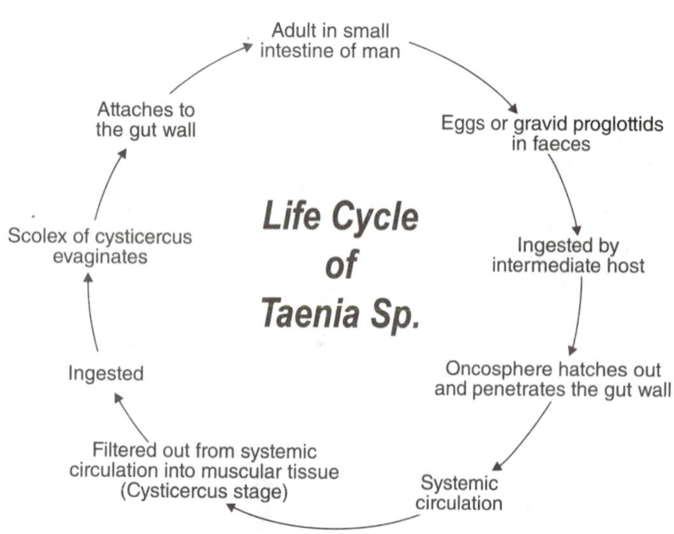

Life cycle of *T. saginata* is same except that the intermediate host is cattle and the larval stage is named as *cysticercus bovis*.

Cysticercus cellulosae (Fig. 44.10)***:*** This is the larval stage of *Taenia solium* developing in the muscles of its intermediate host, i.e., the pig. A mature cyst is an opalescent ellipsoidal body and the long axis of the cyst is parallel to the muscle fibre. A dense milky-white spot is present at the side where the scolex with its hooks and suckers remains invaginated. This cyst develops further when ingested by man, its definitive host.

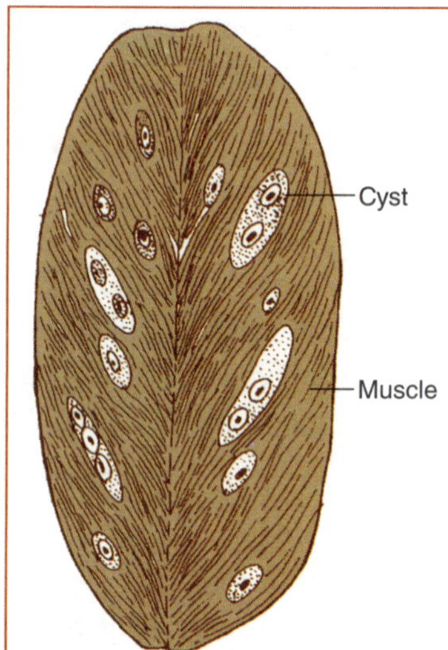

Fig. 44.10 Cysticercus cellulosae

Man sometimes gets infection in the same way as the pig, i.e., either by drinking contaminated water or by eating uncooked vegetables infected with eggs. Apart from this, a man harbouring the adult worm may also auto-infect himself either due to unhygienic personal habits or by a reversal of peristaltic movements of the intestine by which the gravid segments are thrown back to the stomach, equivalent to the ingestion of thousands of eggs. These cysticerci may develop in any organ but are usually present in the subcutaneous tissues and muscles but may be found in the brain leading to epileptic attacks. These cysts have a tendency to become calcified and obsolete over the period of 5 to 6 years.

Cysticercus bovis: This is the larval stage of *Taenia saginata* in the muscles of its intermediate hosts i.e. a cow or a buffalo. It contains a scolex without hooks and rostellum invaginated at one side. It can only develop further into adult worm when ingested by man, its definitive host. *Cysticercus bovis* does not occur in man.

3. Mode of Infection

It is by ingestion of undercooked meat of the intermediate hosts containing larvae.

T. solium—Pork, containing *Cysticercus cellulosae*
T. saginata—Beef, containing *Cysticercus bovis*

4. Clinical Features

They usually do not give rise to any symptom. Occasionally, vague abdominal discomfort, chronic indigestion, anaemia and intestinal disorders may be present.

5. Laboratory Diagnosis

(i) ***Stool examination:*** Naked eye examination of the stool should be made for segments of *Taenia* sp. A microscopic examination of the specimen for the eggs can be carried out by wet preparation. The eggs of *T. saginata* and *T. solium* cannot be differentiated by morphology. Hence, the 'head' and the gravid segment are required to establish a species diagnosis.

(ii) ***Diagnosis of cysticercosis:*** This can be done by following investigations:

(a) Biopsy examination of subcutaneous nodules for cysticerci.
(b) X-ray of skull and soft tissues to reveal calcified cysticerci.
(c) CT scan of brain to show lesions.
(d) Eosinophilia.
(e) Serological tests can be used for demonstration of specific antibodies in serum and CSF. Indirect fluorescent antibody (IFA) and enzyme linked immunoassay (ELISA) are employed for detection of these antibodies.
(f) A history of intestinal taeniasis is another aid in the diagnosis.

6. Treatment

Praziquantel and niclosamide are used for the treatment of human tapewom infactions.

7. Prophylaxis

The preventive measures include:

1. Avoidance of eating raw or undercooked meat.
2. Effective treatment of infected individual to prevent infection of the intermediate hosts.
3. Personal hygiene to prevent the risk of acquiring cysticercosis by autoinfection.

C. Echinococcus granulosus

It is a cestode and is the causative agent of the hydatid disease. Man harbours the larval form of the parasite, while the adult worm is found in small intestine of dog and other canine animals.

1. Morphology

(i) ***Adult worm*** (Fig. 44.11): It measures 3 to 6 mm in length. It contains *scolex* (head), neck and strobila. Strobila consists of three segments. Occasionally, the fourth segment is also present. The first segment is immature, the second one is mature and the third one is gravid. If fourth segment is present, that will also be gravid. The terminal segment is the biggest among all the segments. The scolex bears four suckers and a rostellum which contains two circular rows of hooks. The 'neck' is short and thick.

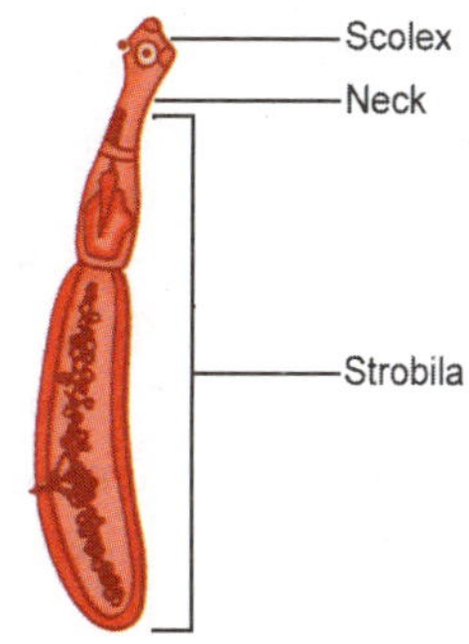

Fig. 44.11 Echinococcus granulosus—Adult worm

(ii) ***Egg*** (Fig. 44.12): It is ovoid in shape and measures 32-36 µm × 25-32 µm. It contains hexacanth embryo with 3 pairs of hooks.

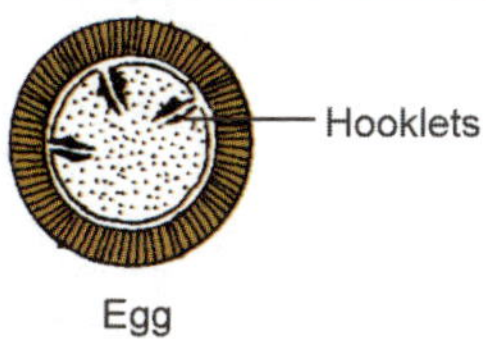

Fig. 44.12 Egg of *Echinococcus granulosus*

(iii) ***Larval form*** (Fig. 44.13): This is found within the hydatid cyst and represents the scolex of the future adult worm. It remains invaginated within a vesicular body. When it enters the definitive host, the scolex with four suckers and hooklets, becomes evaginated and develops into an adult worm.

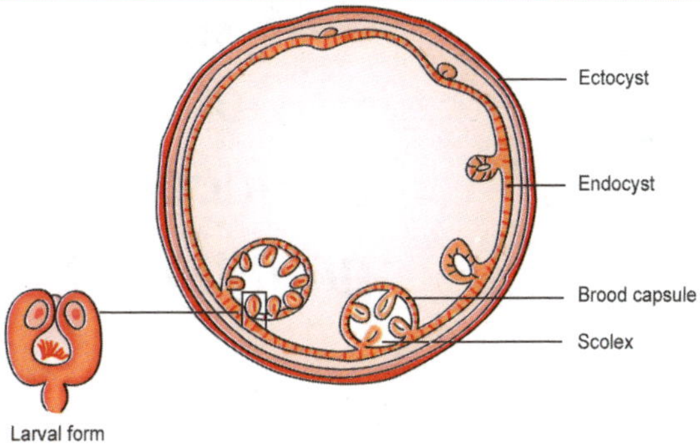

Fig. 44.13 Hydatid cyst

2. Life Cycle

The worm passes its life cycle in two hosts, i.e., definitive host and intermediate host.

(i) ***Definitive hosts:*** The adult worms live in small intestine of these animals and discharge eggs in their faeces. The dog is the optimum definitive host but wolf, fox and jackal may also act as definitive host.

(ii) ***Intermediate hosts:*** The larval stage is present in these animals including man, giving rise to hydatid cyst. Sheep, pig, cattle, horse, goat and man may act as intermediate host.

The eggs are discharged in the faeces of the definitive hosts and are swallowed by the intermediate hosts. The man gets infection due to intimate handling of infected dogs. After ingestion, the hexacanth embryos are hatched out in the small intestine and penetrate its wall. They then enter the radicles of portal vein. The embryos are carried to the liver which acts as the first filter. Some of the embryos enter the pulmonary circulation and thus the lungs act as the second filter. Embryos may lodge in any organ or tissue but most frequently are found in the liver and lungs. The embryo develops slowly into the hydatid cyst. The cyst's wall is differentiated into a thick outer laminated, non-cellular layer and the inner thin germinal epithelium. From the inner layer, brood capsules with a number of scolices develop. A hydatid cyst may contain thousands of scolices. These hydatids when ingested by the dog, are capable of growing into adult worms in the intestine. Hence, the life cycle is repeated.

As the dogs have no access to the hydatid cyst developed in man, the life cycle comes to a dead-end. The natural cycle is thus maintained by dog and sheep.

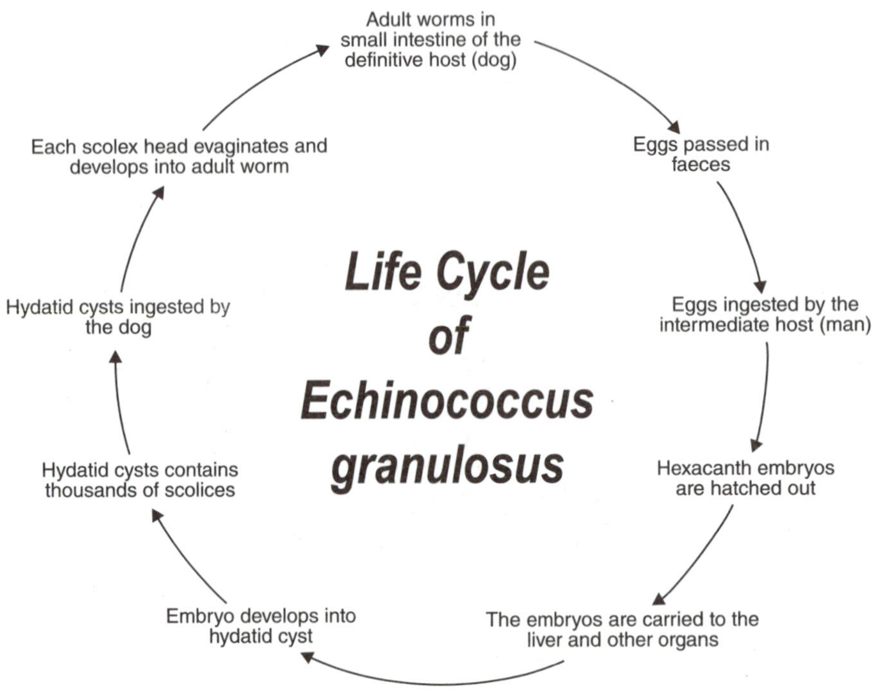

3. Pathogenesis and Clinical Features

In man, the larval form causes unilocular hydatid disease.

(i) Mode of infection

Ingestion of eggs by man may occur in the following ways:

1. by direct contact with infected dogs.
2. by allowing the dog to feed from the same dish.
3. by uncooked vegetables contaminated with infected animals faeces.

Infection is generally acquired in childhood due to their intimate association with dogs.

(ii) Hydatid cyst

The cyst wall secreted by embryo consists of two layers: outer layer (ectocyst) and inner or germinal layer (endocyst) (Fig. 44.13).

Ectocyst: It is elastic but when incised or ruptured, it curls on itself thus exposing the inner layer containing the brood capsules and daughter cysts.

Endocyst: It is inner or germinal layer. It forms the outer layer (ectocyst) and gives rise to brood capsules and scolices on inner side. It also secretes hydatid fluid.

Hydatid cyst may involve liver, lung, brain, heart, kidney, spleen, bone, muscles etc. Liver is the commonest site. The disease remains symptomless for many years.

4. Laboratory Diagnosis

It consists of the following tests:

(i) ***Serological tests:*** Enzyme-linked immunosorbent assay (ELISA), complement fixation test (CFT), indirect haemagglutination assay (IHA) and latex agglutination tests are used for diagnosis of hydatid cyst.

(ii) ***Radiological examination:*** X-ray, ultrasonography and CT scan are useful in the diagnosis of hydatid cyst.

(iii) ***Blood examination:*** Eosinophilia (20-25%) may be present.

(iv) ***Examination of cyst fluid:*** It reveals the typical scolices, brood capsules and hooklets. Leakage of hydatid fluid in the adjoining tissue may lead to anaphylactic shock, therefore, the diagnostic puncture of cyst is not advised. However, the fluid aspirated from surgically removed hydatid cyst should be examined for diagnosis.

(v) ***Casoni test:*** It is an immediate hypersensitivity skin test introduced by Casoni. Sterile hydatid fluid is used as antigen. The hydatid fluid is drawn from unilocular hydatid cysts from human cases (removed by operation) or from animals (obtained from slaughterhouse). It is filtered and made sterile. 0.2 ml of this antigen is injected intradermally in one arm. Sterile normal saline, 0.2 ml, is injected intradermally in the other arm which acts as control. In positive case, tested site develops a large wheal (measuring 5 cm in diameter or more) with multiple pseudopodia. This test has a low sensitivity, thus, gives false positive reactions in other cestode infections.

IV. NEMATODES

A. Ascaris lumbricoides

The common name for *Ascaris lumbricoides* is roundworm. It has a worldwide distribution. It is the largest intestinal nematode parasitising man. The adult worm lives in the small intestine (jejunum) of man.

1. Morphology

(i) ***Adult worm:*** It is elongated and rounded in shape and tapers at both ends. The mouth opens at the anterior end and possesses three lips. Male worm measures about 15-25 cm in length and 3-4 mm in diameter. The tail end is curved ventrally in the form of a hook. Two curved copulatory spicules protrude from the cloaca. The anus along with the ejaculatory duct opens into the cloaca (Fig. 44.14). Female worm is longer and stouter than the male worm. It measures 25-40 cm in length and 5 mm in diameter. The tail end is conical and straight. The anus opens directly on the ventral surface in the form of a transverse slit.

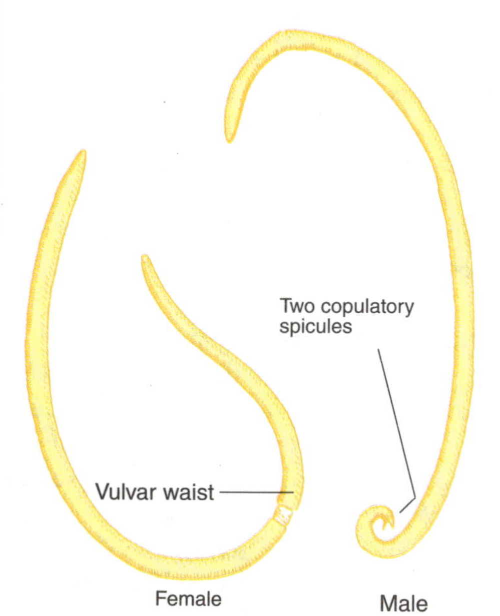

Fig. 44.14 *Ascaris lumbricoides* Adult worms

The vulva opens at the junction of the anterior and the middle thirds of the body. This part of the worm is narrower and is called as vulvar waist (Fig. 44.14). A mature female Ascaris may have enormous egg-laying capacity, liberating about 200,000 eggs daily.

(ii) ***Eggs:*** The eggs are passed out of the human host with the faeces. Eggs are of two types: fertilised eggs and unfertilised eggs.

Fertilised egg (Fig. 44.15)

1. It is round or oval in shape measuring 60-75 μm in length and 40-50 μm in breadth.
2. It is bile stained and thus brownish in colour.
3. It is surrounded by a thick, translucent shell with an outer albuminous coat in the form of rugosities. This outer coat is sometimes lost (decorticated egg).
4. It contains a large unsegmented ovum with a clear crescentric area at each pole.
5. It floats in saturated solution of common salt.

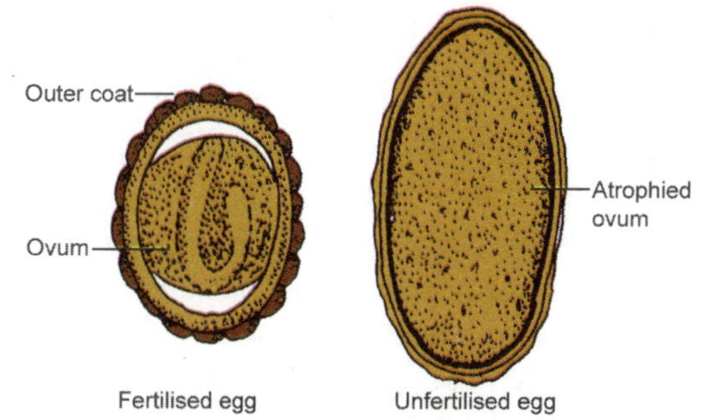

Fig. 44.15 Eggs of Ascaris lumbricoides

Unfertilised egg (Fig. 44.15)

The female, even if not fertilised, can produce unfertilised eggs. These eggs can be produced by female worms when these is an absence of male worm, therefore these are unfertilised eggs.

1. It is narrower and longer measuring 80 μm in length and 55 μm in breadth.
2. It is bile stained and brownish in colour.
3. It has a thinner shell with an irregular coating of albumin.
4. It contains a small atrophied ovum.
5. It does not float in saturated solution of common salt (heaviest of all helminthic eggs).

2. Life Cycle

Ascaris lumbricoides passes its life cycle in only one host, man. No intermediate host is required. Man is the only definitive host. Adult worms live in the jejunum of man. Fertilised eggs containing the unsegmented ova are passed

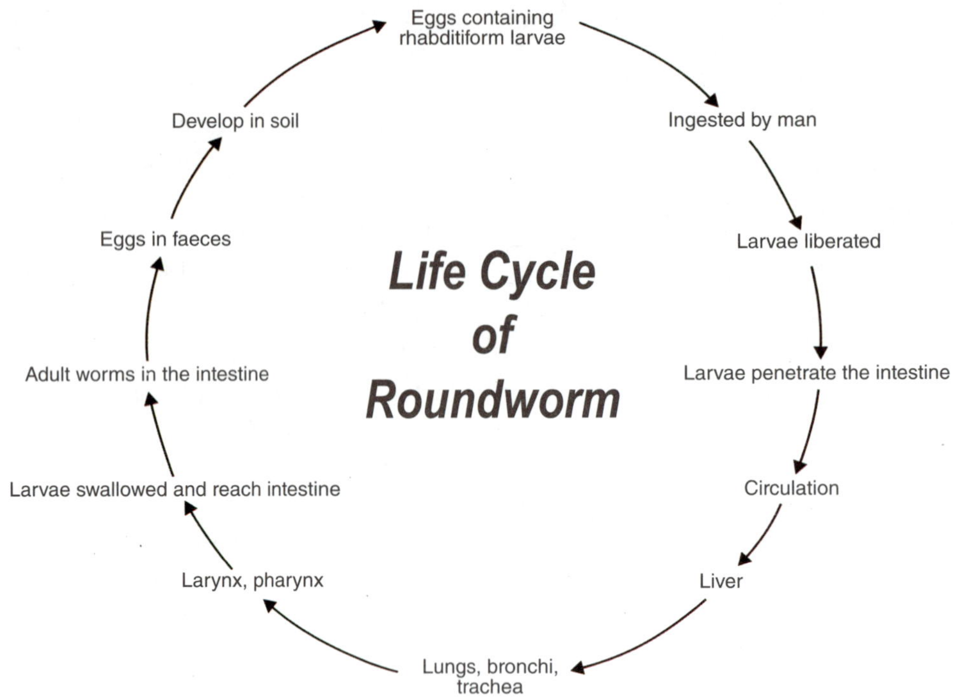

in the faeces. These eggs are not immediately infective to man. Eggs undergo development in soil. A rhabditiform larva is developed from unsegmented ovum and undergoes first moulting within the egg shell. These **eggs containing rhabditiform** larvae are **pathogenic** to man. Man acquires infection by ingestion of food, drink or raw vegetables contaminated with eggs containing rhabditiform larvae (**embryonated eggs**). In the upper part of the small intestine (duodenum), rhabditiform larvae are liberated from the embryonated eggs. These newly hatched larvae then burrow their way through the mucous membrane of the small intestine and are carried by the portal circulation to the liver. They then pass out of the liver and via right heart enter the pulmonary circulation. In the lungs they grow much bigger in size and moult twice. They break through the capillary wall and reach the lung alveoli. From here, the larvae crawl up the bronchi and trachea and are propelled into the larynx and pharynx and are swallowed. They pass down the oesophagus to the stomach and localise in the upper part of the small intestine, their normal abode. Another moulting takes place. The larvae grow into adult worms and sexual maturity occurs. The gravid female begins to discharge eggs in the stool and the life cycle is again repeated.

3. Mode of Infection

Infective form—Embryonated eggs
Portal of entry—Alimentary canal (ingestion)
Site of location—Small intestine

4. Pathogenesis and Clinical Features

Infection of *Ascaris lumbricoides* is known as **ascariasis**. The symptoms may be due to migrating larvae or due to adult worms. Presence of larvae in the lungs may lead to symptoms of pneumonia. If the ascaris larvae reach other organs, they may set up clinical symptoms related to these organs.

5. Laboratory Diagnosis

(i) ***Stool examination:*** Adult worms or eggs may be demonstrated. Eggs can be detected by direct microscopic examination of stool specimen or after concentration of the same.
(ii) ***Barium meal*** may occasionally demonstrate the presence of adult worms in the small intestine.
(iii) ***Serodiagnosis:*** Antibodies against *A. lumbricoides* can be detected. These tests are useful for the diagnosis of extraintestinal ascariasis involving other organs.

Visceral Larva Migrans

Visceral larva migrans is a condition caused by ingestion of embryonated eggs of some nematodes parasitising animals. Larvae are hatched out in the small intestine and are carried out to extraintestinal sites; such as liver, lungs and other organs. Wherever they settle, their progress is arrested by the formation of granulomatous lesion.

Visceral larva migrans is characterised by leucocytosis, eosinophilia (15 to 80%) with or without any constitutional symptoms. Diagnosis can be made by serological tests to detect antibodies in the serum. As dog roundworm (*Toxocara canis*) and cat roundworm (*T. cati*) are commonly involved in this condition, preventive measures include deworming of dogs and cats so that young children are not exposed to the infection.

B. Hookworms

Human hookworms (*Ancylostoma duodenale* and *Necator americanus*) are distributed in all tropical and subtropical countries. Adult worms live in the small intestine of man, mostly in jejunum, less often in the duodenum and rarely in the ileum.

1. *Ancylostoma duodenale*

(i) Morphology

Adult worm: It is small, greyish white and cylindrical in shape. The anterior end is bent dorsally, hence the name *hookworm.* The buccal capsule is provided with 6 teeth, 4 hook like on the ventral surface and 2 knob like on the dorsal surface (Fig. 44.16).

Copulatory bursa: It is present in male worm for attachment with female during copulation. It consists of three lobes, one dorsal and two lateral lobes. Each lobe is supported by chitinous rays. There are total 13 chitinous rays, the dorsal lobe contains 3 and the two lateral lobes contain 10 (Fig. 44.16).

Egg: The egg is oval measuring 65 µm in length and 40 µm in breadth. It is colourless (not bile stained) and is surrounded by a thin transparent hyaline shell-membrane. It contains a segmented ovum with four blastomeres. There is a clear space between the egg shell and the segmented ovum (Fig. 44.17). The egg floats in saturated salt solution.

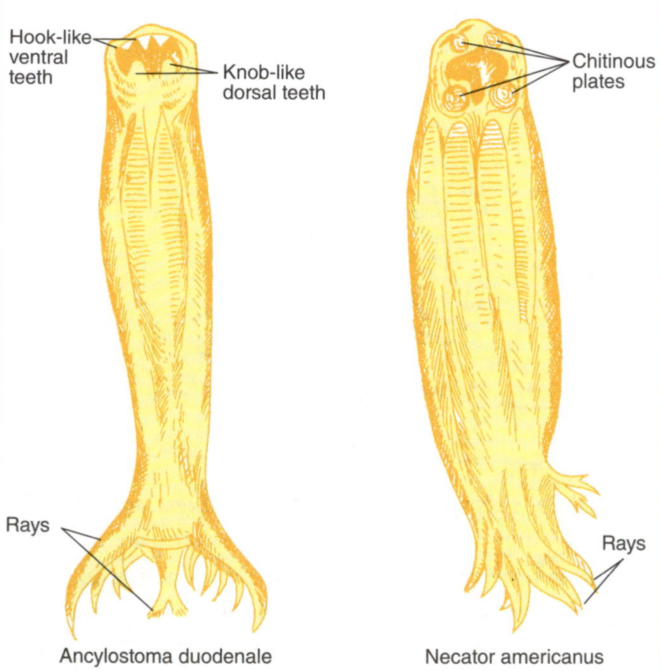

Fig. 44.16 Hook worms—Adult forms

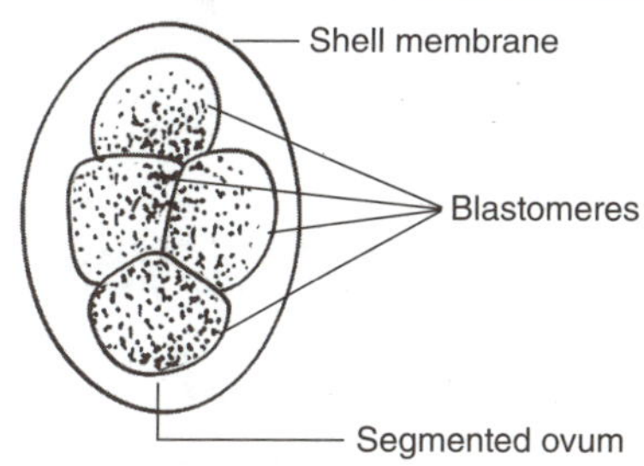

Fig. 44.17 Egg of hookworm

(ii) Life cycle

Man is the only **definitive host**. No intermediate host is required. The eggs containing segmented ova with 4 blastomeres, are passed out in the faeces of infected person. In the soil, from each egg a ***rhabditiform larva*** hatches out. The rhabditiform larva moults twice and then develops into a ***filariform larva***. This is the infective stage of the parasite and is capable of penetrating unbroken skin. When a person walks barefooted on soil containing filariform larvae, they penetrate the skin. On reaching the subcutaneous tissues the larvae enter into the lymphatics or small venules. Through lymph-vascular system they gain entry into the venous circulation and are carried via right heart into the pulmonary capillaries, where they break through the capillary walls and thus enter into the alveolar spaces. From alveoli, the larvae migrate on to the bronchi, trachea and larynx, crawl over the epiglottis to the pharynx and are ultimately swallowed. During migration or on entering the oesophagus they undergo third moulting. The larvae settle down in the small intestine, undergo a fourth moulting and develop into adult worms. They attach themselves to the small intestine by their mouthparts. Male fertilises female and the fertilised female begins to lay eggs in the faeces and the life cycle is thus repeated.

(iii) Pathogenesis and clinical features

Infective agent—Filariform larva
Portal of entry—Skin

The worm causes hookworm disease in man, characterised mainly by anaemia.

Pathogenic effects may be due to migrating larvae or due to adult worms. Migrating larvae may cause three types of lesions:

1. **Ancylostoma dermatitis or ground itch:** It occurs at the site of entry.
2. **Creeping eruption or cutaneous larva migrans:** It is a condition in which the filariform larvae wander about the skin and produce a reddish itchy papule along the path traversed by them.

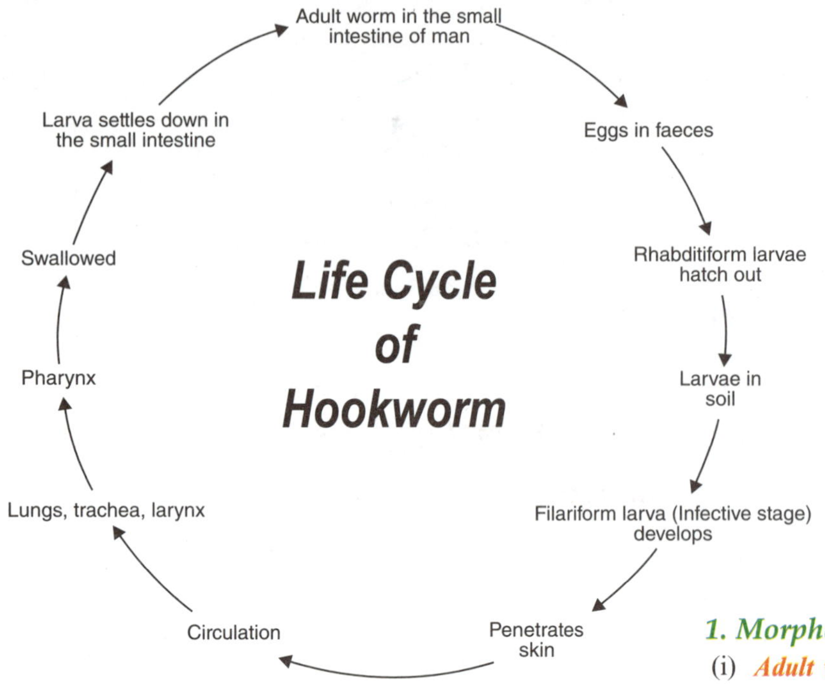

This is particularly seen with filariform larvae of animal hookworms, which are not adapted to man. Occasionally creeping eruptions may be caused by the larvae of *A. duodenale* or *N. americanus*.

3. **Lesions in the lungs:** Bronchitis and broncho-pneumonia may occur when the filariform larvae enter alveolar spaces.

Adult worms are responsible for the disease known as **hookworm disease**. This is characterised by **microcytic, hypochromic anaemia**. Hookworms ingest blood. Adult worm of *A. duodenale* sucks more blood than adult worm of *N. americanus.* Patient develops epigastric pain, dyspepsia, vomiting and diarrhoea. The stool becomes reddish or black in colour. Symptoms and signs of anaemia are present.

(iv) Laboratory diagnosis

The diagnosis of hookworm infection consists of:

Direct methods

1. Examination of stool is done to find the adult worms or characteristic hookworm eggs. Direct microscopy of stool or after concentration of the same can be used to detect eggs. Egg of *A. duodenale* or *N. americans* cannot be differentiated by morphology. Thus specific diagnosis can only be made by studying the morphology of adult worms.
2. Duodenal contents may reveal eggs or adult worms.

Indirect methods

1. Blood examination may be carried out to reveal microcytic, hypochromic anaemia and eosinophilia.
2. Stool examination may show occult blood and Charcot-Leyden crystals in a majority of cases of hookworm disease.

2. Necator americanus

The life cycle, pathogenesis and laboratory diagnosis of *N. americanus* is similar to those of *A. duodenale*.

C. Enterobius vermicularis

It is an intestinal nematode present in the **caecum** and **vermiform appendix** of human beings. Common names for it are **threadworm**, **seatworm** and **pinworm**.

1. Morphology

(i) ***Adult worm:*** Adult worm is small and white in colour. It resembles a short piece of thread. Male measures 2 to 4 mm in length and 0.1 to 0.2 mm across its girth. The posterior third of the body is curved in male but straight in female. The size of female is 8 to 12 mm in length and 0.3 to 0.5 mm across its thickest part.

(ii) ***Eggs*** (Fig. 44.18)***:*** The characteristics of the egg are as follows:

1. Colourless, i.e., not bile-stained.
2. Planoconvex in shape, i.e., flattened on the ventral side and convex on the dorsal side.
3. 50 to 60 µm × 30 µm (length × breadth).
4. Contains a tadpole-like larva.
5. Surrounded by a transparent shell.
6. Floats in saturated solution of common salt.

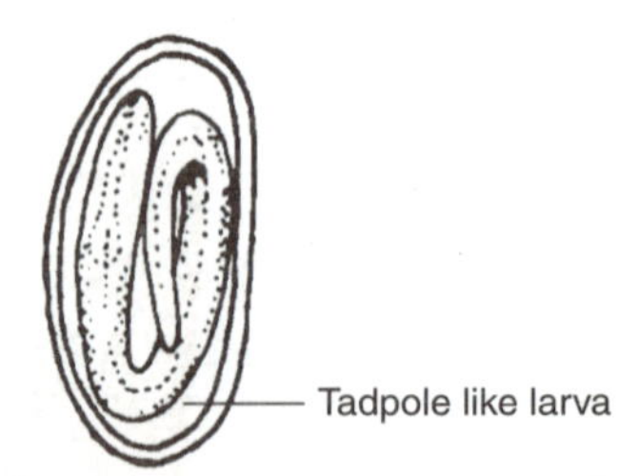

Fig. 44.18 Egg of *Enterobius vermicularis*

2. Life Cycle

Life cycle of this worm is completed in ***single host***.Infection occurs by **ingestion** of eggs which contain larvae. These eggs are laid on perianal skin and contamination of fingers with these eggs occur during scratching.

The egg-shells are dissolved by digestive juices, therefore, the larvae escape in the small intestine and develop into worms. The male worm fertilises the female

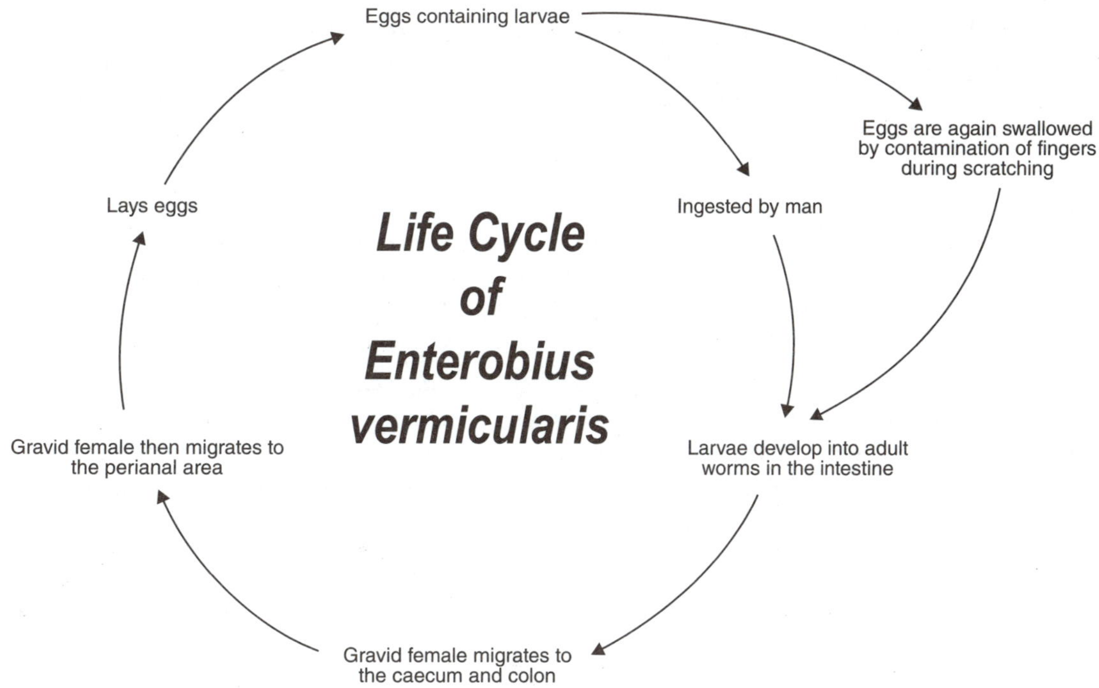

and dies. The gravid female then migrates to the caecum and colon (also the vermiform appendix) and remains there until the eggs develop. The fertilised female then wanders down and comes out of the anus during the night (after the patient has gone to bed) to deposit eggs on the perianal skin. These eggs are again swallowed by contamination of fingers during scratching and the cycle is repeated. Hence, no intermediate host is required.

3. Pathogenesis

Infection of *E. vermicularis* in man is named as **enterobiasis** or **pinworm infection**. Children are usually affected. The first infection is due to contaminated food and drink. **Autoinfection** may occur by carrying the eggs on their fingers while scratching the affected perianal area. Another mode of infection is retroinfection or retrograde infection. In this process, the eggs laid on the perianal skin immediately hatch into the infective-stage larvae and migrate through the anus to develop into worms in the colon.

4. Clinical Features

These include:

(i) Pruritus ani and an eczematous condition around the anus and perineum.

(ii) Nocturnal enuresis (frequency of micturition).

5. Laboratory Diagnosis

(i) ***Finding of adult worms:*** The worms are often detected by the patient himself or by the parents of the children. These worms can be identified as *Enterobius vermicularis* by characteristic features.

(ii) ***Demonstration of eggs:*** Eggs are usually demonstrated in the scrapings from the perianal skin by a **NIH (National Institute of Health)** swab (Fig. 44.19). The swab should be taken immediately after the patient wakes up in the morning. Eggs can also be found under the finger-nails. As oviposition in the bowel is rare, microscopic examination of stool for eggs of *E. vermicularis* may occasionally be successful.

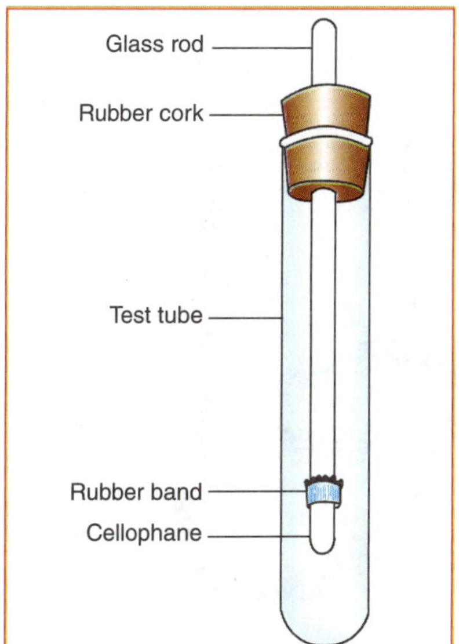

Fig. 44.19 NIH swab

D. Wuchereria bancrofti

Wuchereria bancrofti is mainly confined to the tropics and subtropics. In India, it is distributed along the sea coasts and also along the banks of big rivers.

1. *Morphology*

(i) ***Adult worms:*** Adult worms are transparent, long hair-like structures. They are often creamy-white in colour. They are filiform in shape and both ends are tapering. The sizes of male and female are 2.5–4.0 cm (length) × 0.1 mm (thickness) and 8–10 cm (length) × 0.2-0.3 mm (thickness) respectively. The female is ovo-viviparous (laying eggs with embryos). The life span of adult worms is several years (5 to 10 years).

(ii) ***Embryos (Microfilariae):*** They are colourless and transparent with blunt heads and pointed tails. The embryo measures 290 μm × 6–7 μm in size and is covered by a hyaline sheath (Fig. 44.20). The sheath is much longer than the embryo so that the microfilaria (embryo) can move forwards and backwards within it. The somatic cells or nuclei appear as granules in the central axis of the embryo and extends from the head to the tail-end. The granules do not extend up to the tip of the tail and is a distinguishing feature of *Microfilaria bancrofti*.

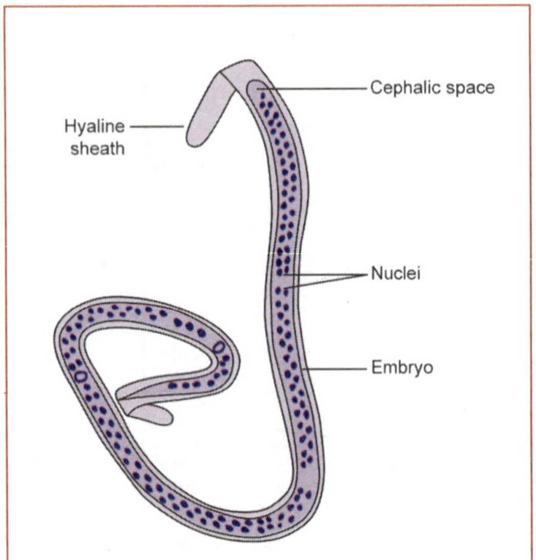

Fig. 44.20 Microfilaria of Wuchereria bancrofti

2. *Life Cycle*

W. bancrofti passes its life cycle in two hosts, i.e., **man (the definitive host)** and **mosquito (the intermediate host)**. The adult worms are harboured in lymphatic system of man. The male fertilises the female. Microfilariae (embryos) are discharged by the gravid female and reach the blood stream. These microfilariae are taken up by the female mosquitoes during their blood meal. The microfilariae undergo further development in a mosquito and become infective to man. Mosquitoes belonging to the genera *Culex*, *Aedes* and *Anopheles* act as intermediate hosts. When the infected mosquito bites a human being, the larvae are deposited on the skin near the site of puncture. The infective larvae penetrate the skin and reach the lymphatic channels and

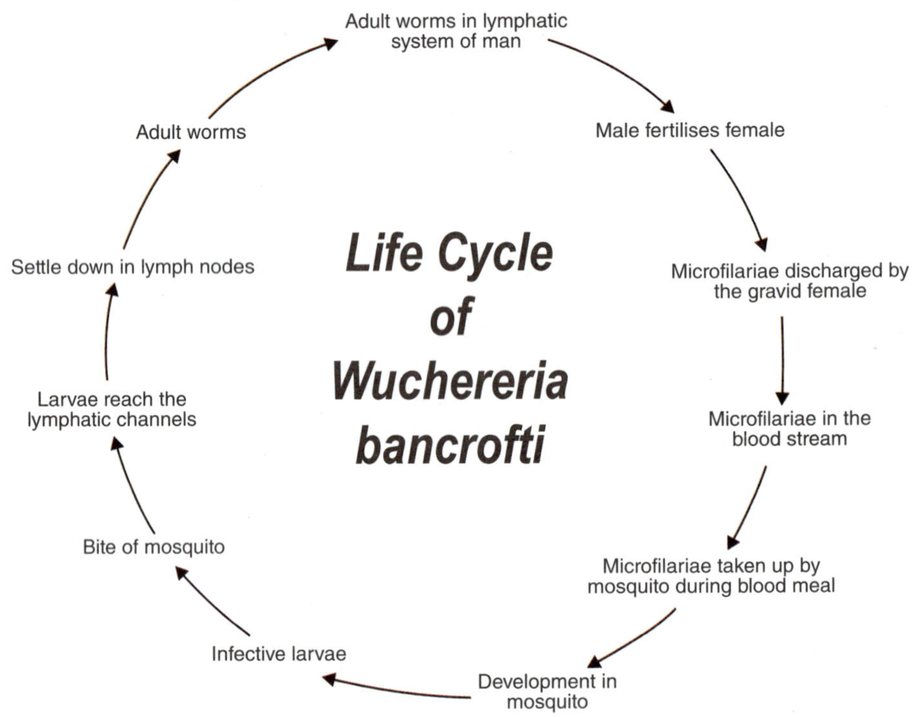

settle down usually in inguinal, scrotal and abdominal lymph nodes, where they develop into adult worms. They become sexually mature. The male fertilises the female, the gravid female gives birth to embryos (microfilariae). Thus the life cycle is repeated.

3. *Pathogenesis*

The infection with this parasite is named wuchereriasis or filariasis. The disease is of two types: classical filariasis (caused by adult worms) and occult filariasis (caused by embryos).

(i) ***Classical filariasis:*** It leads to **lymphangitis**, **lymphadenitis**, **lymphoedema** with hyper-trophy of affected part (**elephantiasis**), lymphangiovarix, hydrocele and chyluria.

(ii) ***Occult filariasis:*** It is due to **hypersensitivity reaction to microfilarial antigens**. Patient develops massive eosinophilia (30-80%), hepatosplenomegaly, generalised lymphadenopathy and pulmonary symptoms. Microfilariae are not found in the peripheral blood. Classical features of lymphatic filariasis are absent.

4. Laboratory Diagnosis

It depends on direct evidence (to search for microfilariae and adult worms) and indirect evidence (serological tests).

(*i*) ***Direct evidence:*** Demonstration of microfilariae in peripheral blood film, chylous urine, exudate of lymph varix and hydrocele fluid. The microfilariae appear in large numbers in peripheral blood at night. Hence, blood film should be made in night between 10 P.M. and 2 A.M.

(*ii*) ***Indirect evidence:*** Eosinophilia (5 to 15%) can be detected due to allergic reaction to antigens. Serological tests like enzyme linked immunosorbent assay (ELISA), indirect fluorescent antibody (IFA) and indirect haemagglutination assay (IHA) can also be used but these tests have low sensitivity and specificity.

KEY POINTS >>>

1. *Parasite* is a living organism which depends on a living host for its survival and derives nutrition from the host, without giving any benefit to the host.
2. *Definitive host* is the host that harbours the adult stage of the parasite or where the parasite replicates sexually.
3. *Intermediate host* is the host that harbours the larval stages of the parasite or where the parasite replicates asexually.
4. *E. histolytica* is the causative agent of amoebic dysentery and hepatic amoebiasis. Man acquires the infection by ingestion of water and food containing cysts of *E. histolytica*. Stool examination for cysts and trophozoites is one important diagnostic test.
5. *Leishmania donovani* causes *visceral leishmaniasis* or *kala-azar.* Infection occurs by bite of infected sandfly. Laboratory diagnosis depends on demonstration of *amastigote forms* in thick blood films and culture.
6. *P. vivax* and *P. falciparum* are very common in India and cause malaria. Man gets infection by the bite of infected anopheles mosquito. The parasite passes its life cycle in two hosts, i.e., *man* (*intermediate host*) and *female anopheles mosquito* (*definitive host*). *Microscopic examination* of a *peripheral blood smear* is the most important diagnostic procedure in malaria.
7. *Taenia solium* and *T. saginata* are cestodes. Common name for these parasites is *tapeworm.*
8. *Echinococcus granulosus* is the causative agent of the *hydatid cyst*. *Man* is the *intermediate host* while *dog* is the *definitive host*. Infection is generally acquired in childhood due to their intimate association with dogs. *Casoni test* is used in diagnosis of hydatid cyst.
9. *Ascaris lumbricoides* (round worm) is the largest intestinal nematode parasitising man. Man acquires infection by ingestion of food, drink or raw vegetables contaminated with eggs containing rhabditiform larvae (*embryonated eggs*). Adult worms or eggs may be demonstrated in stool specimen.
10. Human hookworms (*Ancylostoma duodenale* and *Necator americanus*) cause hookworm disease in man, characterised mainly by anaemia. Infective agent is *filariform larva* and portal of entry is *skin.* Examination of stool is done to find the adult worms or characteristic hookworm eggs which are not bile stained.
11. The infection with *Wuchereria bancrofti* is named *Wuchereriasis* or *filariasis*. The parasite passes its life cycle in two hosts, i.e., *man* (*the definitive host*) and *mosquito* (*the intermediate host*). Man gets the infection by bite of the infected mosquito. Laboratory diagnosis depends on *demonstration* of *microfilariae* in *peripheral blood film* or other specimens.

STUDY QUESTIONS

1. Describe the laboratory diagnosis of amoebic dysentery.
2. Write short notes on:
   (i) *Giardia lamblia* (ii) *Trichomonas vaginalis*
3. Describe the life cycle of *Plasmodium vivax* and the laboratory diagnosis of malaria caused by this parasite.
4. Describe briefly about:
   (i) *Plasmodium falciparum* (ii) Laboratory diagnosis of Kala-azar
5. Describe the life cycle of *Echinococcus granulosus* and the laboratory diagnosis of hydatid cyst.
6. Write short notes on:
   (i) Cysticercus cellulosae (ii) *Enterobius vermicularis*
   (iii) Larva migran (iv) NIH swab

7. Describe the life cycle of *Ancylostoma duodenale*.
8. Write short notes on:
   (i) Life cycle of *Ascaris lumbricoides* (ii) Differences between *Taenia solium* and *Taenia saginata*
   (iii) Microfilaria (iv) *Wuchereria bancrofti*

MULTIPLE CHOICE QUESTIONS (MCQs)

1. Mature cyst of *Entamoeba histolytica* contains:
   (a) Four nuclei
   (b) Eight nuclei
   (c) Two nuclei
   (d) None of the above
2. The infective form of *E. histolytica* is:
   (a) Uninucleate cyst
   (b) Binucleate cyst
   (c) Quadrinucleate cyst
   (d) None of the above
3. Extraintestinal amoebiasis may occur in:
   (a) Liver
   (b) Lung
   (c) Brain
   (d) All of the above
4. How many nuclei are there in cyst of *G. lamblia*?
   (a) One
   (b) Two
   (c) Four
   (d) Eight
5. *Leishmania donovani* causes
   (a) Sleeping sickness
   (b) Kala-azar
   (c) Malaria
   (d) Chaga's disease
6. Culture medium used for growing *L. donovani*:
   (a) Chick embryo
   (b) Chocolate agar
   (c) NNN medium
   (d) Diamond medium
7. Which of the following is intermediate host in malaria?
   (a) Man
   (b) Female anopheles mosquito
   (c) Culex mosquito
   (d) None of the above
8. Which of the following is definitive host in malaria?
   (a) Man
   (b) Female anopheles mosquito
   (c) Culex mosquito
   (d) None of the above
9. The infective form of malarial parasite is:
   (a) Merozoite
   (b) Sporozoite
   (c) Gametocyte
   (d) None of the above
10. In malaria, pre-erythrocytic schizogony occurs in:
    (a) Blood
    (b) Liver
    (c) Kidney
    (d) None of the above
11. Erythrocytes size increase in size when they are infected with:
    (a) *Plasmodium vivax*
    (b) *Plasmodium falciparum*
    (c) *Plasmodium malariae*
    (d) *Plasmodium ovale*
12. Gametocytes of which plasmodium sp. are sickle shaped?
    (a) *Plasmodium vivax*
    (b) *Plasmodium falciparum*
    (c) *Plasmodium malariae*
    (d) *Plasmodium ovale*
13. Pernicious malaria may occur in:
    (a) *Plasmodium vivax*
    (b) *Plasmodium falciparum*
    (c) *Plasmodium malariae*
    (d) *Plasmodium ovale*
14. Malaria can be diagnosed in the laboratory by:
    (a) Peripheral blood smear examination
    (b) Quantitative buffy coat (QBC) test
    (c) Detection of parasite lactate dehydrogenase (PLDH)
    (d) All of the above
15. The common name for *Taenia saginata* is:
    (a) The beef tapeworm
    (b) The pork tapeworm
    (c) The armed tapeworm
    (d) None of the above
16. The larval form of *Taenia saginata* is named as:
    (a) *Cysticercus cellulosae*
    (b) *Cysticercus bovis*
    (c) Hydatid cyst
    (d) None of the above
17. The common name for *Taenia solium* is:
    (a) The pork tapeworm
    (b) The beef tapeworm
    (c) The unarmed tapeworm
    (d) None of the above
18. The larval form of *Taenia solium* is named as:
    (a) *Cysticercus cellulosae*
    (b) *Cysticercus bovis*
    (c) Hydatid cyst
    (d) None of the above
19. Humans acquire *Cysticercus cellulosae* infection by:
    (a) Contaminated vegetables
    (b) Reversal of peristaltic movement of the intestine
    (c) Autoinfection
    (d) All of the above
20. In humans, Cysticercus cellulosae can occur in following tissues:
    (a) Subcutaneous tissues
    (b) Brain
    (c) Muscles
    (d) All of the above

21. The adult worm of *Echinococcus granulosus* contains:
    (a) 3 to 4 segments
    (b) 100 to 200 segments
    (c) 400 to 800 segments
    (d) 1000 to 2000 segments
22. Which skin test is useful for diagnosis of hydatid disease?
    (a) Casoni test
    (b) Dick test
    (c) Schick test
    (d) Tuberculin test
23. The common name for *Ascaris lumbricoides* is:
    (a) Roundworm
    (b) Hookworm
    (c) Threadworm
    (d) None of the above
24. The largest intestinal nematode infecting humans is:
    (a) *Ascaris lumbricoides*
    (b) *Necator americanus*
    (c) *Enterobius vermicularis*
    (d) None of the above
25. The common name for *Ancylostoma duodenale* is:
    (a) Roundworm
    (b) Hookworm
    (c) Threadworm
    (d) None of the above
26. Hookworm infection occurs by:
    (a) Eggs present in food
    (b) Auto infection
    (c) Penetration of skin by infective larvae
    (d) All of the above
27. Hookworm infection may lead to:
    (a) Ground itch
    (b) Anaemia
    (c) Creeping eruption
    (d) All of the above
28. The common name/s for *Enterobius vermicularis* is/are:
    (a) Threadworm
    (b) Pinworm
    (c) Seatworm
    (d) All of the above
29. *Enterobius vermicularis* infection in humans may occur by:
    (a) Raw or inadequately cooked pork
    (b) Autoinfection
    (c) Penetration of skin by infective larvae
    (d) None of the above

ANSWERS (MCQs) ...✓

1. (a)	2. (c)	3. (d)	4. (c)	5. (b)	6. (c)	7. (a)	8. (b)	9. (b)	10. (b)
11. (a)	12. (b)	13. (b)	14. (d)	15. (a)	16. (b)	17. (a)	18. (a)	19. (d)	20. (d)
21. (a)	22. (a)	23. (a)	24. (a)	25. (b)	26. (c)	27. (d)	28. (d)	29. (b)	

Unit VII

Hospital Infection Control and Safety

Healthcare Associated Infection

45

HEALTHCARE ASSOCIATED INFECTION

A. Definition

The terms *health care associated infection, health associated infection, hospital acquired infection, hospital-associated infection, hospital infection or nosocomial infection* (*nosocomion*, meaning hospital) is defined as infection developing in patients after admission to the hospital, which was neither present in the incubation period nor at the time of hospitalisation. Such infections may become evident during their stay in the hospital or, sometimes, after their discharge. The infection is acquired 48 hours after admission and patient was not admitted in hospital for management of that infection.

B. Factors Influencing Infection

Health associated infection is probably a great problem today despite advances in hygiene and treatment of infecting organisms. Several factors contribute to the occurrence and severity of these infections. These include:

1. Susceptible Patients

Many patients in hospitals have impaired defence mechanisms due to pre-existing diseases, such as diabetes, immunosuppression and patients with prosthetic implants. They are, therefore, more susceptible to infection.

2. Hospital Environment

The hospital environment is heavily laden with a wide variety of pathogens. These pathogens may be present in air, dust, water, food or antiseptic lotions. Equipment may be contaminated. Bedding, linen and utensils may act as fomites. Patients shed the organisms from their bodies while hospital personnel spread these organisms through their hands and clothes.

3. Diagnostic or Therapeutic Procedures

During diagnostic or therapeutic procedures such as insertion of urethral or intravenous catheters, the slightest lapse in asepsis may lead to infection.

4. Drug Resistance

Hospital infections are generally refractory to treatment as the infecting agents are usually multidrug resistant.

5. Transfusion

Blood, blood products and intravenous fluids used for transfusion, if not properly screened, can transmit many infections.

C. Sources of Infection

1. Exogenous

Hospital-infection is mostly exogenous from another patient or member of the staff or from the environment in the hospital. Patients and hospital personnel suffering from infection, or asymptomatic carriers are the most important sources. Environmental sources include inanimate objects, air, water and food in the hospital. Inanimate objects in the hospital are medical equipments (endoscopes, cystoscopes, catheters etc.), bed pans, surfaces contaminated by patient's secretions, excretions, blood and body fluids.

2. Endogenous

Patients own flora may invade the patient's tissue during some surgical operation or instrumental manipulations.

D. Microorganisms

Almost any microorganism can sometimes cause hospital acquired infection but those that survive in the hospital environment for long periods and develop resistance to antibiotics and disinfectants are particularly important. *Staph. aureus* strains, resistant to multiple antibiotics spread globally in the 1950's and 1960's, colonising hospitals and continue to be very common agents in nosocomial infection. *Staph. epidermidis* and Group D streptococci also are sometimes responsible for health-associated infections.

In recent decades, *Esch. coli, Klebsiella pneumoniae, Enterobacter, Proteus* and *Serratia* have become the most important hospital pathogens, particularly because of dissemination among them of R factor conferring multiple drug resistance.

Pseudomonas aeruginosa and other *Pseudomonas* species have always been important hospital pathogens because of their intrinsic resistance to most antibiotics and ability to survive and even multiply in disinfectant solutions. *Acinetobacter baumannii* is another very important organism responsible for healthcare associated infections.

Tetanus spores can survive in dust and may sometimes contaminate items used in hospitals. Hospital tetanus is usually due to faulty sterilisation techniques or other lapses in asepsis.

HIV and hepatitis B and C viruses are transmitted by contaminated blood or blood products. Screening of blood donors has reduced the risk to a large extent.However, HIV escapes detection during the window period.

Viral diarrhoea and chickenpox may spread in hospitals. Cytomegalovirus, influenza, herpesvirus, enteroviruses and arenaviruses are some other viruses which may cause hospital infection.

Candida albicans, Aspergillus, Mucor, Entamoeba histolytica, Pneumocystis carinii and *Toxoplasma gondii* may also sometimes cause hospital infection.

E. Modes of Transmission

There are four main routes of transmission of infection:

1. Contact

It is the principal route of transmission of nosocomial pathogens.

(i) Hands or clothing

The hands of hospital staff are an important vehicle of spread of infection. There is adequate scope of transmission of microorganisms from one person to another by contact of hands and clothings of attendants. *Staph. aureus* and *Str. pyogenes* are two important pathogens spread by hand contact.

(ii) Inanimate objects

Certain instruments (endoscope, bronchoscope, cystoscope), if not properly disinfected, may transmit pathogenic organisms (e.g. *Pseudomonas aeruginosa*).

2. Airborne

(i) Droplets

Droplets of respiratory infection is transmitted by inhalation.

(ii) Dust

Dust from bedding, floors, exudates dispersed from a wound during dressing and from skin by natural shedding of skin scales (measles, staphylococcal sepsis), may contribute in spread of infections e.g. *Pseudomonas aeruginosa, Staph. aureus.*

(iii) Aerosols

Aerosols produced by nebulizers, humidifiers and air conditioning apparatus transmit certain pathogens to the respiratory tract. Occurrence of legionellae in hospital water supply has led to outbreaks of infections mainly with *Legionella pneumophila*.

3. Oral Route

Hospital food may contain antibiotic-resistant bacteria (*Pseudomonas aeruginosa, Esch. coli*, Klebsiella spp. and others), which may colonise the intestine and later cause infection in susceptible patients.

4. Parenteral Route

With the introduction of disposable syringes and needles, transmission of infection by parenteral route has been infrequent. However, certain infections may be transmitted by blood transfusion or tissue donation, contaminated blood products (factor VIII) and contaminated infusion fluids. Hepatitis B and HIV are two viruses which may be transmitted in this way.

F. Types of Healthcare Associated Infection (HAI) (Table 45.1)

Major healthcare associated infections (HAIs) include:

1. Catheter Associated Urinary Tract Infection (CAUTI)
2. Ventilator Associated Pneumonia (VAP)
3. Central Line Associated Blood Stream Infection (CLABSI)

} These are associated with devices used hence named as Device associated infections (DAIs)

4. Surgical Site Infection (SSI)

1. Catheter Associated Urinary Tract Infection (CAUTI)

Urinary tract infection (UTI) accounts for the majority of healthcare associated infections (HAIs). This is usually associated with catheterisation. Infection rate increases in case of indwelling urinary catheter. Urinary tract infection associated with catheterisation is named as ***catheter associated urinary tract infection* (CAUTI)**. Infection is caused by *Esch. coli, Klebsiella, Proteus,* Pseudomonas and enterococci. *Esch. coli* is the most common organism implicated. Infection can be prevented by strict asepsis during catheterisation. Indwelling catheter should be used only when its use is unavoidable.

Predisposing risk factors for hospital acquired UTI include:

(i) extreme of age
(ii) females
(iii) catheterisation for > 2 days
(iv) severe underlying disease

Table 45.1 Common Healthcare Associated Infections

Healthcare associated infection	Causative organisms
CAUTI	*Esch. coli, Klebsiella, Proteus, Pseudomonas,* and enterococci.
Ventilator associated pneumonia (VAP)	*Staph. aureus, Klebsiella, Enterobacter, Serratia, Proteus, Esch. coli, Pseudomonas aeruginosa, Acinetobacter, Legionella pneumophila and respiratory viruses*
Surgical site infections (SSI)	*Staph. aureus, Pseudomonas aeruginosa, Esch. coli, Proteus,* enterococci and coagulase negative staphylococci
Gastrointestinal infection	*Salmonella, Shigella sonnei* and *viruses*
Burns	*Staph. aureus, Pseudomonas aeruginosa, Acinetobacter and Str. pyogenes*
Central line associated blood stream infections (CLABSI)	Gram negative bacilli, *Staph. epidermidis*

2. *Ventilator Associated Pneumonia (VAP)*

It is the second common cause of HAIs after UTI. Aspiration in unconscious patients and pulmonary ventilation may lead to nosocomial pneumonia. It is called ***ventilator associated pneumonia (VAP)***. The major pathogens include *Staph. aureus, Klebsiella spp., Enterobacter, Serratia, Proteus, Esch. coli, Pseudomonas aeruginosa, Acinetobacter*, *Legionella pneumophila* and respiratory viruses.

Risk factors includes:

- Device related: Endotracheal intubation
- Prolonged ICU stay: More risk of hospital acquired multidrug resistant organisms.
- Semiconscious state: Aspiration of oropharyngeal flora.
- Poor infection control practices e.g. poor hand hygiene.

3. *Central Line Associated Blood Stream Infection (CLABSI)*

It is the fourth common cause of HAIs. It may be due to consequences of infection at any site but is generally caused by infected intravenous cannulae. These infections are also named as **central line associated blood stream infections (CLABSI)**. Gram negative bacilli are common pathogens. Infection can be prevented by proper skin toilet before 'cut-down'. Intravenous rehydration in diarrhoea should be replaced by oral fluids as early as possible.

Staph. epidermidis bacteraemia is found commonly in patients with artificial heart valves. Bacteraemia in patients with valvular defects may lead to endocarditis.

Risk factors include:

- Extreme of age
- Low immunity
- Malnutrition
- Burns or bed sore
- Prolonged ICU stay
- Presence of central line
- Poor infection control practices e.g. poor hand hygiene

4. *Surgical Site Infection (SSI)*

Infection that develops at surgical site within 30 days of surgery (within 90 days of cardiac, breast and joint surgeries) is called **Surgical site infections (SSI)**. The incidence of post-operative infection is higher in elderly patients. *Staph. aureus* is the predominant pathogen, followed by *Pseudomonas aeruginosa* and then *Esch. coli, Proteus,* enterococci and coagulase negative staphylococci.

Surgical site wounds are classified as clean wound, clean-contaminated wound and contaminated or dirty wound. The skin flora is the major pathogen for clean wound. This skin flora may be from surgical team or from the environment. The most common pathogen in clean wound is *Staph. aureus*. For other two types of wounds, the patient's endogenous flora are the common pathogens.

Other HAIs

(i) Gastrointestinal Infections

Food poisoning and neonatal septicaemia in hospitals have been reported. *Salmonella* and *Shigella sonnei* are mainly associated with these infections.

(ii) Burns

Staph. aureus (may be MRSA), *Pseudomonas aeruginosa, Acinetobacter* and *Str. pyogenes* are responsible for hospital associated infections in cases of burns.

G. Diagnosis and Control

Healthcare associated infection may occur sporadically or as outbreaks. Diagnosis is by the routine bacteriological methods such as direct smear examination, culture and sensitivity testing. This requires the samples from possible sources of infection such as hospital personnel, inanimate objects, water, air or food. Typing of isolate (phage typing, bacteriocin typing, biotyping or antibiogram) may indicate a causal connection.

Control of hospital infection should be a permanent ongoing activity. Examples of sources of hospital outbreaks are nasal carriage of staphylococci in hospital staff or Pseudomonas growing in lotions. Carriers should be suitably treated.

The cause of infection may be a defective autoclave, therefore, sterilisation techniques have to be tested.

Unfortunately, in many hospitals, infection control is attempted by use of more and more antibiotics. This may lead to selective colonisation by multiresistant pathogens and has a harmful effect.

Concerns about transmission of the hepatitis B virus (HBV) and human immunodeficiency virus (HIV) led to the introduction of '**universal precautions**', to minimise the infections in medical laboratory workers and health care personnel.

H. Prevention

The health associated infections can be prevented by following means:

1. Transmission of infection can be controlled by regular proper washing of hands, disinfection of equipments and change of working clothes.
2. Administration of antibiotic therapy to the carrier staff or source patient to destroy the pathogenic agents.
3. Proper sterilisation and disinfection of the inanimate objects should be done. This helps to control the source of infection.
4. Disinfection of excreta and infected material is necessary to control the exit point of infection.
5. The use of sterile dressings, surgical gloves, face-masks and I/V fluids further contribute in control of infection.
6. Preoperative disinfection of the patient's skin.
7. Rational antibiotic prophylaxis.
8. Proper investigation of hospital-associated infection and the treatment of such cases.

Broadly prevention can be done by

(i) Standard precautions (Chapter 46)

(ii) Transmitted based precautions

KEY POINTS

1. The terms health associated infection, healthcare associated infection, hospital acquired infection or nosocomial infection is defined as infection developing in patients after admission to the hospital, which was neither present nor in the incubation period at the time of hospitalisation.
2. Healthcare associated infection is mostly exogenous from another patient or member of the staff or from the environment in the hospital.
3. Almost any microorganism can, on occasion, cause healthcare associated infection but those that survive in the hospital environment for long periods and develop resistance to antibiotics and disinfectants are particularly important.
4. *Staph. aureus, Pseudomonas aeruginosa, Esch. coli, Klebsiella* are some important agents responsible for health associated infections.
5. Diagnosis of hospital associated infection is done by the routine bacteriological methods. This requires the samples from possible sources of infection such as hospital personnel, inanimate objects, water, air or food.
6. Every hospital must have an effective infection control committee (ICC) which should be responsible for the control of healthcare associated infection (HAI).

STUDY QUESTIONS

1. Define healthcare associated infection. Enumerate the microorganisms causing it. What are the factors which contribute in development of this infection?
2. Write short notes on:
   (a) Modes of transmission of healthcare associated infection
   (b) Diagnosis and control of healthcare associated infection
   (c) Prevention of healthcare associated infection
   (d) Infection control policy

MULTIPLE CHOICE QUESTIONS (MCQs)

1. What are different modes of transmission of healthcare associated infections?
   (a) Through contact
   (b) Airborne
   (c) Parenteral route
   (d) All of the above
2. Which of the following bacteria can cause hospital acquired urinary tract infection?
   (a) *Escherichia coli*
   (b) *Klebsiella species*
   (c) *Proteus* species
   (d) All of the above
3. Which of the following bacteria can cause infection in hospitalised burn patients?
   (a) *Pseudomonas aeruginosa*
   (b) *Staphylococcus aureus*
   (c) *Acinetobacter* species
   (d) All of the above
4. Which of the following bacteria can cause hospital acquired respiratory infections?
   (a) *Staphylococcus aureus*
   (b) *Klebsiella* species
   (c) *Enterobacter* species
   (d) All of the above

ANSWERS (MCQs) ...✓

1. (d) 2. (d) 3. (d) 4. (d)

46

Standard Precautions

I. UNIVERSAL PRECAUTIONS

1. Assume that all specimens/patients are potentially infectious for HIV and other blood borne pathogens.
2. All blood specimens or body fluids should be placed in a leak-proof impervious bags for transportation to the laboratory.
3. Use gloves while handling blood and body fluid specimens and other objects exposed to them. If there is a likelihood of spattering, use face masks with glasses or goggles.
4. Wear laboratory coats or gowns while working in the laboratory. Wrap-around gowns should be preferred. These should not be taken outside.
5. Never pipette by mouth. Mechanical pipetting devices should be used.
6. Decontaminate the laboratory work surfaces with an appropriate disinfectant after the spillage of blood or other body fluids and when the procedures are completed.
7. Limit use of needles and syringes to situations for which there are no other alternatives.
8. Biological safety hoods should be used for laboratory work.
9. All the potentially contaminated materials of the laboratory should be decontaminated before disposal or reprocessing.
10. Always wash hands after completing laboratory work and remove all protective clothings before leaving the laboratory.

Most common agents which are associated with laboratory acquired infections include hepatitis B virus, *Coccidioides immitis, Bacillus anthracis,* Brucella species, *Mycobacterium tuberculosis, Francisella tularensis* and shigella species.

II. STANDARD PRECAUTIONS

Universal precautions were used in the past for the infection control while handling patient's body fluids. Now it is replaced by "**standard precautions**" which include a set of infection control practices to prevent transmission of diseases which can be acquired by contact with blood, body fluids, non-intact skin (including rashes) and mucous membranes. Unlike 'Universal precautions', 'Standard Precautions' are not restricted to body fluids only. These standard precautions apply to all patient care regardless of patient status i.e. whether infective or not.

The components of standard precautions include:

1. **Hand hygiene** (For details see chapter 47)
2. **Personal protective equipment (PPE)**
   - Wear gloves while handling blood and body fluids.
   - Wear other PPEs such as gown, mask, glasses or goggles, shoes etc. whenever indicated.
3. **Biomedical waste management** (For details see chapter 52)
4. **Spillage cleaning**
   - Clean up any spill of infective material and disinfect promptly.
5. **Disinfection**
   - Patient care equipment, linen contaminated with infective material should either be discarded or disinfected/sterilised between each patient care.
6. **Safe injection practices**
   - Aseptic techniques should be used while preparing and administering medicines or fluids.
7. **Environmental cleaning**
   - Surface and floor should be cleaned especially in operation theaters, ICUs etc.
8. **Sharp handling**
   - All sharps including needles should be handled with extreme care.
9. **Respiratory hygiene (cough etiquette)**
   - Covering the nose/mouth when coughing or sneezing.

1. Personal Protective Equipment (PPE)

Personal protective equipment (PPE) are used to protect Health Care Workers (HCWs) from exposure to blood and/or body fluids which may contain pathogens. PPE also protects the patient by preventing the transmission of organisms from HCWs hands to patient during sterile and invasive procedures.

(i) Components of PPE (Fig. 46.1)

- **Gloves (Non-sterile):** They are used when the risk of infection is to HCW only e.g. touching blood, body fluids.
- **Gloves (Sterile):** They are used when the risk of infection is to both HCW and patient e.g. during invasive procedure or surgery.
- **Plastic apron:** It is used during surgery.
- **Gown:** It is used when soiling is expected during surgery.
- **Coverall:** Coverall are designed to cover the whole body and provides 360° protection. By using appropriate protective clothing it is possible to eliminate or reduce contact and droplet exposure.
- **Surgical mask:** It is used during surgery and for droplets precautions while handling patients. It is triple layered mask, fluid resistant, provide protection from droplets of infection. It is also named as medical mask.
- **N95 mask:** It is used when handling or examining patients with airborne infections e.g. tuberculosis, H1N1 virus, Ebola virus, SARS-CoV-2 etc. It is respiratory protective device with high filtration efficiency to airborne particles. These masks are cup-shaped structured design which does not collapse against the mouth. If correctly worn, the filtration capacity of these masks exceeds that of surgical mask. Since these masks have a much tighter air seal than surgical masks, they protect wearer from inhaling airborne particles.
- **Cap, goggles, face shield:** It is used when spillage of blood is likely to be expected e.g. cardiac surgery. Contamination of mucous membranes eye, nose and mouth may occur during droplets generated by cough, sneeze of an infected person or during aerosol generated procedure. Hence goggles/face shields are an integral part of standard and contact precautions. The flexible frame of goggles should provide good seal with the skin of the face, covering the eyes and other areas.
- **Surgical shoes:** It is used in operation theaters and intensive care units (ICUs) to prevent transmission of organisms to HCW and as well as to environment.

(ii) Selection of appropriate PPE

- It is based on the level of risk associated during a specific patient care procedure or intervention (as a part of standard precautions).
- Route of transmission of suspected pathogen e.g. contact, droplet, airborne (as a part of transmission based precautions).

(iii) Donning and Doffing of PPE (Fig 46.2 and 46.3)

Donning (wearing) and Doffing (removing) of PPE must be done in a particular sequence mentioned below, to minimise the risk of infection.

Donning	**Doffing**
Perform hand hygiene	Gloves
↓	↓
Gown	Goggles or face shield
↓	↓
Mask or respirator	Gown
↓	↓
Goggles or face shield	Mask or respirator
↓	↓
Gloves	Perform hand hygiene

During doffing, discard PPE components into appropriate biomedical waste bins.

- **Yellow bin:** Gown or coverall, mask or respirator, cap, shoecover.
- **Red bin:** Plastic apron, goggles or face shield, gloves.

Note: During doffing, perform hand hygiene in between the steps also if hands get contaminated.

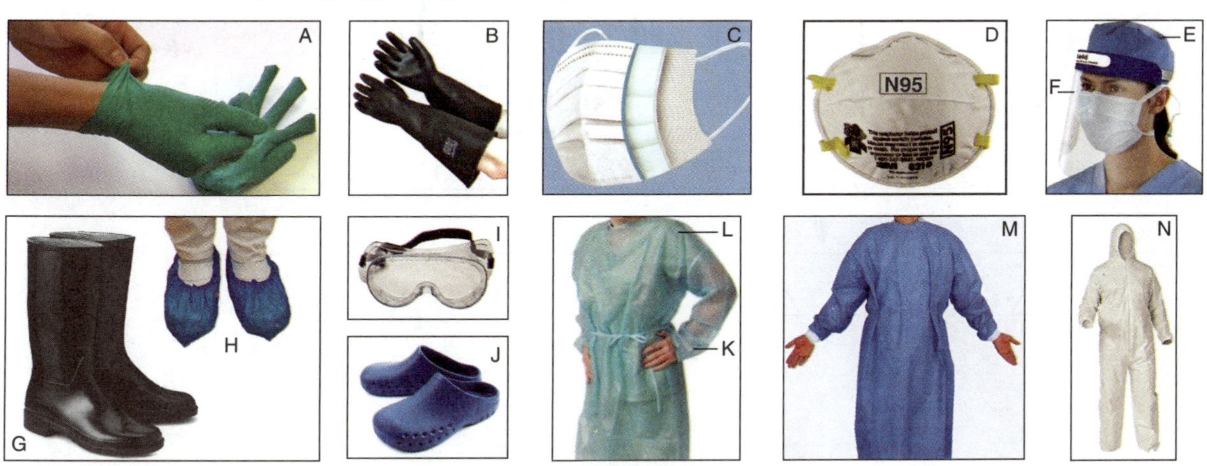

Fig. 46.1 A to N Personal protective equipment
A. Gloves; B. Heavy-duty gloves; C. Surgical mask; D. N95 respirator; E. Cap; F. Face shield; G. Gumboot; H. Shoe cover; I. Goggles; J. Shoes; K. Plastic apron; L. Linen gown; M. Disposable gown; N. Coverall

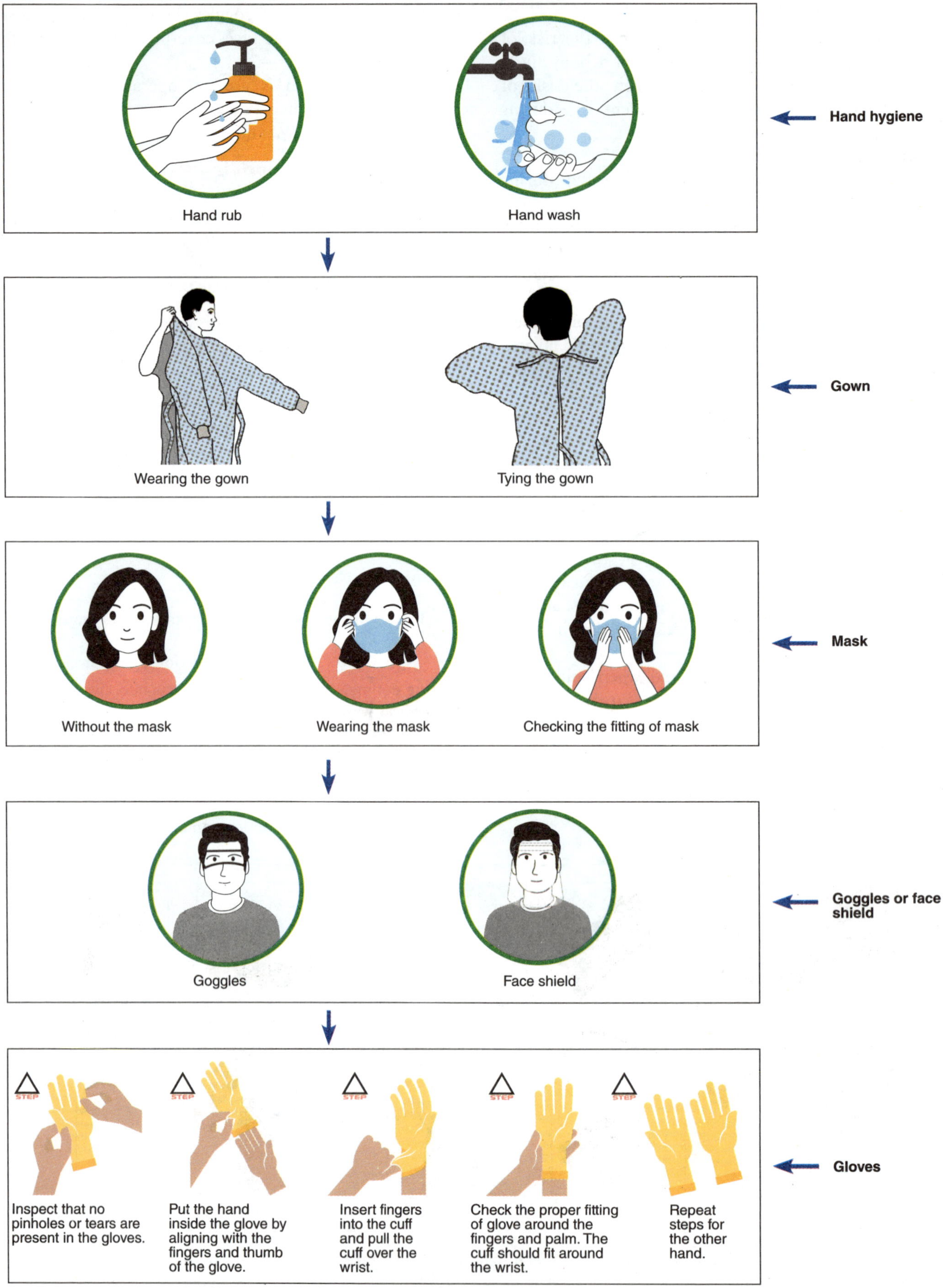

Fig. 46.2 Donning of PPE

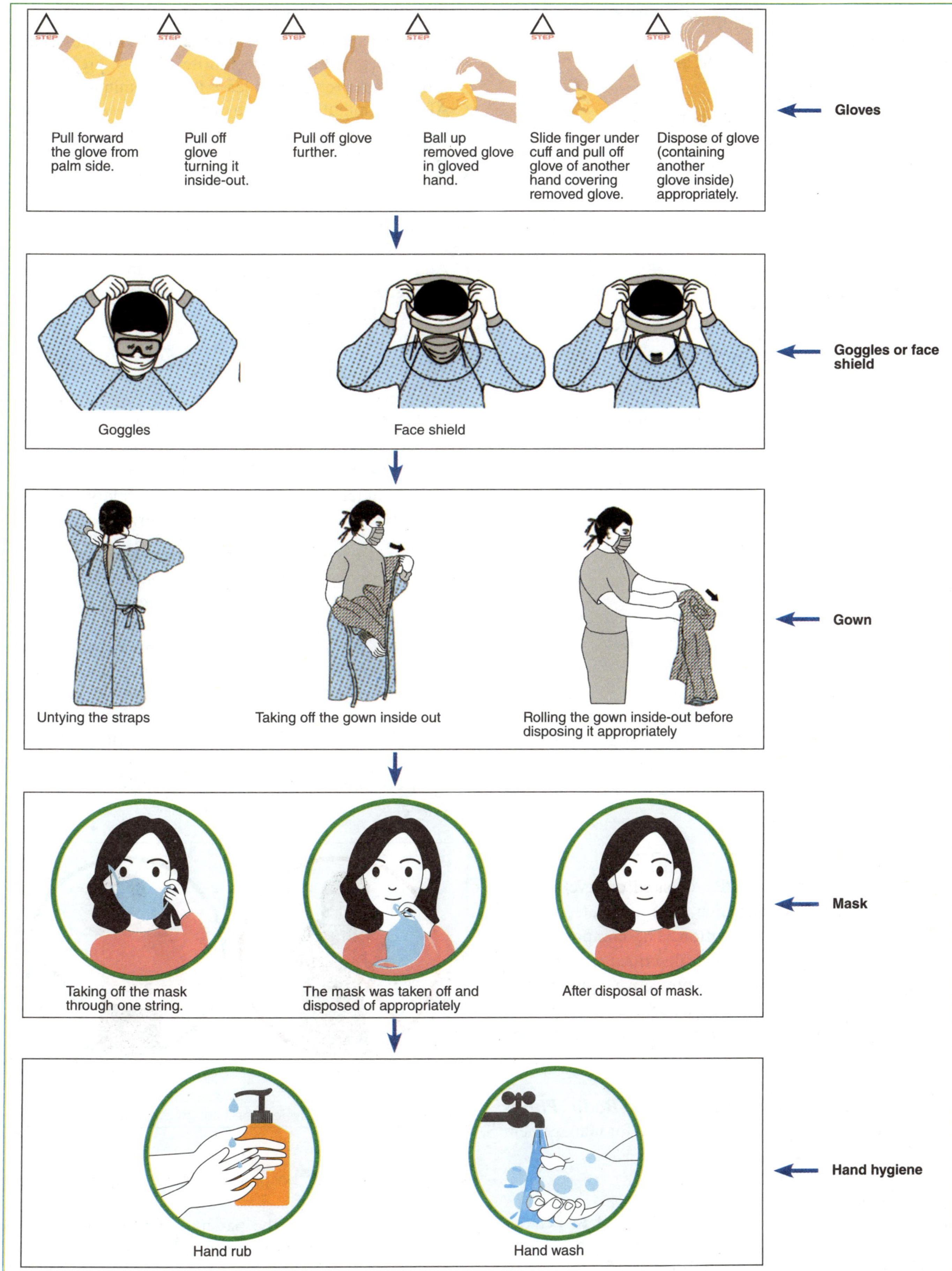

Fig. 46.3 Doffing of PPE

2. *Personal Protective Equipment (PPE) in COVID-Care*

The following components of PPE are used.

(i) Goggles and faceshield.

Both goggles and faceshield should be used.

(ii) Mask

- N-95 mask
- Triple layer medical mask
  If N-95 mask is not available, triple layer medical mask can be used.

(iii) Gloves

- Nitrile gloves
- Latex groves
  Two pair of gloves, one over the other, may be used.

(iv) Coveralls/Gowns

Coveralls are designed to cover the whole body and provides 360 degree protection. By using protective clothing, it creates a barrier to eliminate or reduce contact and droplet exposure.

Gowns can also be used instead of coveralls. Both gowns and coveralls can also be worn.

(v) Shoe covers

Shoe covers should be made of impermeable fabric similar to fabric of coveralls. These are used over shoes to facilitate personal protection and decontamination.

(vi) Head covers

Coveralls usually cover the head. When using gowns, head cover should be used to cover the head and neck. Hair and hair extensions should fit inside the head cover. Cap may be used as head over.

Selection of PPE

The selection of appropriate PPE is based on level of risk (low risk, moderate risk and high risk) associated during a specific procedure or intervention. The components of PPE may be selected accordingly as described earlier under heading 'components of personal protective equipment'. The complete PPE mentioned above is used at high risk area e.g. microbiology laboratory for RT-PCR testing, COVID-19 patient care ward.

3. *Spill Management of Blood and Body Fluids*

The following basic steps are to be followed for management of blood and body fluids.

- Spillage should be attended immediately.
- Mark the spill area.
- Entry to the spill area should be restricted to persons who are involved in management.
- Bring the spill kit containing all material to the site of spillage.
- Wear appropriate PPE (gloves and gown).
- Cover the spill with paper towels to absorb the spillage.
- Pour 0.5% sodium hypochlorite (freshly prepared) on top of paper towels and leave it for 15 minutes.
- After 15 minutes, remove the paper towels; put fresh paper towels to clean the area. Then all these towels are to be discarded as infectious waste.
- Wipe the area with 0.5% sodium hypochlorite (freshly prepared)
- Wash the area with soap and water.
- Remove PPE.
- All PPE material and paper towel etc. are to be discarded as infectious waste in appropriate waste container.
- Perform hand hygiene.
- Record the incident.

Note: The above steps are basic. However hypochlorite solution percentage and its period of contact may vary according to recommendations of various agencies (WHO, CDC etc). CDC recommends 0.5% hypochlorite for large spill (>10 mL) and 0.05% hypochlorite for small spill (<10 mL) for contact time of 10 minutes in both large and small spill. WHO recommends 0.5% hypochlorite.

4. *Respiratory Hygiene and Cough Etiquette*

Persons with signs and symptoms of respiratory tract infection should follow respiratory hygiene and cough etiquette:

- Cover the nose/mouth with tissue paper (single time use) while coughing, sneezing, wiping and blowing noses.
- If tissues are not available then cough or sneeze into inner elbow but not on the hand (Fig 46.4).
- Follow hand hygiene after contact with respiratory secretions.
- Keep contaminated hands away from mucous membranes especially those of the eyes and nose.

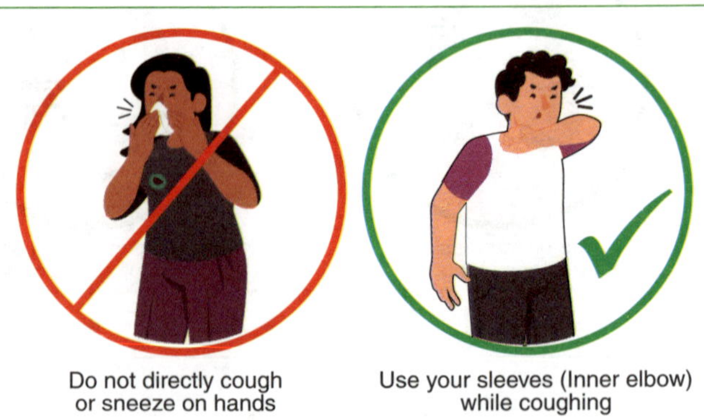
Do not directly cough or sneeze on hands
Use your sleeves (Inner elbow) while coughing

Fig 46.4 Respiratory hygiene and cough etiquette.

In high risk areas of hospitals such as pulmonary medicine department:

- Give face masks to the patients with cough and make separate queue away from general queue.
- Sputum should be collected in an open space or in a well ventilated room.

KEY POINTS »»

1. Standard precautions include a set of infection control practices to prevent transmission of diseases which can be acquired by contact with blood, body fluids etc.
2. Hand hygiene, personal protective equipment (PPE) and biomedical waste management are some important components of standard precautions.

STUDY QUESTION

1. Write short notes on:
   - (i) Universal precautions
   - (ii) Standard precautions
   - (iii) Personal protective equipment (PPE)
   - (iv) Spill management

47

Hand Hygiene

I. INTRODUCTION

Hands have been known to be involved in many infectious disease outbreaks especially in nurseries, neonatal units, intensive care units and other hospital settings. This happens because hands of medical personnel may be transiently infected with pathogenic organisms from infected patients or environment, and thus these can be transmitted to other patients. Therefore, hand hygiene is very important in keeping the health care associated infections at minimum. The World Health Organisation (WHO) has published the standard guidelines when hand hygiene should be performed. There are five moments for hand hygiene which are as follows:

Five moments for hand hygiene (Fig. 47.1)

1. Before touching a patient
2. Before any aseptic procedure
3. After a procedure or body fluid exposure risk
4. After touching a patient
5. After touching patient's surroundings.

II. TYPES OF HAND HYGIENE TECHNIQUES

1. Routine hand washing
2. Hygienic hand care
3. Surgical hand washing or hand scrub

1. Routine Hand Washing

It involves washing of hands with soap and water. It removes most transient microorganisms from the hands. Routine hand washing should be performed in the following conditions.

(a) Before and after contact with patients,
(b) Before wearing and after removing gloves,
(c) After wound dressing,
(d) After contact with body fluids of patients,
(e) After handling devices for patient care or having contact with inanimate objects in and around patient.

2. Hygienic Hand Care

(i) Hand wash method

- Wash hands with soap and water by rubbing hands in the six movements by covering all surfaces of hands as shown in Fig. 47.2.

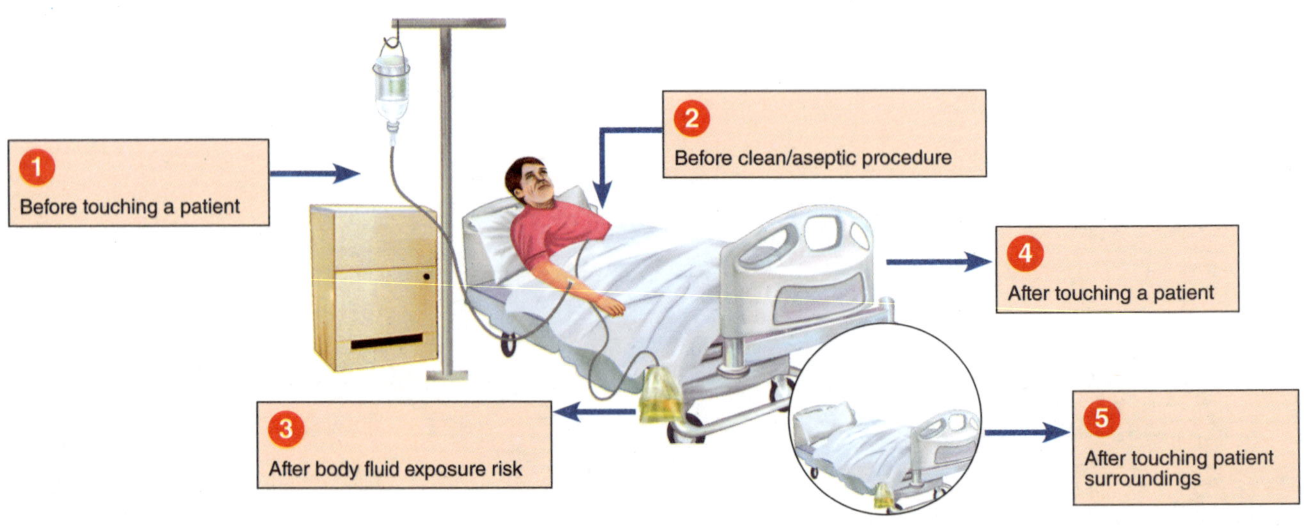

Fig. 47.1 Five moments for hand hygiene

- Rinse hands with water.
- Dry hands with single-use towel.
- Duration of hand wash method is 20–30 seconds.

(ii) Hand rub method

- When alcohol-based hand rub solution is used instead of soap, dry hands are required. Rest of the procedure is same as above with the difference that no towel is required for drying as alcohol evaporates in the environment.
- Duration of hand rub method is 40–60 seconds.

3. Surgical Hand Washing or Hand Scrub

- It requires more time for washing than hygiene hand care.
- Besides hands, wrists and forearms are also included for washing.
- For drying, sterile towels are used.

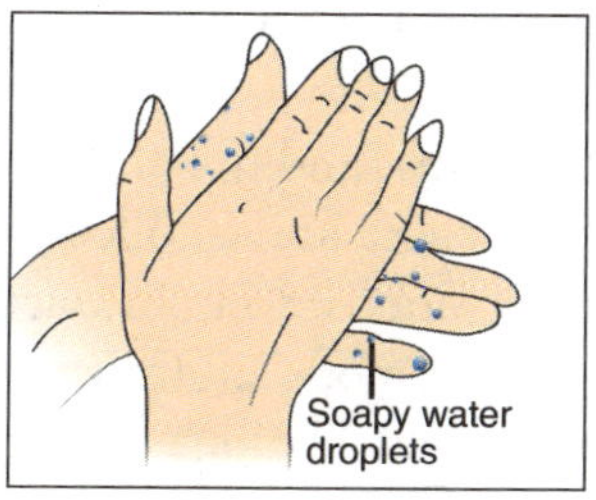

Step 1: Wet hands and apply soap. Rub hands palm to palm

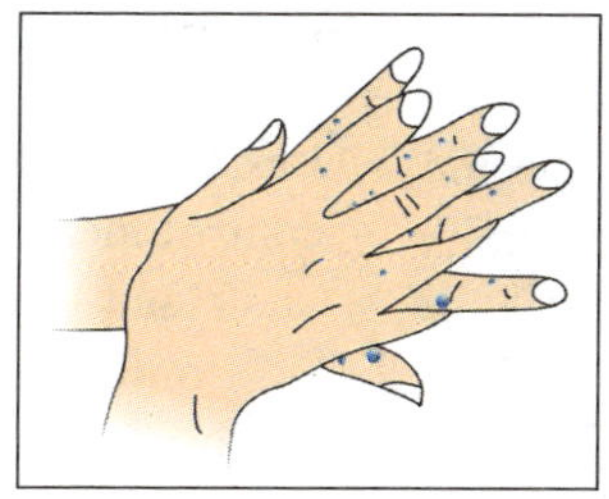

Step 2: Rub each palm over the back of the other palm with interlaced fingers.

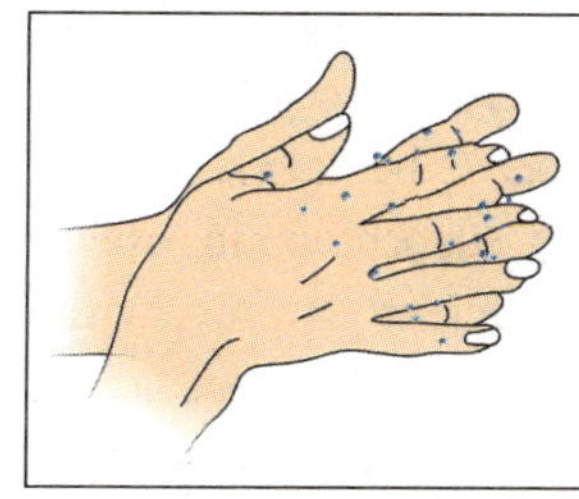

Step 3: Rub palm to palm with fingers interlaced.

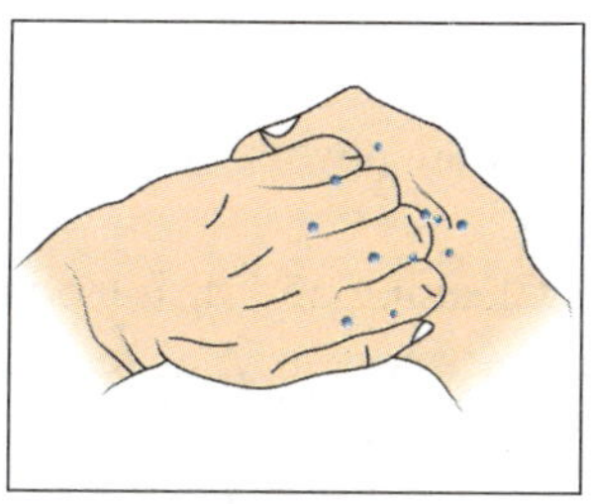

Step 4: Rub backs of your fingers to opposing palms with fingers interlocked.

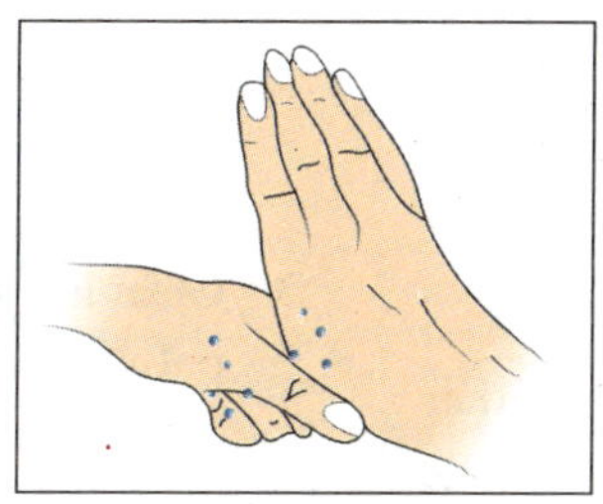

Step 5: Rotational rubbing of your thumb in opposite palm and vice-versa.

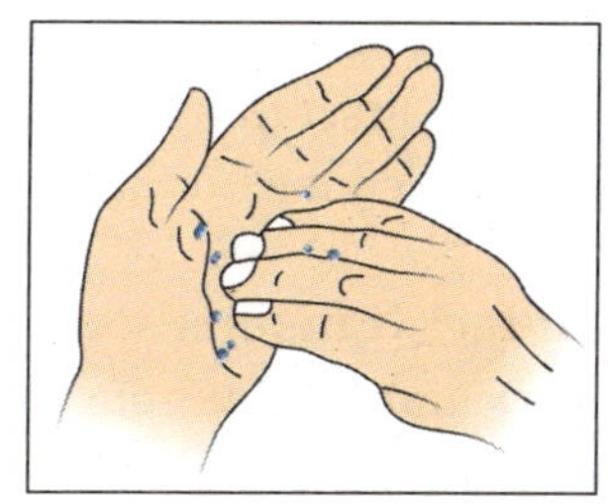

Step 6: Rub in circles, backwards and forwards with clasped fingers of right hand in left palm and vice-versa; on and then rinse and dry your hands.

Fig. 47.2 Hygienic hand care – standard method

KEY POINTS >>>

1. Hands have been known to be involved in many infectious disease outbreaks.
2. Hand hygiene is very important in keeping the health care associated infections at minimum.
3. There are three types of hand hygiene techniques namely routine hand washing, hygienic hand care, surgical hand washing or hand scrub.
4. Six steps are involved in standard method of hygiene hand care.
5. When alcohol-based hand rub solution is used instead of soap, dry hands are required. Rest of the procedure is same except that no towel is required for drying as alcohol evaporates in the environment.

STUDY QUESTIONS

1. Name various blood group systems and describe Rh blood group system.
2. Write short notes on:
   (i) Haemolytic disease in newborn
   (ii) Complications of blood transfusion

Transmission-Based Precautions

48

I. INTRODUCTION

Besides standard precautions, sometimes additional precautions are to be taken when a disease of a specific transmission is suspected, in which standard precautions may not be sufficient to prevent the transmission of that infection. Based on the specific modes of transmission, there are three types of precautions.

II. CONTACT PRECAUTIONS

Contact precautions should be followed whenever it is definitive or suspected that certain infectious organisms may be transmitted by contact during patient care. Transmission may occur by direct contact or indirect contact

A. Direct contact transmission

Transmission occurs directly from one person to another person without any intermediate object or person. The common example of direct contact transmission is through contaminated hands. The another example is direct contact with blood or body fluids of an infectious person.

B. Indirect contact transmission

Transmission occurs indirectly by involving some intermediate objects which are contaminated. Examples are clothes, fomites, environmental surfaces or instruments/ equipments used for patient care.

Some of the infectious organisms transmitted by contact mode of transmission are shown in Table 48.1.

C. Infection Control Measures for Contact Transmission

Besides standard precautions, some additional infection control measures are also taken. These are as follows:

1. **Hand hygiene:** It is of utmost importance as contaminated hands are major mode of transmission by contact. Hand hygiene should be done before and after contact with the patient and on leaving the room.
2. **Personal protective equipment (PPE):** Gloves and gowns are the essential PPE components as these will act as barrier between healthcare worker (HCW) and the patient, thus preventing contact transmission. HCW must remove gloves and gowns before leaving the patient-care area.
3. **Cleaning and disinfection:** Cleaning and disinfection of patient rooms must be done frequently, at least daily and definitely before use by another patient. This helps in environment cleaning (floor, toilet etc.) and thus prevents the infection by contact transmission.
4. **Isolation:** Isolation of the patient in a separate room with a bathroom is preferred. If not available then cohorting may be carried out as follows.
   - Keeping the patients with the same pathogen together in the same room or in the same cubicle is cohorting.
   - Patients' beds may also be separated by a minimum of 3 feet distance between the beds with curtains.
5. **Dedicated equipment:** Equipments (e.g. blood pre-ssure cuffs, thermometer) should be used for single patient. If not possible then these instruments must be disinfected before using it for another patient.

Table 48.1: Organisms transmitted through different modes

Contact	Droplets	Aerosols
• Methicillin resistant *Staphylococcus aureus* (MRSA)	• *Corynebacterium diphtheriae*	• *Mycobacterium tuberculosis*
• Vancomycin resistant enteroceri (VRE)	• Haemophilus influenzae type B	• Measles virus
• Multidrug resistant *Acinetobacter* species	• *Bordetella pertussis*	• Varicella zoster
• *Pseudomonas* species	• *Mycoplasma pneumoniae*	• Monkeypox virus
• *Clostridioides difficile*	• *Streptococcus pyogenes*	
• Adenovirus	• SARS-CoV2	
• Rotavirus	• Influenza virus	
• Hepatitis A virus	• Rhinovirus	
• Hepatitis E virus		

6. **Patient movement:** Patient movement should be restricted only for medically essential procedures. During movement of patient, appropriate PPE must be used by HCWs and also cover the infected part of the patient's body to contain the infection.

III. DROPLET PRECAUTION

Droplet precautions are used to prevent the spread of infectious organisms which are transmitted through respiratory droplets. These precautions are used in addition to standard precautions.

- Respiratory droplets (> 5 μm in size) are generated by a person during coughing, sneezing or talking. As these are large droplets therefore they do not remain suspended in the air and travel only shorter distances (within one meter). These droplets settle on the surfaces and inanimate objects within a distance of 1 meter.
- Droplet transmission occurs by contact mode (direct or indirect) when other persons touch the contaminated objects and then touch the contaminated hands to their own mouth, nose or conjunctiva.

Some of the Infectious organisms transmitted by droplet mode of transmission are shown in Table 48.1.

A. Infection Control Measures for Droplet Transmission

Besides standard precautions, some additional infection control measures are also applied. These are as follows:

Hand hygiene

Droplet transmission also occurs by contact as described earlier. Hence, hand hygiene becomes very important measure for control of droplet transmission.

PPE

- Healthcare workers should wear a surgical mask while entering in patient's room and also when anticipating close contact (< 1 meter) with the patient. The surgical mask will protect HCW from larger droplets in the environment. N95 mask should not be used for this purpose as it does not provide any additional protection. Gown and gloves should also be worn for prevention of contact transmission.
- However, HCWs should wear N95 mask during procedures which generate aerosols especially when doing these procedures in patients with influenza or COVID -19.
- Patient should wear a surgical mask all the time to prevent the transmission of droplets from the patient to the environment.

Isolation

Isolation of the patient in a separate room is essential.

Patient movement

Patient movement is restricted. However, patient should wear a surgical mask when leaving the room.

IV. RESPIRATORY HYGIENE AND COUGH ETIQUETTE

Persons with signs and symptoms of respiratory tract infection should follow respiratory hygiene and cough etiquette.

1. Cover the nose/mouth with tissue paper (single time use) while coughing, sneezing, wiping and blowing noses.
2. If tissues are not available then cough or sneeze into inner elbow but not on the hand (Fig. 48.1).
3. Follow hand hygiene after contact with respiratory secretions.
4. Keep contaminated hands away from mucous membranes especially those of the eyes and nose.
5. Patients with respiratory symptoms should be segregated separately and provided with masks.
6. **Distancing:** At least distance of 1 meter should always be maintained from persons with respiratory symptoms. The following measures are also applied.
   - **Cleaning and disinfection** of patient rooms and patient-care items.
   - **Isolation** of the patient in a separate room is preferred if not available then cohorting or spatial separation between beds of > 3 feet similar to control measures in contact transmission.
   - **Patient movement** should be limited only for medically essential purposes as there is high risk of transmission. If it is unavoidable then the following precautions are to be taken.
     - While being transferred, patients should wear a surgical mask.
     - Patients should also follow respiratory hygiene and cough etiquette.
     - During transport of these patients, HCWs should wear PPE especially surgical mask, gloves, gowns and protective eye goggles.

V. AIRBORNE PRECAUTIONS

Airborne precautions are used to prevent the spread of infectious organisms which are transmitted through respiratory aerosols.

Aerosols are small particles (< 5 μm in size) generated during coughing, sneezing or talking. The aerosols are also generated during certain procedures such as intubation. These procedures are named as aerosol generated procedures. Aerosols being smaller particles remain suspended in the air for longer period and thus may travel to a distant place along with the air current.

Some of the infectious organisms transmitted by airborne mode of transmission are shown in Table 48.1.

A. Aerosol-generating Procedures

Aerosol-generating procedures (AGPs) generate higher concentration of aerosols and thus poses a higher risk of transmission of infectious agents.

- Due to higher risk of transmission by these procedures, air-borne precautions should be followed such as isolating the patient in a negative pressure room and wearing N95 mask during AGPs.

B. Infection Control Measures for Airborne Transmission

Infection control measures should be applied whenever there is a clinical suspicion of airborne infection. However, these airborne precautions may be discontinued later on when the diagnosis is confirmed with a disease which does not require airborne precautions.

1. PPE

Healthcare workers should wear N 95 mask properly fitted. Gloves, gowns and protective eye goggles may be required when there is any exposure risk. Patient may also wear the surgical mask all the time.

2. Isolation

Isolation of patients in a separate room with adequate ventilation, ultraviolet germicidal irradiation (UVGI) and filtration is needed.

3. Ventilation

Adequate ventilation reduces the risk of infection by diluting the infectious aerosols with introduction of fresh air into the room. It also removes the infectious aerosols due to continuous entry of fresh air in the room. Ventilation may be of two types: natural and mechanical.

Natural Ventilation

Natural ventilation occurs through fresh air which enters and leaves through windows and doors of the room.

- Natural ventilation is very effective when windows and doors are placed opposite to each other. When these doors and windows are open, then cross ventilation occurs.
- To minimise the risk of exposure to doctors and patients, doctors should sit away from direction of natural airflow and similarly patients' beds should be placed away from airflow.

Mechanical Ventilation

Mechanical ventilation system maintains the pressure of the room lesser than the pressure at the entry area outside the room, thus creating a negative pressure inside the room. Air naturally flows from areas with higher pressure to areas with lower pressure, hence prevents the contaminated air escaping from the room. The negative pressure room should have the following properties:

- Air changes per hour (ACH): High risk area should have a minimum of 12 ACH while 6 ACH in a low risk area for airborne transmission. Tuberculosis / Chest department, MDR-TB wards, bronchoscopy rooms are examples of high risk areas.
- The door should be kept closed all the times.
- Anteroom: A small outer waiting room (anteroom) should be there before entering the patient room (negative pressure room).
- Ultraviolet Germicidal Irradiation (UVGI): UVGI kills the infectious organisms by irradiation. These devices can be used in addition to negative pressure ventilation when there is not adequate ventilation.
- Filtration: By filtration, the room air is directly exhausted outside either through an exhaust fan or through high-efficiency particulate air (HEPA) filter.

4 Patient Movement

The patient movement to outside the negative pressure room should be done only when it is absolutely necessary. In such cases, the following precautions should be taken.

- The patient should wear a surgical mask and follow respiratory hygiene and cough etiquette.
- HCWs must wear N95 mask and other PPE components as per indications.
- If patient has some associated skin lesions in any part (e.g. chickenpox), these should be covered.

VI. VISITORS AND STAFF

Entry of visitors and staff should be absolutely restricted. Before entering the room, they should wear the PPE.

KEY POINTS

1. Transmission based precautions (TBPs) are infection control practices which should be followed in certain conditions.
2. According to mode of transmission there are three types of TBPs such as contact precautions, droplet precautions and airborne precautions.

STUDY QUESTION

1. Write short notes on:
   (i) Contact precautions
   (ii) Droplet precautions
   (iii) Airborne precaution

MULTIPLE CHOICE QUESTION (MCQ)

1. All of the following are infection control measures for contact transmission except.
   (a) Hand hygiene
   (b) Personal protective equipment (PPE)
   (c) Disinfection
   (d) Adequate ventilation equipment

ANSWER (MCQ) ...✓

1. (d)

Major Healthcare Associated Infection Types

49

I. INTRODUCTION

Any infection which develops in the patient 48 hours after admission and patient was not admitted in hospital for management of that infection is labelled as healthcare associated infection (HAI). There are four major HAIs which include:

1. Catheter Associated Urinary Tract Infection (CAUTI)
2. Ventilator Associated Pneumonia (VAP)
3. Central Line Associated Blood Stream Infection (CLABSI)
4. Surgical Site Infection (SSI)

(Items 1–3: These are associated with devices used hence named as Device Associated Infections (DAIs))

II. CATHETER ASSOCIATED URINARY TRACT INFECTION (CAUTI)

Urinary tract infection (UTI) accounts for the majority of HAIs. This is usually associated with catheterisation. Infection rate increases in case of indwelling urinary catheter. Urinary tract infection associated with catheterization is named as **catheter associated urinary tract infection (CAUTI)**. When significant bacteriuria is present with symptoms or signs related to the urinary tract, it is called CAUTI. When significant bacteriuria is present without symptoms or signs related to the urinary tract, it is called **catheter associated asymptomatic bacteriuria (CA-ASB).**

A. Causative Organisms

A number of bacteria can cause CAUTI, most of these bacteria are multidrug-resistant.

1. In short-term catheterised patients.

Gram negative bacilli

Esch coli – Predominant

Klebsiella spp.

Pseudomonas spp.

Acinetobacter spp.

Gram positive cocci

Enterococcus spp.

2. In long-term catheterised patients

Esch. coli

Klebsiella spp.

Pseudomonas spp.

Acinetobacter spp.

Enterococcus spp.

(These are same organisms also responsible for short-term catheterised patients as above.)

Proteus spp.

Providencia spp.

Morganella spp.

B. Risk of Catheterisation

Approximately 20% of indoor patients in hospital require catheterization during their stay in the hospital.

- The risk of developing CAUTI increases with duration of catheterization and risk may be 100% in one month duration of catheterization. However, only one fourth of these patients progress to CAUTI.
- The CAUTI rate varies from 0 to 5 per catheterized patients depending upon the location of hospital e.g. wards, ICU.

C. Pathogenesis

The risk factors for developing CAUTI are shown in Table 49.1.

- The source of infection in catheterized patient may be patient's normal flora, hands of healthcare workers or inanimate objects.
- When aseptic precautions are not taken at the time of insertion or during maintenance of the catheter, there is a risk of migration of bacteria from one of these sources into the urinary bladder.

D. Laboratory Diagnosis

1. Collection of Specimen

- Urine should never be collected from the urine collecting bag.
- Urine should be collected through the port of catheter using all aseptic techniques or by puncturing the catheter tube with a needle and syringe.

Table 49.1: Risk factors for developing CAUTI

Risk Factors		
Device Related	**Patient Related**	**Caregiver Related**
1. Duration (i) Long term catheterisation (≥ 30 days) – Higher risk (ii) Short term catheterization (< 30 days) – lesser risk than long term **2. Material of Catheter** (i) Latex catheter – Higher risk	1. Female 2. Older age (> 50 years) 3. Diabetes mellitus 4. Poor hygiene 5. Incomplete emptying of urinary bladder e.g. prostate enlargement	1. No adherence to aseptic technique while inserting as well as during maintenance of catheter

2. Diagnosis

The clinical diagnosis of CAUTI depends on the following criteria.

- **Catheter Criteria:** History of catheterization within 48 hours.
- **Clinical Criteria:** Presence of at least one symptom or sign of urinary tract infection such as urinary urgency, frequency, dysuria (pain during micturition), suprapubic tenderness or fever.
- **Culture Criteria:** On urine culture, significant bacteriuria should be present depending upon colony count.
  In symptomatic patients: ≥ 10^3 colony forming units (CFU)/mL
  In asymptomatic patients: 10^5 CFU/mL.

E. Treatment

1. Management of CAUTI

It includes:

- Removal of catheter
- Appropriate antibiotic therapy based on antibiotic susceptibility testing of the bacteria isolated

2. Management of CA-ASB

Treatment is **not recommended** except in the following conditions.

- After removal of catheter if bacteriuria persists for > 48 hours.
- In pregnancy, as there is increased risk of developing pyelonephritis and risk of premature delivery.
- Prior to transurethral resection (TUR) of prostate where mucosal bleeding may occur and thus may cause bacteraemia.

F. Prevention

Prevention of CAUTI is described under "Care bundle approach" later in this Chapter.

III. VENTILATOR ASSOCIATED PNEUMONIA (VAP)

It is the second common cause of HAIs after CAUTI. Aspiration in unconscious patients and pulmonary ventilation may lead to nosocomial pneumonia. It is called ventilator associated pneumonia.

It is the most common cause of death among HAIs and is the primary cause of death of patients in intensive care units (ICUs).

A. Causative Agents

VAP can be divided into early-onset and late-onset VAP.

- **Early-Onset VAP**
  It occurs during first 4 days of mechanical ventilation. Causative agents of early onset VAP include *Streptococcus pneumoniae, Haemophilus influenzae, methicillin sensitive Staphylococcus aureus* (MSSA) etc.
- **Late-Onset VAP**
  It develops ≥ 5 days after mechanical ventilation. Causative agents include multidrug resistant hospital organisms such as *Pseudomonas aeruginosa, Acinetobacter spp., Staphylococcus aureus* (MRSA). Due to multidrug resistant organisms, it is associated with high mortality.

Risk factors

1. **Endotracheal intubation:** It is the most important risk factor. Due to this procedure, oropharyngeal bacteria gets direct access to the lower respiratory tract. It is due to impairment of mucociliary clearance caused by endotracheal tube.
2. **Biofilm:** The microorganisms form a biofilm both inside and outside endotracheal tube, which acts as a reservoir of infection. It also prevents the entry of antimicrobials.
3. **Subglottic secretions:** Subglottic suctioning should be done to remove these secretions which may be present on and above the endotracheal (ET) tube cuff. Pooling of secretions on ET tube cuff can also be prevented by maintaining the ET tube cuff pressure at 20–30 cm of H_2O.
4. **Supine position** may facilitate aspiration therefore elevate the head of patient bed to 30–45° (semi-recumbent position) which may prevent VAP.
5. **Sedation:** Sedation, unconsciousness may increase the risk of aspiration, due to inhibition of patient natural ability to clear secretions.
6. **Nasogastric tube:** Ventilated patients are very often on nasogastric tubes. This will increase the risk of aspiration of gastric contents.

7. **Critical illness**, poor nutrition and immobilisation are also some factors which make the patient more susceptible to infections.
8. **Stress ulcer prophylaxis:** Intubated patients are at high risk to develop stress ulcers. Hence, stress ulcer prophylaxis is a common practice in these patients. Sucralfate is given for stress ulcer prophylaxis. However, sucralfate is also associated with a low risk of VAP.

B. Diagnosis

The clinical pulmonary infection score (CPIS) system is used for diagnosis of VAP. It is based on scores assigned to six parameters. These include body temperature, leucocyte count, tracheal secretions, oxygenation PaO2/FiO2 mm Hg, chest X-ray, culture report of tracheal aspirate. Each parameter is given a score ranging from 0 to 2. The score > 6 is diagnostic of VAP.

The diagnosis depends upon microbiological criteria and radiological criteria as follows:

1. Microbiological Criteria

(i) Specimens

- Endotracheal aspiration—The most common
- Broncho alveolar lavage (BAL)
- Protected specimen brush (PSB)
- Lung biopsy

(ii) Processing

Specimens should be processed immediately. If delay occurs, it should not be more man 2 hours.

(iii) Gram staining

Gram staining should be done from the mucopurulent portion of the specimen. Demonstration of higher number of bacteria, intracellular bacteria or fibrin strands is suggestive of VAP.

(iv) Culture

Culture of specimens is done either quantitative or semi-quantitative.

- **Quantitative culture**

The following counts are significant in different specimens.

Endotracheal aspirate — ≥ 105 CFU/mL
BAL — ≥ 105 CFU/mL
PSB — ≥ 103 CFU/mL

- **Semi quantitative culture**

Moderate to heavy growth may be suggestive of ≥ 105 CFU/mL

2. Radiological Criteria

Chest X-ray or CT scan is done. These may show infiltrate, consolidation or cavitation, without underlying pulmonary or cardiac disease.

C. Treatment

Empirical treatment is started on clinical diagnosis of VAP, which can be modified later based on culture and susceptibility testing of the bacteria isolated.

D. Prevention

Prevention of VAP is described under "care bundle approach" later in this Chapter.

IV. CATHETER RELATED BLOOD STREAM INFECTIONS (CRBSI)

Blood stream infections (BSI) in hospitalized patients associated with a central line as a source of infection is called catheter related blood stream infections (CRBSI). A central line is a catheter (tube) that is often placed in a large vein for administration of drugs or fluids, parental nutrition etc. Central line can be inserted into subclavian vein, internal juglar vein, or femoral vein. Central line-associated blood stream infection (CLABSI) is another term used only for surveillance purpose.

The CLABSI rate in hospitalized patients depend upon the location *i.e.,* wards (or ICUs). Infection rate is more in ICUs than wards.

A. Pathogenesis

The microorganisms can reach the extraluminal or intraluminal surface of the central line as described below in the decreasing order of frequency.

1. Patient's own skin flora can migrate along the surface of catheter and colonization of these bacteria occurs at the catheter tip.
2. Contamination of the catheter by the hands of healthcare workers.
3. Haematogenous spread from other focus of infection in body.
4. Contamination of the device at the manufacturing end.

Risk factors

1. Device-related

- Duration of central line: Longer duration (≥ 72 hours) poses a more risk than shorter duration (< 72 hours).
- Site of insertion: Femoral vein has a higher risk than subclavian vein
- Multi lumen central line poses a higher risk compared to single lumen central line.
- Non-tunneled catheters pose a higher risk than tunneled catheters.
- Emergency insertion of central line poses a higher risk than elective insertion.

2. Caregiver-related

- Lack of infection control practices during insertion and maintenance of an central line.
- Use of alcohol for skin asepsis has a higher risk than use of chlorhexidine.

3. Patient-related

- Immunocompromised
- Presence of distant infection in patient's body
- Malignancy especially haematologic.
- Severe illness

B. Source of Infection

It may be extraluminal (contamination during insertion) or intraluminal (contamination occurs during device production and thus acts a source of infection). Extraluminal contamination occurs due to poor hand hygiene and poor aseptic precautions during insertion.

Following events takes place after entry of microorganisms into the central line.

- Colonisation of microorganisms
- Biofilm formation on catheter surface by bacteria such as *Staphylococcus aureus, Pseudomonas aeruginosa* and *Candida spp*.

C. Diagnosis

The diagnosis of CRBSI depends on clinical criteria (signs and symptoms) and microbiological criteria (culture examination). However, there should not be any alternate source of blood stream infection (BSI).

1. Clinical Criteria

Signs and symptoms after insertion of catheter may be present as follows:

- Fever
- Chills
- Low blood pressure
- Signs of catheter site infection such as erythema, swelling, tenderness etc.

2. Microbiological Criteria

Blood culture from the central line and the peripheral line is carried out simultaneously. Central line blood culture should be positive ≥ 2 hours earlier to peripheral line blood culture positivity for the same organism.

D. Treatment

1. Removal of the central line.
2. The empirical treatment should be started whenever there is clinical suspicion of CRBSI. Later on treatment may be modified according to the antibiotic sensitivity testing of the organism isolated.

E. Prevention

Prevention of CRBSI is described under 'Care bundle approach' later in this Chapter.

V. SURGICAL SITE INFECTION (SSI)

Surgical site infections (SSIs) are infections that occur within 30 days of surgery in the part of body where surgery took place (or within 90 days of surgeries for breast, heart and joint including implant).

A. Causative agents

Causative agents involved in SSI depends upon the site of surgery and the source of infection, *i.e.,* endogenous or exogenous source.

1. Endogenous source

- **Skin flora of the patient:** *Staphylococcus aureus* (The most common causative organism of SSI), Coagulase negative staphylococci (CoNS)
- **From mucosal surfaces of the patient:** These may be from gastrointestinal tract (GIT) respiratory tract or genitourinary tract. Organisms involved may include *Escherichia coli, Klebsiella spp., Enterobacter spp.* or anaerobic bacteria *e.g.*, *Bacteroides spp.*

2. Exogenous source

These organisms come in contact with patient from healthcare persons present in operation room, or instruments or environment. Some examples of these organisms include *Staphylococcus aureus*, *Pseudomonas spp.* and *Acinetobacter spp.*

The risk of developing SSI depends on the inoculum load and virulence of these organisms.

Large inoculum of organisms lodging into the wound during surgery has a higher risk of developing SSI. Surgery sites (*e.g.* vagina, intestines) which are heavily colonised with bacteria have a higher risk.

Infection with organisms of a **higher virulence** has more chance of developing SSI and thus higher risk.

B. Pathogenesis

Due to the presence of innate immunity of host, most patients do not develop infection at surgical site. However, when host immunity to eliminate the microorganisms fail due to greater load and higher virulence of these organisms, it leads to development of SSI.

C. Risk factors:

The risk is higher in the following conditions:

1. **Patient related**
   - Older age (>60 years)
   - Immunocompromised
   - Longer hospital stay
   - Patient is MRSA carrier at the time of surgery.
   - Higher wound class – most Important risk factor

2. **Procedure related**
   - Inadequate skin asepsis
   - Improper infection control practices
   - Inadequate antimicrobial prophylaxis
   - Emergency procedures
3. **Environment related**
   - Presence of blood/clot and foreign bodies at the surgical site
   - Contaminated medications
4. **Microorganism related**
   - Higher inoculum size *e.g.*, in bowel surgery
   - Higher virulence of bacteria
   - Biofilm formation by the organism

D. Types of wounds

Wounds are classified according to degree of microbial contamination as follows:

1. Class I, Clean wound
2. Class II, Clean-contaminated wound
3. Class III, Contaminated wound
4. Class IV, Dirty wound

The class III and class IV have a higher risk of developing surgical site infection.

E. Classification

SSIs are classified into three types as follows:

- **Superficial SSI:** Infection develops at superficial incision site *i.e.,* skin and subcutaneous level.
- **Deep SSI:** Infection develops at deep incision site *i.e.*, muscle and facial level.
- Organ space site.

F. Diagnosis

Diagnosis of SSI is based on different criteria as described in Chapter on HAI surveillance and HICC.

G. Treatment

- Removal of suture
- Incision and drainage of pus
- Antimicrobial therapy

H. Prevention of SSI

Preventive measures of SSI may include as follows:

1. **Handwashing:** Surgeon and other surgery staff should scrub their hands and arms with soap.
2. **Incisional Site:** Incisional site should be cleaned with an antiseptic solution.
3. **Sterile clothing and drapes:** The surgical team must wear sterile surgical gowns, masks, gloves, caps and shoe covers. Sterile drapes (sheets) should be used on the patient body.
4. **Environment cleaning:** Operation rooms should have special air filters to prevent unfiltered air from entering the room.
5. **Surgical antimicrobial prophylaxis:** It must be provided for all except clean surgeries.
6. **Hair removal:** Hair removal should not be done but if necessary then remove with clipper and not to be shaved with a razor.
7. **Blood sugar levels:** High blood sugar level delays wound healing hence blood sugar level should be within normal range.
8. **Wound dressing:** Daily would dressing should be done and removal of any discharge if present. Perform hand hygiene and use sterile gloves before dressing the wound.

VI. PREVENTION OF DEVICE ASSOCIATED INFECTIONS (DAIs)

- Strict aseptic precautions must be followed during insertion of devices and also during daily maintenance of these devices later on.
- These preventive measures for DAIs are named as 'Care bundle approach'.

Care Bundle Approach

Care bundle approach must be followed during insertion and daily maintenance of devices to prevent the occurrence of infection. There are different components under 'Care bundle approach'.

1. Bundles for Prevention of Catheter Associated Urinary Tract Infection (CAUTI)

The implementation of care bundles before and after placement of urinary catheters can prevent CAUTI. These include:

- Avoiding use of urinary catheters by considering alternative methods such as condom catheters, intermittent catheterisation.
- Appropriate use of catheter if required.
- Aseptic insertion of catheter and its maintenance.
- Early removal of catheter.
- Hand hygiene during the procedures.

Implementation of care bundles should accompany with approaches such as hand hygiene practices, healthcare worker education, feedback of catheter use and CAUTI rates.

2. Bundles for Prevention of Ventilator Associated Pneumonia (VAP)

Care bundles of ventilator care processes may reduce VAP rates. These include:

- Elevate the head of bed between 30 to 45 degrees. It will prevent the aspiration of gastric content.

- Daily assessment of readiness to extubate.
- Daily oral care should be done with chlorhexidine.
- Prophylaxis of peptic ulcer disease
- Prophylaxis of deep venous thrombosis

Besides implementation of care bundles, standard precautions as well as adequate disinfection and maintenance of equipment and devices should also be done.

3. Bundles for Prevention of Central Line Associated Infections

Implementation of care bundles during insertion of central line and their maintenance reduces the incidence of central line associated infections in patients.

Insertion care bundle

The following steps should be adapted during insertion of central line.

- Use of sterile mask, sterile gloves, cap, sterile gown and sterile drape.
- Clean the skin with chlorhexidine (rather than iodine).
- Skin must be completely dry after using antiseptics.
- Avoid use of the femoral vein for central line in adult patients; use of subclavian vein (rather than juglar vein).
- Use semi-permeable dressing.

Maintenance of care bundle

- Daily review of central line should be done.
- Remove unnecessary lines promptly.
- Disinfect catheter hubs, ports etc.
- Change dressings and disinfect sites with 2% chlorhexidine

All these activities should also include hand hygiene, clinician and nurse education, and performance of surveillance alongwith feedback of CLABSI.

KEY POINTS

1. Any infection which develops in the patient 48 hours after admission and patient was not admitted in hospital for management of that infection is labelled as healthcare associated infection (HAI).
2. There are four major HAIs which include catheter associated urinary tract infection (CAUTI), Ventilator associated pneumonia (VAP), Catheter related blood stream infection (CRBSI) and Surgical site infection (SSI).

STUDY QUESTION

1. Write short notes on:
   (i) CAUTI (ii) VAP
   (iii) CRBSI (iv) SSI

MULTIPLE CHOICE QUESTION (MCQ)

1. All of the following are device associated infections (DAIs) except:
   (a) Catheter associated urinary infection (CAUTI)
   (b) Ventilator associated pneumonia (VAP)
   (c) Catheter related blood stream infection (CRBSI)
   (d) Acute tonsilitis

ANSWER (MCQ)

1. (d)

Healthcare Associated Infection (HAI) Surveillance (Including HICC)

50

I. INTRODUCTION

Healthcare associated infections (HAIs) surveillance monitors the HAIs in a hospital. The objectives of HAI surveillance are as follows:

- To provide baseline HAI rate in hospital.
- To identify the types of HAIs.
- To know HAI rates in different units of a hospital and thus to identify the problem area.
- On the basis of above information, root cause analysis of problem area can be conducted and thus corrective measures can be implemented.
- To provide feedback to clinicians so that they may adopt best practices to control the infection.
- All the above information and actions contribute in controlling the healthcare associated infections in hospital.

II. TARGETED SURVEILLANCE

The National Healthcare Safety Network (NHSN) division of Centers for Disease Control and Prevention (CDC) provides the following guidelines for HAI surveillance.

1. **High risk locations:** HAI surveillance should be done only in high risk locations *e.g.* intensive care units (ICUs).
2. **Types of HAIs:** Only the major types of HAIs are to be monitored such as CAUTI, CLABSI, VAP and SSI. As monitoring is technically difficult hence only major HAIs are included.
3. **Persons involved in conduction:** The infection control nurses (ICNs) conduct HAI surveillance under the supervision of office in-charge of Hospital Infection Control Committee (HICC).
4. **HAI surveillance diagnostic criteria:** The NHSN has provided the diagnostic criteria for four major types of HAIs. The criterias are very objective so that the uniformity of data collection between hospitals can be maintained.

The surveillance criteria should strictly be used for surveillance only and not for clinical diagnosis and treatment.

III. CONDUCTION OF HAI SURVEILLANCE

The HAI surveillance is conducted by Data Collection and then its analysis, interpretation, dissemination is done.

Data Collection	→	Data Analysis
		↓
Data dissemination	←	Data Interpretation

1. **Data collection:** The ICNs visit daily to high risk areas and collect the clinical data of patients who are on devices (urinary catheter, central line, ventilator) and also from patients who have undergone surgery. These nurses also prospectively check the laboratory investigations for confirmation of diagnosis.
2. **Data analysis:** The types of HAIs are diagnosed according to criteria of HAI by NHSN/CDC (Tables 50.1 to 50.4). The surveillance HAI rates are then calculated according to formulae shown in Table 50.5. The monthly report of HAI rates (location wise) of the hospital is prepared.
3. **Data interpretation:** HAI rates are compared for same location or different locations.
   - HAI rates of the same location are compared across different time frames.
   - HAI rates of different locations of the same or different hospitals are compared during the same time frame.
4. **Data dissemination:** The monthly HAI surveillance report is presented during HICC meetings. This report should also be shared with all clinical departments and administrators. On the basis of monthly report the appropriate corrective actions are planned for the problem areas if any.

Table 50.1: NHSN Surveillance Diagnostic Criteria for Symptomatic Catheter Associated Urinary Tract Infection (CAUTI)
1. Urinary catheter had been in place for more than 2 consecutive days.
2. Presence of any one symptom such as (i) fever (iv) dysuria (ii) suprapublic tenderness (v) frequency (iii) urgency
3. Patient has a urine culture positive for urinary pathogen with $\geq 10^5$CFU/mL

Table 50.2: NHSN Surveillance Diagnostic Criteria for Central Line-Associated Blood Stream Infection (CLABSI)

LCBI-1
Patient of any age has • One or more blood culture positive for healthcare associated pathogens. • No additional signs or symptoms such as fever are required. • Catheter present for more than two calendar days.
LCBI-2
Patient of any age has at least any one of the following signs or symptoms. • Fever (>38°C) • Chills • Hypotension **AND** • Two or more blood culture positive for commensals • Catheter present for more than two calendar days
LCBI-3
Patient ≤ 1 year of age has at least any one of the following signs or symptoms. • Fever (>38°C) • Hypothermia • Apnoea • Bradycardia **AND** • Two or more blood culture positive for commensals. • Catheter present for more than two calendar days.
LCBI: Laboratory confirmed blood stream infection

Table 50.3. NHSN Surveillance Diagnostic Criteria for Ventilator-Associated Event (VAE)

I. Ventilator-Associated Condition (VAC)
• Patient is on a mechanical ventilator at least for 2 calendar days. • Baseline period of stability/improvement on ventilator for 2 days by daily minimum FiO_2 and PEEP value followed by worsening oxygenation with at least one of the following indicators. – Increase in daily minimum FiO_2 of ≥ 0.20 over daily minimum FiO_2 of first day in the baseline period and sustained for ≥2 calendar days or – Increase in daily PEEP value of ≥3 cm water over daily minimum PEEP of first day in the baseline period and sustained for ≥2 calendar days
II. Infection-related Ventilator-Associated Complication (IVAC)
VAC plus the following criteria: Patient has any one of the following: • Fever > 38 °C (> 100.4 °F) • Hypothermia < 36 °C (<96.8 °F) • Leukocytosis ≥12,000 luckocytes/mm^3 **AND** • A new antimicrobial agent is started and continued for ≥4 days.
III. Possible Ventilator-Associated Pneumonia (PVAP)
IVAC plus the following criteria: • Positive culture (quantitative or semi-quantitative) from one of the specimens such as endotracheal aspirate, bronchoalveolar lavage, lung tissue, protected specimen brush. • Organism identified from pleural fluid.

IV. HOSPITAL INFECTION CONTROL COMMITTEE (HICC)

Every hospital must have an effective hospital infection control committee (HICC) which should be responsible for the control of healthcare associated infection (HAI). The Medical Superintendent (MS) constitutes the HICC. The HICC is advisory to the MS and submit its recommendations to the MS.

A. HICC Constitution

Chairperson: Medical Superintendent
Secretary: Most often Head of Department, Microbiology
Hospital infection Control officer: Representative from Department of Microbiology
Members:

- Head of all clinical departments
- Nursing superintendent
- Hospital infection control nurses
- Officer incharge of biomedical waste management
- Incharge of Central Sterile Supplies Department (CSSD)
- Incharge of pharmacy
- Incharge of laundry
- Incharge of hospital kitchen
- Chief of operation theaters (OTs)
- Incharge of engineering department of the hospital
- Incharge of house keeping
- Epidemiologist

B. Functions of HICC

The HICC supervises and implements the hospital infection control programme. The functions of the committee include:

1. **HAI surveillance**
2. **Investigating and controlling healthcare associated infections**
3. **Antimicrobial stewardship programme (AMSP).**
   - Antibiotic policies are developed to monitor the antibiotic usage.
   - To advise the MS about the rational use of antibiotics in the hospital.
4. **Hospital infection control policies**
5. **Conduction of teaching sessions for various healthcare workers**
6. **Staff health**
   - Monitor needle stick injury in healthcare workers and, its preventive measures.
   - Hepatitis B vaccination of staff.
7. **Outbreak investigation and its management.**

Table 50.4: NHSN Surveillance diagnostic criteria for Surgical Site Infection (SSI)

Superficial SSI
The following criteria must be met: • Infection occurs within 30 days at the level of superficial incisional site (skin and superficial level) irrespective of type of surgery **AND** Patient has at least **one** of the following: • Purulent discharge from the superficial incision. • A positive culture from aseptically collected discharge from the superficial incision or subcutaneous tissue. • Patient has at least one of the following signs or symptoms: – Localised pain/tenderness – Localised swelling – Heat – Erythema • Diagnosis of a superficial incisional SSI by a surgeon.
Deep SSI
The following criteria must be met: • Infection occurs within 30 days of operative procedure (within 90 days for breast, cardiac and joint surgeries etc.) It involves deep incisional site (*e.g.* Fascial and muscle layers) **AND** Patient has at least **one** of the following: • Purulent discharge from the deep incision. • A positive culture from the discharge from deep soft tissues. • Patient has at least **one** of the following signs or symptoms: – Fever (>38 °C) – Localised pain/tenderness • Histological, gross anatomical or imaging evidence of an abscess/infection involving the deep incision.
Organ/Space SSI
The following criteria must be met: • Infection occurs within 30 days at the level of organ/space for all operative procedures (within 90 days for breast, cardiac and joint surgeries etc.). It involves part of body deeper than the fascial/muscle layers. **AND** Patient has at least **one** of the following: • Purulent discharge from a drain placed into organ/space. • A positive culture from fluid or tissue in the organ/space. • Histological, gross anatomical or imaging evidence of an abscess/infection involving the organ/space.

8. **Communication with other departments of the hospital such as:**
   - CSSD
   - Laundry department
   - Pharmacy
   - Biomedical waste management committee
   - Antimicrobial usage committee
   - Blood transfusion committee
   - **Review** of infections risks associated with new devices, products and technologies, prior to their approval for use.
   - **HICC meetings:** HICC meeting is held regularly not less then once a month. However, during any emergency such as hospital outbreak, this meeting must be held as and when required.

Table 50.5: Device Specific and Procedure Specific Infection Rates

$$\text{CAUTI rate} : \frac{\text{Number of CAUTI cases}}{\text{Number of urinary catheter days}} \times 1000$$

$$\text{CLABSI rate} : \frac{\text{Number of central line related BSI Cases}}{\text{Number of central line days}} \times 1000$$

$$\text{VAP rate} : \frac{\text{Number of ventilator associated event (VAE) cases}}{\text{Number of ventilator days}} \times 1000$$

$$\text{SSI rate} : \frac{\text{Number of surgical site infection}}{\text{Number of surgical operations done}} \times 100$$

C. Role and responsibility of HICC

1. Hospital Administration

The hospital administration has a main role for implementation of hospital infection control programme. The responsibilities include:

- To formulate a multidisciplinary HICC
- To provide adequate resources (financial and human) for implementing the hospital infection control programme.
- To make available hand hygiene products, personal protective equipment (PPE), disinfectants, vaccines etc. for healthcare workers.
- To review and approve the policies and guidelines for hospital infection control practices formulated by HICC and update periodically.
- Organises and conducts regular infection control training activities for healthcare workers.
- Conducts regular surveys to monitor all infection control measures.
- Performs Antimicrobial resistance (AMR) surveillance and also prepares antibiogram.
- Participates in implementing antimicrobial stewardship programme.
- Prepares the annual budget of HICC and is involved in purchase activities related to infection control.
- Organises regular HICC meetings.

2. Infection Control Nurse (ICN)

A full time nursing staff should be appointed as the ICN. She/he should have practical training in infection control.

- ICNs should undergo competency assessment tests at the beginning and then periodically.
- **Recommendation:** A minimum of 0.8–1.0 fulltime ICN is required per 100 beds in acute-care centres and one per 150–250 beds in long-term-care facilities.

Duties of ICN

The ICN is responsible for liaising between the HICC and the hospital wards, ICUs, OTs etc. to identify problems and implement solutions. She/he conducts infection control rounds daily at all hospital locations and tracks all infected cases and monitors the compliance of healthcare workers to infection control measures in the hospital.

- ICN carries out data collection for HAI surveillance, have hygiene audit, PPE audit, care bundle audit etc.
- Monitors the implementation of infection control practices and SOPs, including hand hygiene, care bundles, sterilisation and disinfection and antimicrobial stewardship.
- Identifies the high risk areas for conducting environmental surveillance.
- Imparts education and training to healthcare workers.
- Maintains data of sharp/needle stick injuries and postexposure prophylaxis (PEP).
- Conducts immunisation programme for hepatitis B virus, influenza etc. for healthcare workers.
- Facilitate provision of first aid and appropriate consultation in case of suspected exposure of any healthcare worker.

Infection Control Link Nurse

In case of inadequate ICNs, the existing nursing staff working in ICUs can be trained and engaged in infection control activities of their concerned ICUs. Infection control link nurses can motivate ward staff for adopting effective hospital control practices.

3. Hospital infection control officer

The hospital infection control offices (HICO) is usually a clinical microbiologist or physician specialising in infectious diseases or any other physician working full time in infection control. HICO is responsible for monitoring day-to-day activities of HICC and reports directly to the member secretary and chairperson of HICC.

Duties of HICO

- Planning and implementation of hospital infection control measures such as hand hygiene, effective use of PPE, care bundles etc.
- Initiate and maintain activities of HAI surveillance and analysis of the data.
- Investigate an outbreak, and advise on control measures.
- Supervises the activities of biomedical waste management.
- Nodal officer for management of occupational exposures such as needle stick injury.
- To ensure immunisation (hepatitis B vaccine, influenza vaccine) of all healthcare workers.
- To ensure the implementation of safe work practices.
- To formulate and implement guidelines for sterilisation policy, disinfection policy, house keeping.

KEY POINTS

1. Healthcare associated infections (HAIs) surveillance monitors the HAIs in a hospital.
2. Every hospital must have an effective hospital infection control committee (HICC) which should be responsible for the control of healthcare associated infection (HAI).

STUDY QUESTION

1. Write short notes on:
   (i) Healthcare associated infection (HAI) surveillance
   (ii) Hospital infection control committee (HICC).

Sterilisation and Disinfection

51

I. INTRODUCTION

Some definitions

Sterilisation

It is a process by which an article, surface or medium is made free of all microorganisms either in the vegetative or spore form.

Disinfection

It means the destruction of all pathogens or organisms capable of producing infections but not necessarily spores. All organisms may not be killed but the number is reduced to a level that is no longer harmful to health.

Uses of Sterilisation/Disinfection

1 Sterilisation of materials, instruments used in surgical and diagnostic procedures.
2. For media and reagents used in the microbiology laboratory.

II. METHODS OF STERILISATION

A. *Physical Methods*

1. Sunlight
2. Heat:
   (a) Dry heat
   (b) Moist heat
3. Ozone
4. Filtration
5. Radiation

B. *Chemical Methods*

1. Alcohols
2. Aldehydes
3. Phenols
4. Halogens
5. Oxidising agents
6. Surface active agents
7. Dyes
8. Gases

A. Physical Methods

1. Sunlight

Sunlight has an active germicidal effect due to its content of ultraviolet rays. It is a natural method of sterilisation in cases of water in tanks, rivers and lakes.

2. Heat

Heat is the **most reliable and commonly employed method of sterilisation**. Two types of heat are used, dry heat and moist heat.

Principle

(i) Dry heat kills the organisms by denaturation of bacterial protein, oxidative damage and by the toxic effect of elevated levels of electrolytes.
(ii) Moist heat kills the microorganisms by denaturation and coagulation of proteins.

Dry heat sterilisation

The following procedures are used for sterilisation by dry heat.

(i) Red heat
(ii) Flaming
(iii) Incineration
(iv) Hot air oven

(i) Red heat

Inoculating wires or loops, tips of forceps and needles are held in the flame of a Bunsen burner till they become red hot.

(ii) Flaming

Glass slides, scalpels and mouths of culture tubes are passed through bunsen flame without allowing them to become red hot.

(iii) Incineration

By this method, infective material is reduced to ashes by burning. Instrument named incinerator may be used for this purpose. Soiled dressings, animal carcasses, bedding and pathological materials are dealt with this method. It is also one of the methods for treatment of biomedical waste and disposal.

(iv) Hot Air Oven

It is the most widely used method of sterilisation by dry heat. The oven is electrically heated and is fitted with a fan to ensure adequate and even distribution of hot air in the chamber (Fig. 51.1). It is also fitted with a thermostat that maintains the chamber air at a chosen temperature.

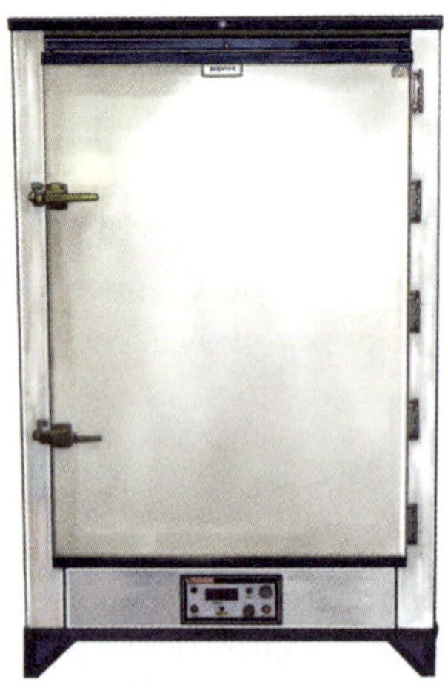

Fig. 51.1 Hot air oven

Temperature and time

160°C for two hours (holding time) is required for sterilisation.

Uses

It is used for sterilisation of

(i) Glass-wares like glass syringes, petridishes, flasks, pipettes and test tubes.
(ii) Surgical instruments like scalpels, scissors, forceps etc.

Precautions

(i) It should not be overloaded.
(ii) The material should be arranged in a manner which allows free circulation of air.
(iii) Material to be sterilised should be perfectly dry.
(iv) Test tubes, flasks etc. should be fitted with cotton plugs.
(v) Petridishes and pipettes should be wrapped in craft paper.
(vi) Rubber materials (except silicone rubber) or any inflammable material should not be kept inside the oven.
(vii) The oven must be allowed to cool for two hours before opening the doors, since the glasswares may crack by sudden cooling.

Sterilisation control

(i) The spores of nontoxigenic strain of *Clostridium tetani* are kept inside the oven. These spores should be destroyed if the sterilisation is proper.
(ii) Thermocouples may also be used.
(iii) Browne's tube with green spot is available. After proper sterilisation a green colour is produced (after two hours at 160°C).

Moist heat sterilisation

This method of sterilisation may be used at different temperatures as follows.

(i) At a temperature below 100°C
(ii) At a temperature of 100°C
(iii) At a temperature above 100°C

(i) At a Temperature below 100°C

(a) ***Pasteurisation of milk***—Two types of method, holder method (63°C for 30 minutes) and flash method (72°C for 20 seconds followed by cooling quickly to 13°C or lower) are used.
(b) ***Inspissation***—Some serum or egg media, such as Lowenstein-Jensen's and Loeffler's serum, are rendered sterile by heating at 80-85°C temperature for half an hour daily on three consecutive days. This process of sterilisation is called inspissation. The instrument used is called inspissator.
(c) ***Low temperature steam formaldehyde (LTSF) sterilisation***—Items which cannot withstand the temperature of 100°C may be sterilised by a method known as low temperature steam formaldehyde (LTSF) sterilisation. In this method steam at subatmospheric pressure at the temperature of 75°C with formaldehyde vapour is used. ***Geobacillus stearothermophilus*** has been used as biological control to test the efficacy of LTSF sterilisers.

(ii) At a Temperature of 100°C

(a) ***Boiling***—Boiling for 10 to 30 minutes may kill most of the vegetative forms but many spores withstand boiling for a considerable time. When better methods are not available, boiling may be used for glass syringes and rubber stoppers. **It is not recommended for the sterilisation of instruments used for surgical procedures.**
(b) ***Tyndallisation or Intermittent sterilisation***—Steam at 100°C for 20 minutes on three successive days is used. This is known as tyndallisation or intermittent sterilisation. The principle is that the first exposure kills all the vegetative forms, in the intervals between the heatings the remaining spores germinate into vegetative forms which are killed on

subsequent heating. It is used for sterilisation of egg, serum or sugar containing media which are damaged at higher temperature of autoclave.

(iii) At a Temperature above 100°C (under pressure)

Water boils when its vapour pressure equals that of the surrounding atmosphere. When the atmospheric pressure is raised then the boiling temperature is also raised. At normal pressure water boils at 100°C but when pressure inside a closed vessel increases, the temperature at which water boils also increases. This principle has been applied in *autoclave* and *pressure cooker*.

Autoclave

Principle

Steam above 100°C or saturated steam has a better killing power than dry heat. Bacteria are more susceptible to moist heat as bacterial protein coagulates rapidly. Saturated steam can penetrate porous material easily. When steam comes into contact with a cooler surface it condenses to water and liberates its latent heat to that surface, for example, 1600 ml of steam at 100°C and at atmospheric pressure condenses into one ml of water at 100°C and releases 518 calories of heat. The large reduction in volume sucks in more steam to the same site and the process continues till the temperature of the article is raised to that of steam. The condensed water produces moist conditions for killing the microbes present.

Components of autoclave

Autoclave is a modified pressure cooker or boiler. It consists of a vertical or horizontal cylinder of gunmetal or stainless steel in a supporting iron case. The lid is fastened by screw clamps and rendered air tight by an asbestos washer. The lid bears a discharge tap for air and steam, a pressure gauge and a safety valve. Heating is generally done by electricity. The steam circulates within the jacket and is supplied under high pressure to the inner chamber where materials are kept for sterilisation (Figs. 51.2 and 51.3).

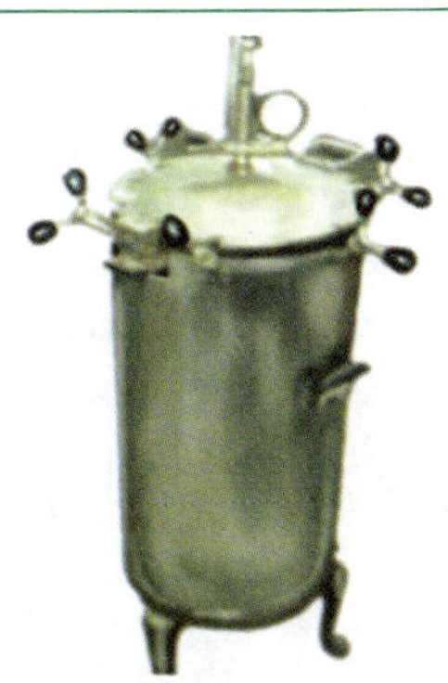

Fig. 51.2 Vertical autoclave

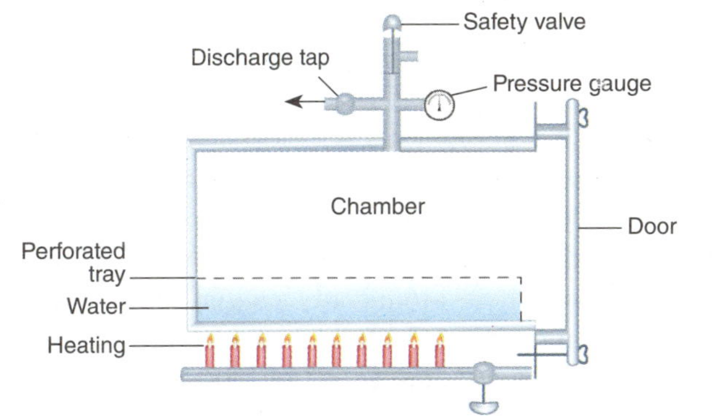

Fig. 51.3 Autoclave (inner view)

Sterilisation conditions

Temperature—121°C
Chamber pressure—15 pounds (lbs) per square inch
Holding time—15 minutes

These conditions are generally used, however, sterilisation can also be done at higher temperatures, at 126°C (20 lbs/square inch) for 10 minutes or at 133°C (30 lbs/square inch) for 3 minutes.

Uses

(i) To sterilise culture media, surgical instruments, dental instruments, rubber material, gowns, dressing, gloves etc.
(ii) It is particularly useful for materials which cannot withstand the higher temperature of hot air oven.
(iii) Treatment of biomedical waste.

Precautions

(i) The air must be allowed to escape from the chamber as temperature of air-steam mixture is lower than that of pure steam.
(ii) Materials should be arranged in such a manner as to ensure free circulation of steam inside the chamber.

Sterilisation control

(i) **Thermocouple**—It is to record the temperature directly by a potentiometer.
(ii) **Biological indicator**—Spores of **Geobacillus stearothermophilus** are used as the test organism. The spores of this organism are killed in 12 minutes at 121°C. An envelope containing a filter paper strip impregnated with 10^6 spores is placed inside the autoclave during sterilisation. Spores are destroyed if sterilising conditions of autoclave are proper.
(iii) **Chemical indicators**—Browne's tube contains red solution which turns green, when exposed to temperature of 121°C for 15 minutes in autoclave.
(iv) **Autoclave tapes**

3. Ozone

Low temperature sterilisation by ozone

Ozone steriliser uses oxygen, water and electricity to produce ozone within the steriliser and provide sterilisation without producing toxic chemicals. It runs at lower temperature, i.e., 25°C–35°C. In this device, oxygen molecules (O_2) are separated into atomic oxygen (O) in the preence of intense electrical field. These atomic oxygen (O) combines with other oxygen molecules (O_2) to form ozone (O_3). The ozone provides a steriligy assurance of 10^{-6} in approximately 4 hours.

4. Filtration

This method of sterilisation is useful for substances which get damaged by heat process e.g. sera, sugars, antibiotic solutions etc.

Uses of filtration

(i) To sterilise sera, sugars and antibiotic solutions.
(ii) Separation of toxins and bacteriophages from bacteria.
(iii) Sterilisation of hydatid fluid.

Types of filters

(i) ***Earthenware candles***—These filters are usually made in the form of hollow candles. The liquid to be filtered is passed through the candle. They are available in different grades of porosity.
(ii) ***Asbestos disc filters (Seitz filter)***—These are no longer used due to carcinogenic property of asbestos.
(iii) ***Sintered glass filters***—These are prepared by fusing finely powdered glass particles. These are available in different pore sizes.
(iv) ***Membrane filters***—Membrane filters are made up of cellulose esters. **Nitrocellulose (Millipore)** membrane filters are widely used. Membrane filters are available in pore sizes of 0.015 to 12 µm.
(v) ***Air filters***—These filters are used to deliver clean bacteria-free air to a cubicle or a room. High efficiency particulate air (HEPA) filters are used in air filtration in laminar air flow system in microbiology laboratories. HEPA filters can remove particles of 0.3 µm or larger.

5. Radiations

Two types of radiations are used for sterilisation: ionising and non-ionising.

(i) ***Ionising radiations***—Ionising radiations include gamma rays, X-rays and cosmic rays. They are highly lethal to all cells including bacteria. They damage DNA by various mechanisms. Gamma radiations are commercially used for sterilisation of disposable items such as plastic syringes, swabs, culture plates, cannulas, catheters etc. This method is also known as **cold sterilisation** because there is no appreciable increase in temperature.
(ii) ***Non-ionising radiations***—These include infrared and ultraviolet (UV) radiations. Infrared is used for rapid mass sterilisation of syringes and catheters. Ultraviolet radiation has marked bactericidal activity. It acts by denaturation of bacterial protein and interference with DNA replication. UV radiation is used for disinfecting enclosed areas such as bacteriological laboratory, inoculation hoods, laminar flow and operation theatres.

B. Chemical Methods

A variety of chemical agents are used as antiseptics and disinfectants.

1. Alcohols

Ethyl alcohol and isopropyl alcohol are the most frequently used. They act by denaturing bacterial proteins. They are used mainly as skin antiseptics. To be effective, they should be used at a concentration of 60-70 per cent in water.

2. Aldehydes

Formaldehyde

It is used both as aqueous solution and in gaseous form. A 10% aqueous solution of formalin is routinely used.

Uses

(i) To sterilise bacterial vaccines.
(ii) To prepare toxoid from toxin.
(iii) For killing of bacterial cultures and suspensions.

Formalin gas has been described under "Gases".

Glutaraldehyde

It is used as 2% buffered solution. It is available commercially as 'cidex'. It can be used for delicate instruments having lenses.

Uses

(i) For sterilisation of cystoscopes, endoscopes and bronchoscope.
(ii) To sterilise plastic endotracheal tubes, face masks, corrugated rubber anaesthetic tubes and metal instruments.

3. Phenols

Phenol (1%) has bactericidal action. Certain phenol derivatives like cresol, chlorhexidine, chloroxylenol and hexachlorophane are commonly used as antiseptics.

(i) ***Cresols***—Lysol is a solution of cresols in soap. It is most commonly used for sterilisation of infected glass wares, cleaning floors, disinfection of excreta.

(ii) ***Chlorhexidine***—Savlon (chlorhexidine and cetrimide) is widely used in wounds, pre-operative disinfection of skin, as bladder irrigant etc.

(iii) ***Chloroxylenol***—It is an active ingredient of dettol.

4. Halogens

Chlorine and iodine are two commonly used disinfectants.

Chlorine is used in water supplies and swimming pools. Chlorine compounds in the form of bleaching powder, sodium hypochlorite and chloramine are also used. The disinfection action of all the chlorine compounds is due to **release of free chlorine**. Bleaching powder or **hypochlorite solution are the most widely used for human immunodeficiency virus (HIV) infected material**. The hypochlorites have a bactericidal, fungicidal, virucidal and rapidly sporicidal action. Hypochlorite solution decays rapidly and should be prepared daily.

Iodine in alcoholic and aqueous solutions is used as a skin disinfectant. Betadine (povidine iodine) is one example of commonly used iodine compound.

5. Oxidising Agents

(i) Hydrogen peroxide

Hydrogen peroxide (H_2O_2) is effective against most organisms at concentration of 3-6%, while it kills all organisms including spores at higher concentration (10-25%). Mode of action is by liberation of free hydroxyl radical on decomposition of H_2O_2. These free radicals are the active ingredient in the disinfection process. H_2O_2 is used to disinfect contact lenses, surgical prostheses and plastic implants. It is used for high level disinfection and sterilisation.

(ii) Peracetic acid

Peracetic acid is an oxidising agent. It is one of the high level disinfectants. The end products (acetic acid and oxygen) of this agent are non°-toxic. It is also used in plasma sterilisation procedure. It is effective in the presence of organic matter. It is a more potent germicidal agent than hydrogen peroxide.

(iii) Plasma sterilisation

Plasma sterilisation is an example of **low temperature sterilisation** as there is no increase in temperature during the process. Hydrogen peroxide is used for sterilisation. Plasma is the fourth state of matter (solid, liquid, gas and plasma). Plasma is created when a gas is heated sufficiently or exposed to a strong electromagnetic field. It is an unstable state of matter. Plasma steriliser is a special instrument used to create the plasma state. Plasma distrupts the metabolism of microorganisms and eventually kills them. Two commercial plasma sterilisers available are *Sterrad 100S steriliser* and *Plazlyte steriliser*. It is used for sterilisation of surgical instruments.

6. Surface Active Agents

surface active agents or surfactants are classified into anionic, cationic, nonionic and amphoteric compounds. Of these, the cationic surfactants have been the most important antibacterial agents. Quaternary ammonium compounds are the most important surfactants. The common compounds used are acetyl trimethyl ammonium bromide (cetavalon or cetrimide) and benzalkonium chloride.

7. Dyes

Two groups of dyes, aniline dyes and acridine dyes have been used extensively as skin and wound antiseptics. Aniline dyes include crystal violet, brilliant green and malachite green. Acridine dyes include acriflavine, euflavine, proflavine and aminacrine.

8. Gases

Formaldehyde gas

This was employed for fumigation of operation theatres, wards etc. However, this method is no longer preferred and is being replaced by other methods. Glutaraldehyde, quaternary ammonium compounds are now used for operation theaters.

Ethylene oxide (ETO)

Ethylene oxide (ETO) is one of the widely used gaseous chemical method for sterilisation. It is specially used for sterilising plastic and rubber articles, plastic syringes, respirators, heart-lung machines, sutures, dental equipments and clothing. It is unsuitable for fumigation of rooms because of its explosive nature.

Recommended concentrations of some commonly used disinfectants are given in Table 51.1. Methods of sterilisation and disinfection of some important materials are shown in Table 51.2.

Table 51.1: Recommended Concentrations of Some Disinfectants

Disinfectant	Concentration
Ethyl alcohol	70%
Glutaraldehyde	2%
Lysol	2.5%
Savlon (chlorhexidine and cetrimide)	2%, 5%
Dettol (chloroxylenol)	4%
Bleaching powder (calcium hypochlorite)	14 gm in one litre of water
Sodium hypochlorite	1%, 0.1%
Betadine (Iodophore)	2%

Table 51.2: Methods of Sterilisation and Disinfection of Some Important Materials

S. No.	Materials	Methods
1.	Inoculating wires or loops	Red heat
2.	Glasswares—syringes, petridishes, test tubes, flasks, universal container, oily fluids (Paraffin)	Hot-air oven
3.	Disposable syringes and other disposable items	Ethylene oxide, Gamma radiations
4.	Culture media	Autoclaving
5.	Culture media containing serum, egg	Tyndallisation
6.	Toxin, serum, sugar and antibiotic solutions	Filtration
7.	Milk	Pasteurisation
8.	Cystoscope and endoscope	Glutaraldehyde
9.	Infective material like soiled dressings, beddings, animal carcasses	Incineration
10.	Skin	Tincture iodine, 70% ethanol, savlon
11.	Aprons, gloves, catheters, surgical instruments except sharp instruments	Autoclaving
12.	Rubber, plastic and polythene tubes	Glutaraldehyde

KEY POINTS

1. *Sterilisation* is a process by which an article, surface or medium is made free of all microorganisms either in the vegetative or spore form.
2. *Disinfection* means the destruction of all pathogens or organisms capable of producing infections but not necessarily spores.
3. *Hot-air oven* and *autoclave* are two commonly used methods of sterilisation. Hot-air oven is a *dry heat sterilisation* method while autoclave is a *moist heat sterilisation.*
4. Temperature and time period for hot-air oven is *160°C for two hours* (*holding time*) whereas it is *121°C for 15 minutes at pressure of 15 pounds per square inch* for autoclave.
5. Filtration is used to sterilise sera, sugars and antibiotic solutions.
6. *Gamma radiations* and *ethylene oxide* (ETO) are the methods commercially used for sterilisation of disposable syringes and other disposable items.
7. *Glutaraldehyde* is used for sterilisation of cystoscopes, endoscopes and bronchoscopes.

STUDY QUESTIONS

1. Define sterilisation. How does it differ from disinfection? Classify the various agents used in sterilisation. Add a note on the principle of autoclave.
2. Write short notes on:
   (i) Hot air oven (ii) Autoclave
3. Write briefly about:
   (i) Sterilisation by moist heat (ii) Tyndallisation

MULTIPLE CHOICE QUESTIONS (MCQs)

1. The process by which an article, surface or medium is made free of all microorganisms either in the vegetative or spore form is known as:
   (a) Sterilisation
   (b) Disinfection
   (c) Asepsis
   (d) None of the above
2. Chemical disinfectants which can be safely applied to living tissues to prevent infection are known as:
   (a) Antiseptics
   (b) Formaldehyde
   (c) Ethylene oxide
   (d) None of the above

3. Temperature and time period used in hot air oven is:
   (a) 160°C for two hours
   (b) 140°C for two hours
   (c) 160°C for one hour
   (d) None of the above
4. Temperature and time period used in holder method of Pasteurisation is:
   (a) 63°C for 30 minutes
   (b) 63°C for 50 minutes
   (c) 72°C for 20 seconds
   (d) 72°C for 40 seconds
5. Steam sterilisation at 100°C for 20 minutes on three successive days is known as:
   (a) Tyndallisation
   (b) Inspissation
   (c) Pasteurisation
   (d) Vaccine bath
6. Which of the following sterilisation conditions are used in autoclave?
   (a) 121°C, 15 pounds pressure/sq inch, 15 minutes
   (b) 160°C, 20 pounds pressure/sq inch, 20 minutes
   (c) 140°C, 10 pounds pressure/sq inch, 15 minutes
   (d) None of the above
7. Which bacterial spores are used as sterilisation control in autoclave?
   (a) *Clostridium perfringens*
   (b) *Bacillus cereus*
   (c) *Bacillus stearothermophilus*
   (d) *Pseudomonas aeruginosa*
8. Gamma radiations can be used for sterilisation of:
   (a) Plastic syringes
   (b) Catheters
   (c) Swabs
   (d) All of the above
9. Glutaraldehyde is used for sterilisation of:
   (a) Cystoscopes
   (b) Endoscopes
   (c) Bronchoscopes
   (d) All of the above
10. The most widely used disinfectant for human immunodeficiency virus (HIV) infected material is:
    (a) Hypochlorite solution
    (b) Lysol
    (c) Formaldehyde
    (d) Mercuric chloride
11. Which of the following is used commercially for sterilisation of disposable plastic items?
    (a) Ethylene oxide
    (b) Autoclave
    (c) Glutaraldehyde
    (d) Ethyl alcohol

ANSWERS (MCQs) ...✓

1. (a) 2. (a) 3. (a) 4. (a) 5. (a) 6. (a) 7. (c) 8. (d) 9. (d)
10. (a) 11. (a)

Biomedical Waste Management

52

Hospital waste is defined as all waste generated from medical facilities including office and kitchen wastes. Only a small fraction of the total waste generated by health care institutions is actually infectious. In contrast to radioactive or chemical wastes, *infectious waste* cannot be identified objectively. It can be defined as the waste that is capable of causing an infectious disease. Hospital waste management is of utmost importance for the safety of laboratory personnel as well as for the community. **Biomedical waste** is a broader term which includes waste generated in the diagnosis, treatment and immunisation of human animals, or in research activities or in the production of biologicals.

Concerns about transmission of the hepatitis B virus (HBV) and human immunodeficiency virus (HIV) led to the introduction of ***universal precautions***, to minimise the infections in medical laboratory workers and health care personnel.

UNIVERSAL PRECAUTIONS

1. Assume that all specimens/patients are potentially infectious for HIV and other blood borne pathogens.
2. All blood specimens or body fluids should be placed in a leak-proof impervious bags for transportation to the laboratory.
3. Use gloves while handling blood and body fluid specimens and other objects exposed to them. If there is a likelihood of spattering, use face masks with glasses or goggles.
4. Wear laboratory coats or gowns while working in the laboratory. Wrap-around gowns should be preferred. These should not be taken outside.
5. Never try to pipette by mouth. Mechanical pipetting devices should be used.
6. Decontaminate the laboratory work surfaces with an appropriate disinfectant after the spillage of blood or other body fluids and when the procedures are completed.
7. Limit use of needles and syringes to situations for which there are no other alternatives.
8. Biological safety hoods should be used for laboratory work.
9. All the potentially contaminated materials of the laboratory should be decontaminated before disposal or reprocessing.
10. Always wash hands after completing laboratory work and remove all protective clothings before leaving the laboratory.

I. CATEGORIES OF BIOMEDICAL WASTE

The new "Biomedical waste rules BMW 2016" has been notified on 28th March 2016 to replace the earlier rules (1998) and the amendments thereof. According to new rules, four categories of biomedical waste have been described according to the colour coding of bag (Table 52.1)

Categories

1. Yellow
2. Red
3. White (Translucent)
4. Blue

Table 52.1: Categories and colour coding of bags for segregation of biomedical waste

Category	Type of container
Yellow	Yellow coloured non-chlorinated plastic bag or container
Red	Red coloured non-chlorinated plastic bag or container
White (Translucent)	Puncture proof, leak proof, temper proof container
Blue	Blue coloured puncture proof and leak proof container

II. SEGREGATION OF WASTE

Prior to treatment and disposal of *waste,* it is important to segregate the *infectious waste* from *non-infectious waste* and to collect these in appropriate receptacles. The wastes are segregated preferably at the point of generation. This is the most important step to safeguard the occupational health of health care personnel.

Infectious waste includes microbiological wastes (cultures etc.), blood and body fluids, contaminated laboratory wastes, used sharps, pathological wastes (samples, tissues etc.), bedding and other wastes like bandages and used cotton swabs, and animal carcasses used in laboratory experiments. Besides infectious waste, *chemical waste* is also a hazardous waste.

Covered containers should be used for waste segregation. Proper segregation will minimise the waste stream needing special treatment i.e. infectious waste. This practice also helps in safe handling and transportation of waste. Segregation of waste in bags of different colours is shown in Table 52.1.

III. WASTE TREATMENT AND DISPOSAL

Waste Treatment

Following techniques are in use for treatment of infected materials:

1. Double chambered incineration
2. Autoclaving
3. Microwaving
4. Hydroclaving
5. Plasma pyrolysis
6. Chemical treatment
7. Effluent treatment plant (ETP)

1. Double chambered incineration

Incineration burns the waste at very high temperatures and thus reduces its volume. The double chambered incinerator contains two chambers. Waste is burnt in one chamber at 800°C. The second chamber has a high temperature of 1000°C.

Body parts, animal waste, microbiological waste and soiled dressings can be treated with this technique. The *disadvantage* of incinerator is that it generates highly toxic gases (e.g. dioxins and furans, if PVC plastics are present).

2. Autoclaving

Autoclaving is used for microbiological waste, blood and blood products, body fluids and used sharps. It is not recommended for pathological waste. Autoclaved material is typically land-filled, therefore, it has a large strain on land fill capacity.

3. Microwaving

Radiations produced by the microwave are involved to break apart molecular chemical bonds and thus disinfect infectious waste. The microwaves heat the waste to temperatures of 97° to 100°C. Cycle time is 40-45 minutes. It has advantage of disinfecting the waste and there are no hazardous emissions. However, it cannot be used to treat body parts and tissues.

4. Hydroclaving

The hydroclave is an expansion of the autoclave technology. Unlike in the autoclave, steam is introduced into the hollow walls of the hydroclave. The steam does not come in direct contact with the waste. Volume reduction of waste is much more than autoclave. Cycle time is one hour.

Hydroclave contains a series of large rotating rods, which spin slowly, putting the material into steam chamber as it is loaded. The rods continue to spin and rupture the waste bags and ensure complete exposure to the heat. After the sterilisation, the material is passed into a shredder. The waste can then be safely recycled or land filled. All items including pathological waste can be treated.

5. Plasma Pyrolysis

Plasma pyrolysis is an innovative technology which disintegrates organic compound into gases and non-leachable solid residues in an oxygen starved environment. Plasma torches are used in this technique, to generate high temperature. Plasma is the state of matter obtained by breaking down atoms into ions and electrons by ionisation. Plasma can easily reach temperature of 10,000°C or above and is used for dissociation of molecular bonds. Plasma pyrolysis can be used to dispose of all types of waste including peastic waste in a safe and reliable manner. The toxic compounds such as dioxins and furans in the emissions are below the prescribed limits. Plasma pyrolysis has been accepted as an alternative to incineration. This is also included in the category of non-burn technology.

6. Chemical Treatment

Chemical treatment ensures disinfection. 1% hypochlorite solution or any other equivalent chemical reagent may be used.

7. Effluent Treatment Plant (ETP)

The liquid waste (effluent) is first subjected to chemical treatment and then it is drained into ETP.

Disposal

Land filling, deep burial and sewage are used for disposal. Infectious waste after treatment can be disposed of by land-filling or deep burial. Besides treatment, incineration is also a method of disposal.

Segregation, collection, treatment and disposal of biomedical waste are shown in Table 52.2.

Table 52.2: Segregation, Collection, Treatment and Disposal of Biomedical Waste as per BMW rules 2016 and its ammendments in 2018 and 2019

Type of bag or container	Type of waste	Treatment and disposal
Yellow coloured non-chlorinated plastic bag or container	(a) Human anatomical waste (b) Animal anatomical waste (c) Soiled waste	Incineration or plasma pyrolysis or deep burial.
	(d) Expired or discarded medicines including cytotoxic drugs	Returned back to the manufacturer or supplier for incineration at temperature >1200°C.
	(e) Chemical waste	Incineration or plasma pyrolysis or encapsulation.
	(f) Chemical liquid waste*	Pretreated before mixing with other waste water and then disposal.
	(g) Discarded linen, mattresses, beddings, contaminated with blood or body fluid, routine mask, cap, gown and shoe cover.	Non-chlorinated chemical disinfection followed by incineration or plasma pyrolysis.
	(h) Microbiology, biotechnology other clinical laboratory waste, blood bags and live vaccines.	Pre-treat to sterilize with non-chlorinated chemicals on-site as per WHO guidelines on safe management of wastes from health care activities and WHO Blue Book 2014 and thereafter sent for incineration.
Red coloured non-chlorinated plastic bag or container	**Contaminated Plastic Waste (Recyclable):** Waste generated from disposable items such as tubing, intravenous tubes, catheters, urine bags, syringes (without needles and fixed needle syringes); vaccutainers with their needles cut, plastic apron, goggles and gloves.	Autoclaving or microwaving/hydroclaving followed by shredding or mutilation. Treated waste to be sent to registered or authorised recycler Plastic waste should not be sent to landfill sites.
White (Translucent) puncture proof, leak proof, temper proof container	**Waste sharps including metals:** Needles, syringes with fixed needles, needles from needle tip cutter or burner, scalpels, blades or any other contaminated sharp object.	Autoclaving or dry heat sterilisation followed by shredding or mutilation or encapsulation in metal container or cement concrete and then sent for final disposal to iron foundries (having consent to operate from the state pollution control boards or pollution control committees) or sanitary landfill or designated concrete waste sharp pit.
Blue coloured Puncture proof and leak proof container	**Glassware:** Broken or discarded and contaminated glass including medicine vials and ampoules except those contaminated with cytotoxic wastes, microscopic slides. **Metallic body implants.**	Disinfection (by soaking washed glass waste after cleaning with detergent and sodium hypochlorite (1%) treatment) or through autoclaving or microwaving or hydroclaving and then sent for recycling.

* Sepatate collection system leading to effluent treatment system is used.

KEY POINTS >>>

1. *Hospital waste* is defined as all waste generated from medical facilities including office and kitchen wastes. Only a small fraction of the total waste generated by health care institutions is actually *infectious*.
2. Prior to treatment and disposal of waste, it is important to *segregate* the infectious waste from non-infectious waste and to collect these in appropriate receptacles.
3. *Infectious waste* includes *microbiological wastes*, *blood* and *body fluids*, *contaminated laboratory wastes*, *used sharps*, *pathological wastes*, *bedding* and other wastes like *bandages* and *used cotton swabs*, and animal carcasses used in laboratory experiments.
4. Double chambered *incineration*, *autoclaving, chemical treatment* and *effluent treatment plant (ETP)* are the various techniques used in treatment of infectious waste.
5. Infectious waste after treatment can be *disposed of.*

STUDY QUESTION

1. Write short notes on:
   (i) Universal precautions
   (ii) Biomedical waste treatment and disposal.

MULTIPLE CHOICE QUESTIONS (MCQs)

1. How many categories of biomedical waste are there?
   (a) Five
   (b) Seven
   (c) Four
   (d) Ten
2. What colour code/s is/are used for plastic bag/s for segregation of biomedical waste?
   (a) Yellow
   (b) Red
   (c) Blue
   (d) All of the above
3. Which of the following methods can be used for treatment of biomedical waste?
   (a) Incineration
   (b) Autoclaving
   (c) Microwaving
   (d) All of the above
4. Which is the most commonly used method for the treatment of microbiological waste?
   (a) Autoclaving
   (b) Microwaving
   (c) Plasma pyrolysis
   (d) None of the above

ANSWERS (MCQs) ...✓

1. (c) 2. (d) 3. (d) 4. (a)

Needle Stick Injury

53

I. INTRODUCTION

Needle stick injury is one type of occupational exposure. An occupational injury is regularly termed as needle stick injury though it also includes injuries with other sharps and splashes besides needle. Needles used on patients may contain infectious agents and thus may transmit it to healthcare workers if needle stick injury occurs. The occupational exposure may be as:

- Percutaneous injury e.g. needle stick injury (NSI) or other sharp injuries.
- Splash injury
  It may occur by following types of contact:
  - Prolonged contact with the intact skin e.g. for several minutes or more.
  - Contact with non-intact skin e.g. abraded skin.
  - Contact with mucous membrane e.g. eye or mouth.

II. ORGANISMS TRANSMITTED

- Hepatitis B Virus (HBV)
- Hepatitis C Virus (HCV)
- Human immunodeficiency virus (HIV)

All these three organisms are blood borne viruses (BBVs) which may be transmitted by NSI. The risk of transmission is 30% (highest) for HBV, 3% for HCV and 0.3% for HIV.

III. SPECIMENS FOR NSI

1. Potentially infectious body fluids

- Blood
- Genital secretions *e.g.* semen, vaginal secretions
- All body fluids *e.g.* cerebrospinal fluid (CSF), pleural fluid, amniotic fluid etc.

2. Specimens not considered as potentially infectious

The following are not considered potentially infectious when these are not visibly contaminated with blood.

- Faeces
- Saliva
- Sputum
- Nasal secretions
- Urine
- Vomitus
- Tears
- Sweat

3. All body fluids containing blood are considered potentially infectious.

IV. RISK OF INFECTION FOLLOWING NSI

The risk of infection depends upon the following:

1. Type of needle *e.g.* injury with hollow bore needle has a higher risk than that of solid needle.
2. Depth of injury *e.g.* risk is directly proportional to depth. Higher the depth, more the risk.
3. Source of injury if visibly contaminated with blood means more risk.
4. Volume of blood involved in exposure e.g. more volume more risk.
5. Viral load present in the blood when exposure has occurred e.g. more viral load more risk.
6. Timely performed first aid will reduce the risk.
7. Appropriate post exposure prophylaxis (PEP) for HBV and HIV: If PEP is started timely, it will reduce the risk.

V. PREVENTION OF NSI

A. Precaution During Handling of Needles

To prevent occupational exposure, the following measures should be adopted while handling needles.

1. **Standard precautions** must be followed while handling blood or body fluids. Appropriate PPE should be used and practise hand hygiene.
2. **Disinfection** of work surfaces with 0.5% sodium hypochlorite solution.
3. **HBV vaccination:** Health care workers (HCWs) must be vaccinated against HBV and protective anti-HBs antibody titre must be documented,
4. **Spill management:** Spillage of blood, other body fluids must be cleaned as per guidelines and surface disinfected with 0.5% sodium hypochlorite solution.
5. **Eliminate** the unnecessary use of needles.
6. **Avoid recapping** of needles.

7. **Disposable needles** should be used. **Never reuse** needles.
8. Avoid the use of needles where safe and effective alternatives are available.
9. Use devices with safety features such as retractable lancets, safety lock syringe with a protective sheath and needleless IV systems.
10. **Dispose of** used needles properly in puncture resistant sharp containers.

B. Precautions during surgery

The following approach should be adopted for every surgical procedure.

1. Sharp instruments should not be passed directly by hands but by non-touch approach.
2. During suturing, forceps or needle holder should be used to hold a needle. Needles must never be picked up with the hands directly while suturing.
3. If a patient is known to have blood borne infections then all members of surgical team must follow appropriate protective measures such as PPE.

VI. POSTEXPOSURE MANAGEMENT

The following steps should be followed when occupational exposure occurs.

1. **First aid:** It should be started as early as possible.
2. **Report** the incident to the nodal centre for the management of occupational exposure / needle stick injury.
3. **First dose** of postexposure prophylaxis (PEP) for HIV should be taken as early as possible. PEP is given as per NACO guidelines.
4. **Testing for blood borne viruses (BBVs):** The following tests are done for both exposure source and healthcare worker.
   - Anti-HIV antibody detection
   - HBs Ag detection
   - Anti-HCV antibody detection

   However Anti-HBs antibody is also done for healthcare worker (HCW) if previously vaccinated with HBV vaccine but antibody titre not tested. The baseline titre of antibody of HCW will also be useful to determine whether the infection was acquired due to this occupational exposure or any other prior exposure.
5. **Decision for PEP** (Table 53.6)
6. **Informed consent and counselling:** Counselling is very important for psychological support.
   - Exposed person should be informed about the risks and benefits of PEP.
   - Person should be informed about the risk of acquiring infection if PEP is not taken.
7. **Recording of exposure**
   - A **performa** is used to record the detailed information related to exposure such as date, time, place, source and type of exposure. Volume, type of specimen involved and duration of exposure is also entered in the performa.
   - **Consent form** must be signed by the exposed person prior to start of PEP. If the individual refuses to take PEP then it should be documented.
8. **Follow up**

   Follow up testing of HCWs is done if the source status is positive or unknown.
   - **HIV testing follow up:** HIV testing is done at 6 weeks, 3 months and 6 months after exposure.
   - **HBV and HCV following up:** For HBV and HCV, testing is done at 6 months after exposure.
   - **Precautions during follow up:** The following precautions should be adopted by HCWs during the follow up period, especially the first 6–12 weeks.
     - Do not donate blood, semen, organ.
     - Abstinence from sexual intercourse or use latex condom till both baseline and 3 months HIV tests are negative.
     - Women not to breast feed infants.
     - Febrile illness of exposed person which occurs within 12 weeks of exposure should be medically evaluated.

A. Postexposure Prophylaxis (PEP) for HIV

Most exposures do not result in infection. Health workers are normally at very low risk of acquiring infection during management of infected patients. Following exposure, postexposure prophylaxis (PEP) may be required depending upon the category of exposure and HIV status of exposure source (Tables 53.1 and 53.2).

Categories of exposure and status of exposure source are given exposure codes (EC) and source codes (SC) respectively (Tables 53.3 and 53.4).

PEP regimen consists of three drug combination (Table 53.5). To be effective these drugs must be started within the first 72 hours and ideally within 2 hours. The PEP should be continued for a period of four weeks.

Other PEP regimen

- Tenofovir 300 mg + Lamivudine 300 mg in fixed dose combination (FDC) in one tablet and Lopinavir 200 mg + Ritonavir 50 mg in FDC in one tablet.

  Doses: One tablet (tenofovir + lamivudine) once a day and two tablets (lopinavir + ritonavir) once a day, for 4 weeks.
- Tenofovir 300 mg + Lamivudine 300 mg + Efavirenz 600 mg in fixed dose combination in one tablet.

  Doses: One tablet once a day (OD) for 4 weeks.

  PEP regimen is recommended on the basis of exposure

Table 53.1: Category of Exposure and its Description

Category of exposure	Description
i. Mild exposure	Mucous membrane/non-intact skin with small volumes
ii. Moderate exposure	Mucous membrane/non-intact skin with large volume or percutaneous superficial exposure with solid needle
iii. Severe exposure	Percutaneous with large volume

Table 53.2: HIV Status of Exposure Source and its Description

HIV status of exposure source	Description
i. HIV negative	Source is not HIV infected*
ii. Low risk	HIV positive and clinically asymptomatic
iii. High risk	HIV positive and clinically symptomatic

*Even if HIV negative, consider HBV and HCV.

Table 53.3: HIV Exposure Code and its Description

Description of exposure	Volume of blood, body fluid etc. or contact duration or severity	Exposure code
i. Mucous membrane or skin integrity compromised (non-intact)	• Small volume/few drops for short duration	EC1
	• Large volume/major splash for long duration	EC2
ii. Percutaneous exposure	• Less severe, solid needle, superficial scratch	EC2
	• More severe, hollow bore needle, deep injury, large volume	EC3

Note: In case of exposure on intact skin, PEP is not required.

Table 53.4: HIV Status Code of Exposure Source

HIV status of exposure source	HIV status code (SC)
1. HIV positive i. • Low titre exposure, • Asymptomatic, • High CD4 count	HIV SC1
ii. • High titre exposure, • Advanced disease, • Low CD4 count	HIV SC2
2. HIV status unknown	HIV SC: Unknown

Note: In case of status of exposure source is HIV negative, PEP is not required.

Table 53.5: Postexposure Prophylaxis (PEP) Regimen in Adults

Drugs for PEP in adults	Dosage and duration
Tenofovir 300 mg + Lamivudine 300 mg + Dolutegravir 50 mg in fixed dose combination (FDC) in one tablet	One tablet immediately within 2 hours of accidental exposure. From next day one tablet once a day (OD) for 4 weeks

Table 53.6: NACO Recommendations of PEP based on Exposure and HIV Source Codes

Combination		
Exposure code (EC)	Source code (SC)	Recommendation for PEP
1, 2 or 3	Negative	Not required
1	1	PEP not required
1	2	PEP* required
2	1	PEP* required
2	2	PEP* required
3	1 or 2	PEP* required
2/3	Unknown	Consider PEP* if HIV prevalence is high in given population and risk categorisation

*Duration of PEP is 28 days.

code and status code combination (Table 53.6). PEP is required in all different combinations of EC and SC except combination of EC1 and SC1. However in combination EC2/3 and SC unknown, PEP is considered if HIV prevalence is high in that population and risk categorisation (Table 53.6).

Both risk of infection and possible side-effects of antiretroviral drugs should be carefully considered when deciding to start PEP. Besides PEP, injured site of the wound should be thoroughly washed with soap and water. Antiseptics may also be used. Before prescribing PEP regimen, counselling of exposed person should be done and also obtain consent for PEP.

Exposed persons should have post PEP HIV testing. If the test at six months is negative, no further testing is required.

B. Postexposure Prophylaxis of HBV

Postexposure prophylaxis of HBV has been shown in Table 53.7.

Table 53.7: Postexposure prophylaxis (PEP) for Hepatitis B

	Source Status	
Status of exposed person	**Positive for HBs Ag or unknown**	**Negative for HBs Ag**
1. Exposed person is completely vaccinated and has protective antibody titre (≥ 10 mIU/mL).	1. No further treatment is required.	–
2. Exposed person is completely vaccinated but the antibody titre is not protective (< 10 mIU/mL).	2.(i) **HBIG** One dose of HBIG should be given immediately; maximum within 7 days. (ii) **Vaccine** three doses of vaccine are given again (second series).	2. **Vaccine** Only three doses of vaccine are given again (second series).
3. Exposed person is either not vaccinated or is partially vaccinated.	3.(i) **HBIG** One dose of HBIG is given immediately; maximum within 7 days. (ii) **Vaccine** Do not restart vaccination but complete the vaccination status from the last dose given.	3. **Vaccine** Do not restart vaccination but complete the vaccination status from the last dose given.
4. **Non responders** (Antibody titre is not protective even after vaccination with 2 series, *i.e.*, 6 doses).	4. **HBIG** Two dose of HBIG is given at 1 month apart (0.06 mL/kg or 10–12 IU/kg).	4. Nothing is required.

HBIG – hepatitis B immunoglobulin, HBs Ag – hepatitis B surface antigen.

- HBIG and HBV vaccine can be given simultaneously but at different sites.
- HBIG which is passive immunisation, gives short protection for 3–6 months.
- Anti-HBs antibody titre should be checked only after 2 months of last dose of vaccine and 6 months after HBIG administration.
- Protective anti-HBs antibody titre is ≥ 10 mIU/mL after three or more doses of vaccination.

KEY POINTS

1. Needle stick injury is one type of occupational exposure. An occupational injury is regularly termed as needle stick injury though it also includes injuries with other sharps and splashes besides needle.
2. Needles used on patients may contain infectious agents and thus may transmit it to healthcare workers if needle stick injury occurs.
3. Hepatitis B virus (HBV), hepatitis C virus (HCV) and human immunodeficiency virus (HIV) can be transmitted by occupational exposure.

STUDY QUESTION

1. Write short notes on:
   (i) Needle stick injury
   (ii) Postexposure prophylaxis of HIV

MULTIPLE CHOICE QUESTIONS (MCQs)

1. Which of the following antiretroviral drugs may be used for postexposure prophylaxis in individuals exposed to potentially HIV infected blood?
   (a) Tenofovir
   (b) Lamivudine
   (c) Dolutegravir
   (d) All of the above
2. After exposure to blood potentially infected with HIV, post exposure prophylaxis with antiretroviral drugs should ideally be started within:
   (a) Two hours
   (b) Four hours
   (c) Six hours
   (d) Eight hours

ANSWERS (MCQs)

1. (d) 2. (a)

54

Environmental Surveillance

I. INTRODUCTION

The environment in the hospital may have an important role in the occurance of healthcare-associated infections. Water, air and environmental surfaces may be important sources for transmission of microorganisms to patients and health care workers. Hence, surveillance of water, air and environmental surfaces for microbiological quality is of utmost importance for safe hospital environment. Rouitine periodic surface surveillance is not recommended. It is used during an outbreak investigation or for research.

II. WATER SURVEILLANCE

A. Water-Borne Pathogens

Hospital water way act as a reservoir of water-borne pathogens. These pathogens may be two types.

1. Enteric pathogens
2. Hospital pathogens

1. Enteric Pathogens

Faecal contamination of drinking water supplies results in presence of enteric pathogens in water. These organisms are transmitted by ingestion of contamination water and may cause diarrhoeal outbreaks. These organisms are more common in community. These pathogens are shown in Table 54.1.

Table 54.1: Water-Borne Pathogens

Bacterial	*Vibrio cholerae, Escherichia coli, Salmonella typhi, S. paratyphi A, B and C, Shigella spp., Yersinia enterocolitica, Campylobacter jejuni and C. coli.*
Viral	Hepatitis A virus, hepatitis E virus, poliomyelitis virus, rotavirus
Protozoal	*Entamoeba histolytica, Giardia lamblia, Balantidium coli, Cryptosporidium, Isospora*
Helminthic	*Ascaris lumbricoides, Enterobius vermicularis, Trichuris trichura*

2. Hospital Pathogens

These organisms include multidrug resistant Gram negative bacilli, legionellae etc. They are commonly present in hospital rather than in community. They can contaminant hospital water such as potable water, sink water, dialysis water etc. They may be transmitted by ingestion, contact, aspiration etc.

B. Bacteriological Examination

1. Testing of drinking water for enteric pathogens

(i) Collection of water samples

Water samples are to be collected in heat sterilised glass bottles of 230 ml with ground glass stoppers protected by Kraft paper. To neutralise the bactericidal effect of chlorine in water, a crystal of sodium thiosulphate is introduced into the bottle prior to sterilisation.

Sampling from a tap

Clean the tap or pump outlet from outside. A tap is turned at maximum flow rate and let the water flow for 5 minutes. Open the stopper, fill the bottle and replace the stopper.

(ii) Transport

Water bottles should be wrapped in a Kraft paper. The water samples should be properly labelled with details of the source, time and date of collection. These should be delivered to the laboratory as quickly as possible. Where delay is anticipated, the bottles should be kept on ice, preferably in an ice box and protected from light. These samples should be processed immediately.

(iii) Methods of analysis

The standard tests usually employed for water bacteriology are:

- Presumptive coliform count
- Differential coliform count
- Detection of faecal streptococci and *Clostridium perfringens*
- Membrane filtration test

Presumptive coliform count

Multiple tube method is generally used for estimation of probable number of coliform bacilli in water. By this method the most probable number (MPN) of coliform organisms are detected in 100 ml water.

(a) Media

Double strength and single strength MacConkey broths in bottles or tubes containing Durham's tube for indication of gas production are used. These media contain bromocresol blue as indicator.

(b) Procedure

Measured amounts of water samples are added by sterile graduated pipettes as under:

- 50 ml of water to one bottle of 50 ml double strength medium.
- 10 ml of water each to five tubes of 10 ml double strength medium.
- 1 ml of water each to five tubes of 5 ml single strength medium.
- 0.1 ml of water each of five tubes of 5 ml single strength medium.

The inoculated tubes/bottles are incubated at 37°C for 48 hours. An estimate of coliform count per 100 ml is made from the tubes/.bottles showing acid and gas production using the probability table (See Appendix). The presumptive coliform count of 0, 1-3, 4-10 and >10 per 100 ml is interpreted as excellent, satisfactory, suspicious and unsatisfactory respectively.

Differential coliform count

Eijkman test

Some spore-bearing organisms give false positive reactions in the presumptive coliform test. The Eijkman test is done to confirm that the coliform bacilli detected in the presumptive test are *Esch. coli*. After the usual presumptive test, subcultures are made from all the positive tubes / bottles to fresh tubes of single strength MacConkey broth with Durham's tube. These are incubated at 44°C in water bath and examined after 24 hours. Those tubes showing gas in Durham's tube contain *Esch. coli*. Confirmation of *Esch. coli* is made by plating on solid media and indole production.

Membrane filtration method

A measured volume of water is filtered through a membrane which retains the bacteria on its surface. The membrane is then placed on a suitable medium and incubated, so that bacteria grows into colonies on its upper surface. The number of colonies is counted and the bacterial content of the water is calculated.

2. Testing of water for hospital pathogens

Hospital pathogenic may also be isolated by 'membrane filtration method' described earlier.

C. Endotoxin Detection

Apart from bacteriological examination, dialysis water is also tested for presence of endotoxin.

Methods

Three methods are available for detection of endotoxin.

1. Limulus amoebocyte lysate assay
2. Turbidometric method
3. Chromogenic method

Permissive Level

Water used for dialysis should contain endotoxin level <0.25 EU/mL.

III. AIR SURVEILLANCE

Since a man respires about 15 cubic meters of air in a day, therefore, the bacterial content of air is important particularly so when the air contains pathogenic organisms. Man is an important source of spreading bacteria in the environment during coughing and sneezing. The bacterial content in air depends on increased density of human and animal population, nature of soil, amount of vegetation and atmospheric conditions.

A. Bacteriological Examination

Bacteriological examination of air is necessary for surgical operation theatres, hospital wards, store house of food and pharmacy. There are two types of method for bacteriological examination of air:

1. Settle plate method
2. Slit sampler method

1. Settle Plate Method

Petri dishes containing nutrient agar and blood agar are left open for one hour. Large bacteria carrying dust particles settle onto the medium. The plates are incubated at 37°C for 24 hours. Colonies are then counted. For pathogenic staphylococci and streptococci, blood agar plates are used. This method is used for testing air in surgical operation theatres and hospital wards.

2. Slit Sampler Method

The number of bacteria in a measured volume of air is determined by slit sampler method. One cubic foot volume of air is directed onto a plate containing culture medium through a slit of 0.25 mm wide. The plate is rotated mechanically so as to allow the organisms to spread out evenly on the medium. The culture media are incubated and the colonies are counted. The number of colonies gives the number of bacteria present in the air.

KEY POINTS

1. The standard tests usually employed for water bacteriology include *presumptive coliform count*, *differential coliform count*, *detection of faecal streptococci* and *membrane filtration test*.
2. *Multiple tube method* is generally used for presumptive coliform count.
3. The *Eijkman test* is done to confirm that the coliform bacilli detected in the presumptive test are *Esch. coli*.
4. Bacteriological examination of air is done by *settle plate method* and *slit sampler method*.

STUDY QUESTION

1. Name various water-borne pathogens. Discuss the bacteriological examination of water.

MULTIPLE CHOICE QUESTIONS (MCQs)

1. Which of the following is/are water-borne pathogen/s?
   (a) Hepatitis E virus
   (b) *Salmonella typhi*
   (c) *Entamoeba histolytica*
   (d) All of the above
2. Which of the following parasites can be water-borne pathogens?
   (a) *Cryptosporidum*
   (b) *Isospora*
   (c) *Giardia lamblia*
   (d) All of the above
3. Which of the following bacteria can act as indicator/s of faecal pollution of drinking water?
   (a) *Escherichia coli*
   (b) *Bacillus subtilis*
   (c) Diphtheroids
   (d) All of the above
4. Drinking water is considered satisfactory if the presumptive coliform count of water is:
   (a) 0/100 mL
   (b) 1-3/100 mL
   (c) 4-10/100 mL
   (d) > 10/100 mL
5. Which test is done to confirm that the coliform bacilli detected in the presumptive test of water are *Escherichia coli*?
   (a) Eijkman test
   (b) Membrane filtration method
   (c) Turbidity test
   (d) Phosphatase test
6. In Eijkman test, MacConkey broth tubes are incubated at:
   (a) 25 °C
   (b) 37 °C
   (c) 44 °C
   (d) 52 °C

ANSWERS (MCQs)

1. (d) 2. (d) 3. (a) 4. (b) 5. (a) 6. (c)

55

Laundry Management

Laundry includes cleaning and disinfection of hospital linens in a healthcare facility (HCF). It includes bed linens, patient clothing, towels, curtains, healthcare workers (HCWs) clothing *e.g.* uniform, coats etc.

I. PURPOSE OF LAUNDRY

To protect the HCWs from exposure to potentially infectious items during the process of collection, handling and sorting of contaminated linen items.

II. CLASSIFICATION OF CONTAMINATED LINEN

For laundry process, the contaminated (*i.e.* used) linen is classified as follows:

1. **Dirty linen:** These are used linen, but are not visibly soiled with blood/blood-tinged body fluids.
2. **Soiled linen:** These are contaminated with blood, excreta or body fluids. These linens have a higher risk of transmitting Infections due to presence of blood, body fluid etc.

III. ROUTE OF TRANSMISSION OF INFECTION

Infections can be transmitted to HCWs from contaminated linens by the following routes.

- **Direct contact:** With contaminated linen.
- **Respiratory route:** Aerosols which are generated during handling of contaminated linen.

IV. COLLECTION AND TRANSPORT OF LINEN

1. Collect used linen at the point of generation *e.g.* wards, OTs etc. and transport it to laundry facility of hospital.
2. **Prevent generation of aerosols:** To prevent the generation of potentially contaminated aerosols, the used linen should be handled with minimum agitation. Linen should not be shaken or sorted in patient care area.
3. **Collection in bags:** Collected linen should be put in bags immediately and not to be placed on the floor for a long time to prevent contamination of surfaces such as floor.
4. **Segregation:** Linen should be segregated into dirty and soiled linen and preferably should be collected in different colour coded trolleys.
5. **Storage:** The collected linen should be stored at a designated place such as dirty utility area of the ward.
6. **Packing in bags:** Linens are packed in bags which are securely tied.
7. **Labelling of bags:** Bags must be labelled or colour coded so that HCWs handling these bags should be aware of the type of contaminated linen. Proper labelling also helps in identification and inventory management.
8. **Inventory of linens:** The inventory record of linens (both receiving and giving) should be kept by the incharge of the area such as sister-incharge.
9. **Transport:** Clean and used linen should be transported separately in dedicated closed trolley or cart. The trolleys should be cleaned and disinfected after transport.

V. LAUNDRY PROCESS

During laundry process, the working staff must wear appropriate personal protective equipment (PPE) such as heavy-duty gloves, gowns and masks.

The laundry process consists of flush, main wash, bleaching, rinsing and souring.

1. **Flush:** Wet the linen with warm water (37°C – 44°C) for 1–3 minutes to remove water soluble soils.
2. **Wash:** Wash the linen with detergents/soap in hot water (57°C – 62°C) for 5 to 8 minutes. Washing removes any stain or dirt and sets the alkaline pH, which is required for the next step i.e. bleach.
3. **Bleach:** Linen is treated with hypochlorite (50–200 ppm) in hot water (60°C–70°C) for about 5 to 8 minutes. The bleach step disinfects the linen and also removes stains.
4. **Rinse:** Rinse the linen in warm water (37°C – 48°C) for 2 to 3 minutes. It neutralises the chlorine of bleach step and also removes the residuals of stain and soiling if any.
5. **Souring:** It is the final rinse step in which warm water mixed with softeners is used for 3 to 5 minutes. It makes the fabrics soft.

VI. POST LAUNDRY PROCESS

The post laundry process involves the following steps.

1. **Sorting:** Sorting of linen into specific product types is carried out.

2. **Drying:** Drying of linen can be carried out either by the mechanical dryer (as in washing machine) or sunlight.
3. **Packing:** The dried linen is ironed and folded to pack.
4. **Storage:** Packed linen are stored in a well-separated clean area.

KEY POINTS

1. Laundry includes cleaning and disinfection of hospital linens in a healthcare facility (HCF).
2. Purpose of laundry is to protect the HCWs from exposure to potentially infectious items during the process of collection, handling and sorting of contaminated linen items.

STUDY QUESTION

1. Write short notes on:
   (i) Collection and transport of linen
   (ii) Laundry process

Immunisation of Healthcare Workers

56

I. INTRODUCTION

Healthcare workers (HCWs) have regular contact with patients in the hospital environment and thus are at increased risk of exposure to infectious agents. Hence they may act as a source of that infection, and may transmit infection to other HCWs, patients, their family members and their contacts in the community. It is thus important to protect them from acquiring healthcare associated infections by immunisation. It is the responsibility of hospital administration to safeguard them by providing appropriate immunisation.

II. IMMUNISATION PROGRAMME FOR HCWs

HCWs should be immunised with vaccines which can prevent the transmission of vaccine preventable diseases.

1. Vaccines strongly recommended for all HCWs.

(i) **Hepatitis B vaccine** *	(i) 3 doses at 0, 1, 6 months.
(ii) **Influenza vaccine**	(ii) Single dose, once yearly, I/M route.
(iii) **Measles, mumps and rubella (MMR) vaccine**	(iii) Single dose, S/C route.
(iv) **Varicella vaccine**	(iv) Single dose, S/c route.
(v) **COVID-19 vaccine**	(v) • **Covaxin:** Two doses, 4-6 weeks apart, I/M route. or • **Covishield:** Two doses, 12-16 weeks apart, I/M route. Precautionary dose is given every year for both covaxin and covishield.

2. Vaccines recommended for those HCWs working in high risk areas.

Vaccine	Recommendation
(i) **Td vaccine (Tetanus toxoid + diphtheria toxoid, adult dose)**	• **HCW > 18 years having complete primary vaccination** Booster dose, every 10 years till 65 years, I/M route. • **HCW > 18 years not having complete vaccination.** Three doses of Td are given at 0, 1 month and 1 year, I/M route. • **Pregnant HCWs** Two doses of Td at interval of 4 weeks during early pregnancy, however only single dose of Td booster is given if she had received two doses of Td in a previous pregnancy within last 3 years. Td is given by I/M route.
(ii) **Meningococcal polysaccharide vaccine**	• Both Men ACWY and Men B vaccines are given to workers who are routinely exposed to isolates of *Neisseria meningitidis*. Single dose is given by I/M route. Booster dose is given every 5 years if risk continues.
(iii) **Rabies vaccine**	• Persons working in a research laboratory are given single dose on days 0, 7 and 28 days by I/M or I/D route.
(iv) **Typhoid-Vi capsular polysaccharide vaccine**	• Workers having moderate to high risk exposure are given single dose by I/M or S/C route. Booster dose is given every 3 years.
(v) **Hepatitis A vaccine**	• Persons working with HAV in a research laboratory are given two doses at 0 and 6–12 months by I/M route.

IM – Intramuscular, I/D – Intradermal, S/C – subcutaneous

* Protective titre of HBV vaccine: Anti-HBS titre of ≥ 10 mIU/mL after three doses of vaccine is protective.

KEY POINTS

1. Healthcare workers (HCWs) have regular contact with patients in the hospital environment and thus are at increased risk of exposure to infectious agents. It is thus important to protect them from acquiring healthcare associated infections by immunisation.
2. HCWs should be immunised with vaccines which can prevent the transmission of vaccine preventable diseases.

STUDY QUESTION

1. Write briefly about immunisation of healthcare workers.

Antimicrobial Stewardship

57

I. INTRODUCTION

Antimicrobial Stewardship Programme (ASP) is a coordinated programme which promotes the rational use of antimicrobials.

A. Definition

Antimicrobial stewardship is defined as use of right antimicrobial agent, with right dose, right route of administration, right frequency, at right time and to right patient, causing the least harm to the patient.

B. Need of ASP

Misuse of antimicrobials leads to delayed recovery, increased length of stay in hospital, recurrent infection and even death of a patient. Hence, antibiotic stewardship programme (ASP) is needed for following reasons:

1. Antimicrobial Resistance (AMR)

Antimicrobial resistance (AMR) is increasing all over the world. Multidrug resistance (MDR) organisms are on the rise and prevalent in every country. Extensive use of antimicrobials is the single foremost factor for development of resistance in bacteria.

2. Misuse of Antimicrobials

Misuse of antimicrobials may occur by using antimicrobials without a prescription or by over prescription; and overuse of antimicrobials for self limiting infections (e.g. diarrhoea), viral infections, and for treatment of colonizers. Misuse is important contributing factor for development of drug resistant organisms including multidrug resistance (MDR) bacteria which are also known as "super bugs".

3. Antimicrobial Usage in Animals

Antimicrobials are widely used in animals for non-therapeutic purposes (70%) followed by therapeutic purposes (15%). Overuse of antibiotics in animals can contribute to the emergence of resistance in bacteria. When these resistant bacteria are passed to humans they can cause serious disease. There is also misuse of antibiotics in farming and agriculture. Stewardship programme would bring down unnecessary use of antimicrobials.

4. Poor Research for Development of Antimicrobials

There is poor research for development of new antimicrobials in pharmaceutical industry. Morever after discovery of a new antimicrobial, the bacteria develop resistance soon and thus wastage of investment.

II. MONITORING OF ANTIMICROBIAL STEWARDSHIP PROGRAMME

Monitoring of the compliance to this programme can be done by two types of indicators namely process indicators and outcome indicators.

1. Process Indicators

It is a policy adherence indicator and can be done by:

(i) Audit of antimicrobial stewardship as described under back-end strategy.

(ii) Prescription compliance.

Prescription compliance can be checked by the following indicators:

- Empirical antibiotic given according to infective syndrome.
- Culture taken before the start of antibiotics.
- Modification of the empirical antibiotic according to antibiotic susceptibility report.
- Surgical antimicrobial prophylaxis according to the formulated policy.

The percentage of how many times these indicators were followed properly should be checked.

(iii) Administrative compliance.

Administrative compliance indicators include:

- Correct administration of antibiotic in terms of dosage, frequency and route (e.g. oral, parentral etc.).
- Similarly correct administration of surgical antimicrobial prophylaxis.

The percentage of how many times these indicators were followed properly should be checked.

2. Outcome Indicators

(i) Antimicrobial usage

This is calculated by drug usage and days of therapy. Two indicators are:

(a) *Defined daily dosage (DDD):* It is the assumed average maintenance dose per day for a drug used for its main indication in adults.
For example, the paracetamol (analgesic) has a DDD of 3 gm, which means that an average patient uses 3 gm of paracetamol per day for its main indication, which is pain relief. This is equivalent to six standard tablets of 500 mg each. If patient consumes 12 such tablets (6 gm of paracetamol) over a certain period, this equals to consumption of two DDDs.
(b) *Days of therapy (DOT):* It is simply the number of days that a patient is on an antibiotic, regardless of dose.

(ii) Antimicrobial resistance (AMR) outcome indicator

AMR pattern is analysed by AMR surveillance conducted periodically. The change in AMR pattern is indicator of outcome.

(iii) Clinical outcome indicator

It can be analysed by:
(a) *Morbidity:* It may be observed by length of patient stay in hospital.
(b) *Mortality:* Deaths related to infectious diseases is another indicator of clinical outcome besides morbidity.

(iv) Financial outcome indicator

It can be analysed by calculating the cost of antimicrobial per patient day or per year or per admission.

III. RATIONAL USE OF ANTIMICROBIALS

Rational use of antimicrobials can be done by considering the following conditions.

1. Prescribe Antibiotics Rationally

- **Viral infections:** Do not use antibiotics in syndromes which are primarily of viral etiology e.g. upper respiratory tract infections.
- **Diarrhoea:** Oral rehydration solution is the main treatment and not antibiotics.
- **Prophylaxis:** Do not use antibiotics routinely to prevent infections except in some situations such as cotrimoxazole prophylaxis in HIV infected persons.

2. Antimicrobial Therapy According to Site of Infection

In urinary tract infection, those antibiotics should be avoided which do not achieve adequate urinary concentration.

3. Correct Administration of Antimicrobials

Right antimicrobial in right dosage, right frequency and for right duration of therapy should be administered.

4. Rational Use of Empirical Therapy

Empirical antibiotic should be given according to the infective syndrome and its causative agent. The local antibiogram of the causative bacterial agent should also be considered to find out antimicrobial resistance patterns.

The empirical therapy should be modified subsequently, when antimicrobial susceptibility test report is available.

5. Antimicrobial Therapy in Some Specific Conditions

In certain conditions such as endocarditis, antibiotic sensitivity testing is to be done by MIC method as treatment given is according to MIC.

6. Drug Monitoring

Therapeutic efficacy of antimicrobial agent depends on its in-vivo activity, which is related to pharmacokinetic and pharmacodynamic parameters of antimicrobial agent and not on in-vitro susceptibility testing (MIC) only. Hence therapeutic drug monitoring is necessary in certain antibiotics such as amikacin and vancomycin. They are more effective if the drug concentration in serum is much higher than the MIC of the drug.

7. Stoppage of Antimicrobial Therapy Appropriately

Antimicrobial therapy should be stopped at appropriate time as determined by clinical improvement or after negative culture report or by report of biomarkers of bacterial infection.

Antibiogram

An antibiogram gives the antimicrobial susceptibility testing results of a specific microorganism to a number of antimicrobial agents. It indicates the antimicrobial resistance patterns within the hospital. Antibiogram guides the clinicians to select the best empirical antimicrobial therapy until culture and susceptibility testing results are available.

KEY POINTS

1. Antimicrobial stewardship programme (ASP) is a coordinated programme which promotes the rational use of antimicrobials.
2. Antimicrobial stewardship is defined as use of right antimicrobial agent, with right dose, right route of administration, right frequency, at right time and to right patient, and causing the least harm to the patients.
3. ASP is required to combat antimicrobial resistance and misuse of antimicrobials. Implementation of ASP will lead to achieve these goals.

STUDY QUESTIONS

1. Define antimicrobial stewardship and describe the need of antimicrobial stewardship programme.
2. Write briefly about core antimicrobial stewardship programme strategies.

MULTIPLE CHOICE QUESTION (MCQ)

1. Which of the following are part of antimicrobial stewardship programme implementation?
   (a) Leadership
   (b) Antimicrobial stewardship team
   (c) Neither (a) nor (b)
   (d) Both (a) and (b)

ANSWER (MCQ)

1. (d)

Patient Safety

58

I. INTRODUCTION

Patient safety refers to preventing and reducing risks and harms that may occur to patients in healthcare facilities during their management. The main aim is to continuously improve, based on learning from errors and adverse events. The improvement is done by capturing incidents and adverse events and doing their root cause analysis (RCA).

II. INCIDENTS AND ADVERSE EVENTS

An incident or adverse event is an event that caused damage to the patient, and which is not due to the patient's underlying condition.

Capturing of Incidents

Capturing of incidents is important for incident reporting. If you don't capture and report incidents that happen, the same type of incident might happen again.

Root Cause Analysis (RCA)

Root cause analysis (RCA) should be carried out for all incidents. It is done to identify underlying problems in systems of work or management systems. Analyse the incident for the root causes and factors involved. Even small incident should be analysed and reported.

Corrective and Preventive Action (CAPA)

Corrective action is taken to eliminate the cause of incident or undesirable situation so as to prevent recurrence. Preventive action is taken to prevent the occurrence of non-confirmities.

CAPA is often undertaken to eliminate causes of non-confirmities or other undesirable situations. Its focus is on investigation of root causes of identified risks so that their recurrences can be prevented (for corrective action) and to prevent occurrence (for preventive action). CAPA is part of quality management system.

Report Writing

Report writing involves completing an incident report form when an incidence occurs. The incident report form should include investigations done to find out the cause of incident and also actions taken to prevent the same type of incident from happening again. An incident report form might be completed by the staff involved in the incident or it may be completed by a safety manager.

The following details should be included in incident report form.

- Type of incident
- Date and time of the occurrence
- Location
- Names of the persons at risk
- Detailed information about the incident
- Names of the supervisors
- Post analysis of the incident

International Patient Safety Goals (IPSG)

International Patient Safety Goals (IPSG) were developed by the Joint Commission International (JCI). The Joint Commission is United-States-based Organisation. It was previously named as Joint Commission of Accreditation of Healthcare Organisation (JCAHO). IPSG were adapted from the JCAHO's National Patient Safety Goals. These goals were established to address specific areas of concern in relation to patient safety. There are seven International Patient Safety Goals (IPSG) which include:

1. Identify patients correctly.
2. Improve effective communication.
3. Improve the safety of high-alert medications.
4. Ensure safe surgery.
5. Reduce the risk of healthcare associated infections.
6. Reduce the risk of patient harm resulting from falls.
7. Reduce the harm associated with clinical alarm system.

III. APPLICATIONS

IPSG 1 Identify Patients Correctly

Always identify patient correctly:

- Before providing treatment.
- Before administering medicines, blood or blood products.
- Before collecting blood and other specimens for testing.
- Before doing any procedure.

IPSG 2 Improve Effective Communication

- The verbal/telephonic order or test result should be written down by the receiver.
- The verbal/telephonic order or test result should be read by the receiver.
- The verbal/telephonic order or test result should be confirmed by the person who gave it.

IPSG 3 Improve the Safety of High-Alert Medications

High-Alert Medications are those:

- which carry a higher risk for adverse outcomes.
- which look-alike or sound-alike.
- which are involved in a high percentage of errors.

To improve the safety with these medicines:

- Policies and/or procedures should be developed and implemented for proper identification, location, labelling and storage of these medicines.

IPSG 4 Ensure Safe Surgery

A checklist or other process should be used to verify preoperatively.

- The correct surgical site.
- The correct procedure.
- The correct patient.
- All documents and equipments needed are available and these are correct and functional. Policies and procedures are developed which ensure the correct surgical site, correct procedure and correct patient, including medical and dental procedures which are done in settings other than the operation theatre.

IPSG 5 Reduce the Risk of Healthcare Associated Infections

- Hand-hygiene guidelines should be adapted.
- Hand-hygiene programme should be implemented.
- Policies and procedures are developed which contribute in continued reduction of health care associated infections.

IPSG 6 Reduce the Risk of Patient Harm Resulting from Falls

- Measures should be implemented to reduce fall risk for those assessed to be at risk.
- Initial assessment of patients for fall risk should be done followed by reassessment of patients after a change in condition or medication, among others.
- Monitor the results of both successful fall injury reduction as well as any unintended related consequences.

IPSG 7 Reduce the Harm Associated with Clinical Alarm System

- Identify the most important alarm systems to manage.
- Establish policies and procedures for managing the alarms which are identified as truly important.
- Educate the staff members about the purpose and proper operation of alarm systems.

KEY POINTS

1. Patient safety refers to prevent and reduce risks and harms that may occur to patients in healthcare facilities during their management.
2. International patient safety goals (IPSG) were established to address specific areas of concern in relation to patient safety.

STUDY QUESTION

1. Write short notes on:
   (i) Patient safety (ii) International patient safety goals (IPSG)

MULTIPLE CHOICE QUESTION (MCQ)

1. All of the following are part of International Patient Safety Goals (IPSG) except:
   (a) Reduce the risk of healthcare associated infections
   (b) Identify patient correctly
   (c) Improve the safety of high alert medicines
   (d) To provide good food to patient

ANSWER (MCQ)

1. (d)

Safety Protocols for Healthcare Workers

59

I. INTRODUCTION

Healthcare workers may face work-related hazards while handling equipment of different nature. These hazards may be physical, chemical and biological. Standard precautions and transmission-based precautions are followed by healthcare workers to reduce the risk of transmission of infection from patients and environment.

Safety protocol deals with workplace safety for healthcare workers and should be followed by all. Various components of the safety protocol are described in this chapter.

II. 5S SYSTEM

The 5S system organises spaces so work can be performed efficiently, effectively and safely. The term 5S comes from five Japanese words *Seiri*, *Seiton*, *Seiso*, *Seiketsu* and *Shitsuke*. These words are translated in English as *Sort*, *Set in order*, *Shine*, *Standardise* and *Sustain*. These 5S steps are described below.

1. Sort

It deals with removal of unnecessary items from each area. This helps in providing the space needed to organise items in next step (set in order). Some of the removed items will need to be thrown away or recycled, other items may belong to another location and hence should be returned to that place.

2. Set in Order

It deals with organising the work area. Each item should be easy to find, use and return *i.e.* a place for everything and everything in its place.

3. Shine

It means 'cleanliness.' The first two steps (Sort and Set in order) cleaned up space and arranged the area of efficiency while this step (Shine) will attack the dirt which builds up underneath the clutter. It involves regular cleaning of every part of the work area. It can be done by routine cleaning *e.g.* brooming.

4. Standardise

This step deals with writing down what is being done, where and by whom. By writing down the decisions made in 5S programme will help ensure that work will be done.

5. Sustain

The 5S approach is not a one time event, but an ongoing cycle. Apply 5S programme over and over as a routine part of normal work.

III. RADIATION SAFETY

Radiation safety is a concern for patients, physicians and hospital staff in many departments including radiology, interventional cardiology and surgery. Any radiation exposure poses a potential risk to patients and health workers alike. In the medical field, ionising radiation is being used for diagnosis and treatment of various medical conditions.

The guiding principle of radiation safety is 'ALARA'. ALARA stands for 'as low as reasonably achievable.' ALARA means avoiding exposure to radiation which does not have a direct benefit to you, even if the dose is small. To achieve this, three basic protective measures can be adapted, *i.e.*, time, distance and shielding.

1. Time

Minimise your time near a radioactive source. Complete your work quickly and then leave the area.

2. Distance

Maximise your distance from a radioactive source. Increasing distance will decrease your exposure dose of radioactivity.

3. Shielding

Put something between you and the radiation source. Commonly used shield for radiation protection from X-rays and gamma rays include 'Lead aprons or Vests'. Wearing lead aprons can reduce health worker's radiation dose.

IV. LASER SAFETY

LASER is an acronym which stands for 'Light Amplification by Stimulated Emission of Radiations'. The laser produces an intense, highly directional beam of light.

Laser radiation safety is important to minimise the risk of laser injuries especially to eyes or skin. Improperly used laser devices are potentially dangerous. The following safety precautions should be considered when working with high power laser and laser system.

1. Wear Laser Safety goggles when operating lasers.
2. Never put yourself into any position where your eyes approach the axis of a laser beam (even with eye protection on).
3. Prevent unprotected personnel from entering the laser area.
4. Ensure new operators are trained in safety procedures for laser.
5. Appoint a laser safety officer (LSO) responsible for ensuring that safety regulations are followed by all the workers.
6. Laser warning symbol **(Fig. 59.1)** should be put outside the room where laser is being used. This will give a warning to persons before entering the room.

Fig 59.1: Laser Warning Symbol

V. FIRE SAFETY

Different fires can have different hazards and risks. Not every fire and its management is the same, therefore, it is necessary to know different types of fire. Using the wrong type of fire extinguisher could do more harm than good.

There are six classes of fire.

1. Class A (Solids)

Class A fires are fires involving solids. This includes paper, cardboard, furniture, fixtures or fittings. It could even be the structure of the building.

This is one of the most common types of fire. The only type of fire extinguisher used on a class A fire is the water extinguisher.

2. Class B (Liquids)

Class B fires include liquids. Many of the liquids and chemicals can be flammable or explosive such as cleaning fluids, solvents, inks, adhesives, paints etc.

These fires are rare but more deadly than other types of fire. The powder fire extinguishers are the best to use in class B fire.

3. Class C (Gases)

Class C fires include gases. This could be natural gas, LPG or other types of gases forming a flammable or explosive atmosphere.

Working with gas is dangerous, and increases fire risk. The only safe method to attack Class C fires is to shut off the gas supply. The best type of fire extinguisher for use is dry powder extinguisher, after shutting off the gas supply.

4. Class D (Metals)

Metals are not often thought of as a combustible material but some metals can be, like sodium. Metals are also good conductors, helping in a fire spread. The dry powder fire extinguishers are developed to tackle metal fires. The powder inside the fire extinguisher may vary depending on the type of metal risk it is designed for.

Electrical Fire

This is not strictly a class (class E) of fire, because electricity is a source of ignition rather than a fuel. Do not use water to attack electrical fires. Carbon dioxide fire extinguisher should be used. Always turn off the power supply if you can.

5. Class F (Cooking fats and oils)

Class F fires are due to deep fat frying and spillages of flammable oils near to heat sources in kitchens. The only type of fire extinguisher approved for Class F fires is the wet chemical fire extinguisher. Fire blanket can be used for small Class F fires.

Fire alarms

Fire alarm helps to provide an early warning on fires. It warns people when smoke, fire, carbon monoxide or other fire-related emergencies are detected. Fire alarms may be activated automatically from smoke detectors and heat detectors or may also be activated by manual fire alarm activation devices. They receive a signal from a fire sensor (smoke, heat or carbon monoxide detector) and transmit it to the fire alarm panel.

Fire Fighting System

A fire fighting system is an activity of prevention during a fire spread with the use of proper safety equipment like extinguisher, hose reels, fire monitors, nozzles and hose pipes. It's aim is to protect human life and property strictly in that order. A fire fighting system consists of three basic parts:

1. a large store of water in tanks, called fire storage tanks.
2. a specialised pumping system.
3. a large network of pipes ending in either hydrants or sprinklers.

VI. HAZMAT SAFETY OR HAZARDOUS MATERIAL SAFETY

Human exposure to chemicals and other hazardous materials can cause simple skin irritation to long term illnesses such as cancer. It is important to create a culture of safety for handling, transporting and storing these materials. To avoid a hazmat incident, follow the rules mentioned below.

1. **Assess the risk**
   This can be done by knowing the materials which represent hazards.
2. **Training**
   Provide training to workers about hazardous materials. They should also be trained on first-aid skills if any co-worker may be injured or experience chemical exposure.
3. **Use of proper personal protection equipment (PPE)**
   Old or damaged PPE should not be used. PPE should be inspected prior to each use.
4. **All hazardous materials to be properly marked**
   All hazmat containers are labelled and chemicals are stored in the appropriate contains.
5. **All hazardous materials to be stored properly**
   Keep chemicals in dry, cool and ventilated areas. Always keep lids closed.
6. **Use hazardous materials for their intended purposes only.**
7. **Always wash hands after using handling or transporting hazardous materials.**
8. **Never eat or drink while handling hazardous materials.**
9. **Report if any damaged container or potential leaks or spills.**

VII. ENVIRONMENTAL SAFETY

Environmental safety includes the practices and procedures which ensure that a surrounding environment including work areas, laboratories or facilities, is free of dangers that could cause harm to a person working in those areas.

A. Environmental risks

1. Chemical pollution
2. Air pollution
3. Climate change
4. Poor water quality
5. Disease causing microbes
6. Lack of access to health care
7. Poor infrastructure

B. Risk Assessment

An environmental risk assessment is the overall process or method to identify hazards and risk factors which have potential to cause harm. Analyse and evaluate the risk associated with that hazard, it is called risk analysis and risk evaluation.

C. Importance of Risk Assessment

The purpose of risk assessments is to improve workplace health and safety.

D. Risk Assessment Process

1. Identify the hazards.
2. Identify who might be harmed and how.
3. Evaluate the risks and decide on control measures.
4. Record the findings
5. Review the risk assessment

E. Temperature and Humidity in Environmental Safety

Temperature is the measure of warmth or coldness. Humidity refers to the amount of water vapour, or moisture, in the air.

When combined with high temperatures, high humidity levels can cause dehydration, muscle cramps, fatigue, fainting, heat exhaustion and heat stroke.

Maintaining a hospital humidity at between 40–60% relative humidity (rH) will reduce the spread of airborne viruses by inhibiting their ability to initially become airborne and the length of time they can survive once in the environment.

The centers for Disease Control and Prevention (CDC) recommends the following temperature ranges for healthcare facilities.

1. Operating rooms, endoscopy rooms and clean workrooms	20°C – 23°C (68°F – 73°F)
2. Hospital patient rooms, delivery rooms	24°C (75°F)
3. Most other healthcare areas	21°C – 24°C (70°F – 75°F)

In some cases, flexibility is needed to ensure thermal comfort and safety. For example, cooler temperatures may be required in operation theatres where specialised operations are being performed.

Humidity level in general should be between 40 – 60% relative humidity (rH). However relative humidity in different settings in hospital is recommended as follows:

1. Maternity and obstetric departments	45 – 65% rH
2. Operation theatres	50 – 60% rH
3. Patient's room	30 – 50% rH

F. Audits for environmental safety

An environmental health and safety (EHS) audit is a systematics objective tool to assess regulatory compliances in the workplace.

There are three main types of environmental audits:

1. Environmental compliance audits
2. Environmental management audits
3. Functional environmental audits

There are 5 stages of environmental audit as follows:

1. Schedule the Audit
2. Plan the Audit
3. Conduct the Audit
4. Develop an Audit Report
5. Audit follow up

VIII. EMERGENCY CODES

Hospital emergency codes are used in hospital worldwide to alert staff to various emergency situations. These emergency codes are often announced over a public address system of a hospital to alert staff for proper action.

Various emergency codes used are as follows:

1. Code Blue – Cardiac arrest
2. Code Pink – Paediatric/Neonatal cardiac arrest
3. Code Red – Fire, smoke or fumes
4. Code Black – Bomb threat/suspicious package
5. Code Brown – Hazardous material spill/leak
6. Code purple – Hostage taking
7. Code Grey – Infrastructure loss/Air exclusion
8. Code Orange – External disaster/Mass casuality
9. Code Green – Facility evacuation
10. Code Yellow – Missing patient
11. Code White – Actual or potential violent behaviour

IX. ROLE OF NURSE IN TIME OF DISASTER

Role of nurse is to ensure the appropriate system procedures and resources are in place to provide prompt effective assistance to disaster victims and thus providing relief measures and rehabilitation services.

Nurse has to intervene immediately after disaster as follows:

1. Establish safety
2. Medical treatment and nursing care by utilising available resources.
3. Life saving measures, first aid.
4. Evacuation and provide shelter
5. Supply of food, water, medicine
6. Psychological support to public.
7. To make voluntary reception for information to relatives
8. To arrange waiting areas for relatives
9. Infection control management

X. ANNUAL HEALTH CHECK-UP

Health check-ups are done to detect medical issues but also to identify risk factors and illnesses before they can cause problems. The aim of health check-ups is to prevent illnesses and its complications. However, it also helps to make changes in the lifestyle for long-term healthy life. Routine health check-up is generally recommended once a year.

During health check-up, a thorough physical examination is done from head to toe. It measures temperature, blood pressure, heart rate alongwith examination of heart, lungs and abdomen. Some important blood tests are also done such as complete blood count, lipid profile, cardiac profile, renal profile, thyroid panel etc. These blood tests will be helpful to detect any illness in heart, liver, kidney, thyroid, blood etc. Early detection of illness means early management including preventive measures.

KEY POINTS

1. Safety protocols deal with workplace safety for healthcare workers and should be followed by all.
2. Various components of safety protocol include radiation safety, laser safety, fire safety, hazmat safety and environmental safety.

STUDY QUESTION

1. Write short notes on:
   (i) Radiation safety (ii) Laser safety (iii) Fire safety
   (iv) Hazmat safety (v) Environmental safety

Unit VIII

APPLIED MICROBIOLOGY

Normal Microbial Flora of the Human Body

60

Normal flora refers to the population of microorganisms that inhabit skin and mucous membranes of normal human body. A healthy foetus in-utero is free from microorganisms. During birth the infant is exposed to vaginal flora. Within a few hours of birth, oral and nasopharyngeal flora develops and in a day or two resident flora of the lower intestine appears. The normal microbial flora is more or less constant for each species of animal.

I. NORMAL FLORA OF THE SKIN

The skin contains 10^2 to 10^4 organisms per cm^2. Bathing has little effect on the resident flora of the skin. *Staph. epidermidis* and *diphtheroids* are numerous and most constant in the skin. Other microorganisms include Peptococcus, *Str. viridans,* Enterococcus, Micrococcus, *Esch. coli,* Proteus, *Candida albicans, and Propionibacterium acne.* Penicillin resistant staphylococci are seen in individuals working in hospitals.

II. NORMAL FLORA OF THE CONJUNCTIVA

The conjunctiva is relatively free from bacteria due to the flushing action of tears and due to the presence of lysozyme in it. The predominant organisms are *Corynebacterium xerosis, Staph. epidermidis,* Moraxella species and non-haemolytic streptococci.

III. NORMAL FLORA OF THE NOSE AND NASOPHARYNX

The flora of nose harbours diphtheroids, staphylococci, streptococci and *Haemophilus* species.

The nasopharynx of the infant is sterile at birth but, within 2-3 days after birth, acquires the flora carried by the mother and the attendants. The nasopharynx is a natural habitat of the common pathogens which cause infections of the nose, throat, bronchi and lungs.

IV. NORMAL FLORA OF THE MOUTH

The mouth contains micrococci, Gram positive aerobic spore bearing bacilli, coliforms, Proteus and lactobacilli. The gum pockets between the teeth have a wide spectrum of anaerobic bacilli, anaerobic micrococci, microaerophilic and anaerobic streptococci, vibrios, fusiform bacilli. Corynebacterium species, actinomyces, mycoplasma and bacteroides are all found in varying extent.

The mouth of infant is not sterile at birth. It generally contains the same organisms as those present in mother's vagina, i.e., a mixture of micrococci, streptococci, coliform bacilli and Doderlien's bacilli. These organisms diminish in number during the first 2-5 days after birth and are replaced by the bacteria present in the mouth of the mother.

V. NORMAL FLORA OF THE UPPER RESPIRATORY TRACT

Within 12 hours after birth alpha haemolytic streptococci are present in the upper respiratory tract. They become the dominant organism of the oropharynx and remain so for life. In the pharynx and trachea, flora is similar to that of the mouth. A few bacteria are present in normal bronchi, but smaller bronchi and alveoli are normally sterile.

VI. NORMAL FLORA OF THE GASTROINTESTINAL TRACT

The gastrointestinal tract of the foetus in-utero is sterile. It becomes contaminated with organisms shortly after birth. In breast fed infants, the intestine contains lactobacilli, enterococci, colon bacilli and staphylococci. In bottle fed infants, the intestine contains *Leptotrichia*, anaerobic lactobacilli, colon bacilli and aerobic and anaerobic spore-bearing organisms.

Due to low pH of the stomach, it is virtually sterile except soon after eating. As the acidic pH of the stomach becomes alkaline in the intestine, the number of bacteria increases progressively beyond the duodenum to the colon. The bacterial count is low in small intestine compared to that in large intestine.

The bacterial count in adult duodenum is 10^3-10^6 per gram, in the jejunum and proximal ileum 10^5-10^8 per gram and in the lower ileum and caecum 10^8-10^{10} per gram of contents. Lactobacilli and enterococci predominate in the duodenum and upper ileum, but in the lower ileum and caecum the flora resemble the faecal flora. Colon and rectum contains about 10^{11} bacteria per gram of contents, constituting 10-20 per cent of the faecal mass. The normal flora of adult colon contains mostly (96-99 per cent) anaerobes and only 1-4 per cent aerobes. The anaerobic flora includes Bifidobacteria, anaerobic lactobacilli, Bacteroides species, anaerobic streptococci, and clostridia. Enterococci, coliforms and small numbers of Proteus, Pseudomonas, mycoplasma, lactobacilli and candida are predominant aerobes present in normal colon.

VII. NORMAL FLORA OF THE GENITOURINARY TRACT

Mycobacterium smegmatis, a harmless commensal, is found in the secretions (smegma) of the genitalia of both males and females. Strains of Mycoplasma and Ureaplasma are frequently present as part of normal flora of genitalia of both sexes. *Gardnerella vaginalis,* Bacteroides species and alpha haemolytic streptococci have been found in penile urethra. The female urethra is either sterile or contains *Staph. epidermidis.*

The vagina of newly born child is sterile. Within 24 hours it is colonised with micrococci, enterococci and diphtheroids. In 2-3 days, the maternal oestrogen induces glycogen deposition in the vaginal epithelium. Glycogen facilitates the growth of a lactobacillus (Doderlien's bacillus) which ferments glycogen to produce acid. The vaginal secretion now becomes acidic and the flora for a few weeks is similar to that of the adult. After the passively transferred oestrogen has been eliminated in the urine, the glycogen disappears, along with Doderlien's bacillus and the pH of the vagina becomes alkaline. Thereafter, the vaginal flora changes to micrococci, alpha and non-haemolytic streptococci, coliforms and diphtheroids.

At puberty, there is again deposition of glycogen and the pH changes to acid due to the metabolic activity of Doderlien's bacilli. The pubertal flora persists throughout the reproductive period till menopause. After menopause, the flora resembles that found before puberty. The normal vaginal flora includes clostridia, anaerobic streptococci, *Bacteroides* species, *Gardnerella vaginalis*, diphtheroids, listeria and *Candida albicans*.

KEY POINTS

1. *Normal flora* refers to the population of microorganisms that inhabit skin and mucous membranes of normal human body.
2. Different bacteria are present as normal flora on different sites e.g. skin, nose, mouth, upper respiratory tract, gastrointestinal tract, genitourinary tract etc.

STUDY QUESTIONS

1. Define normal flora. What is the role of this flora in human body?
2. Write short notes on:
   (i) Normal flora of the gastrointestinal tract (ii) Normal flora of the genitourinary tract

MULTIPLE CHOICE QUESTIONS (MCQs)

1. Which of the following bacteria can be present normally in the conjunctiva?
   (a) *Corynebacterium xerosis*
   (b) *Staphylococcus epidermidis*
   (c) *Moraxella species*
   (d) All of the above
2. Which bacteria is responsible for producing acidic pH in adult vagina?
   (a) *Lactobacillus*
   (b) *Bacteroides* species
   (c) *Diphtheroids*
   (d) *Gardnerella vaginalis*

ANSWERS (MCQs)

1. (d) 2. (a)

Blood Stream Infections

61

I. INTRODUCTION

Blood stream infections (BSI) are infections caused by microorganisms present in the blood. It is a serious condition as microorganisms can travel to any organ in the body and produce disease there. It may also lead to multi-organ failure. Hence, timely detection and identification of the causative agent is very important for proper management.

Some Important Terms

1. **Bacteraemia** is defined as presence of the bacteria in blood without any multiplication.
2. **Septicaemia** is a condition in which bacteria circulate and actively multiply in the blood stream.
3. **Pyaemia** is essentially septicaemia with metastatic infection.
4. **Endotoxaemia** is a condition when bacterial endotoxin circulates in the blood.
5. **Viraemia**, **parasitaemia** and **fungemia** are terms when there is presence of viruses, parasites and fungi in the blood respectively.

II. TYPES OF BACTERAEMIA

1. **Transient bacteraemia:** It is frequent even in healthy persons and may occur during chewing, brushing of teeth. The bacteria are immediately killed by phagocytes and are unable to initiate infection.
2. **Continuous bacteraemia:** It is continuous presence of bacteria in the blood stream. It usually occurs in infected heart valve, CLABSI.
3. **Intermittent bacteraemia:** Bacteraemia is due to same organism which is detected intermittently in the same patient *e.g.* undrained abscess.

III. CAUSATIVE AGENTS OF BSI

Bacteria, viruses, fungi and parasites can cause BSI. Bacterial agents accounts for the majority of BSIs.

1. Bacterial Agents

- Bacterial agents causing **Primary BSI**
  - Salmonella Typhi
  - Salmonella Paratyphi
  - *Brucella spp.*
  - *Leptospira spp.* } spirochetes
  - *Borrelia spp.* } spirochetes
  - HAECK group of organisms
  - Viridans streptococci
  - Rickettsia spp.
- Bacterial agents causing **Secondary BSI**

  These bacteria primarily infect other sites and subsequently may cause BSI.
  - Staphylococci
  - *Streptococcus pneumoniae*
  - *Neisseria meningitidis*
  - *Bacillus anthracis*
  - *Listeria spp.*
  - *Esch coli*
  - *Pseudomonas spp.*
  - *Acinetobacter spp.*
  - *Bacteroides spp.* – Anaerobic bacteria

2. Viral Agents

Many viruses circulate in the peripheral blood in viraemic phase of diseases, however the primary viral infection usually occurs in the target organs. Only a few viruses prefer to infect blood cells and are considered as **primary viral agents of BSI** e.g. human immunodeficiency virus (HIV), viruses causing haemorrhagic fever such as dengue virus, chikungunya virus, Ebola virus etc.

3. Fungal Agents

Fungi in blood stream (fungemia) occurs mainly in immunosuppressed patients, patients on chemotherapy, patients having malignancy etc.

Some fungi which may cause BSI in these patients include:

- *Candida spp.*
- *Cryptococcus spp.*
- *Histoplasma spp.*

4. Parasitic Agents

Parasites which directly infect blood cells.

- *Plasmodium spp.*

- *Babesia spp.*

Both infect erythrocytes

Parasites which may be present in the bloodstream before migrating to target tissues or organs.

- Amastigote forms of *Leishmania donovani*
- Trypomastigotes of *Trypanosoma spp.*

Parasites which are present in the lymphatics but are found in blood transiently.

- Microfilariae of *Wuchereria bancrofti* and some other filarial parasites.

Majority of BSIs are caused by bacteria hence details of bacterial BSIs are described below.

IV. TYPES OF BLOOD STREAM INFECTIONS (BSIs)

1. Intravascular BSIs

These infections occur within the cardiovascular system such as infection of heart (*e.g.* endocarditis etc.) and catheter related BSI (CRBSI).

2. Extravascular BSIs

Most cases of clinically significant bacteremia are extravascular.

- The organisms multiply at the primary site such as genitourinary tract, respiratory tract and then invade the bloodstream.
- The most common portals of entry for bacteria are genitourinary tract, followed by respiratory tract, wound and soft tissue.

V. CLINICAL MANIFESTATIONS

First stage of bloodstream infections is bacteraemia and then followed by septicaemic stage. Clinical manifestations appear only in the septicaemic stage. In septicaemia, the bacteria circulate and actively multiply in the blood stream, thus reaching various organs affecting their functions.

The common sign and symptoms of septicaemia include:

- Fever or hypothermia with/without chills and rigors.
- Dizziness or fainting
- A change in mental state such as confusion or disorientation

Septic Shock

It is the late stage complication of septicaemia and presents as low blood pressure, multiorgan failure etc. along with other signs and symptoms of septicaemia.

SOFA (Sepsis-related Organ Failure Assessment) score or Quick SOFA criteria are used to find the severity and degree of organ failure in septicaemia.

VI. LABORATORY DIAGNOSIS

Diagnosis of blood stream infection is done by isolation of the causative agent from blood by performing a blood culture test.

1. Specimen Collection

- Care should be taken while collecting blood for culture since there is a risk of contamination with normal flora of skin.

2. Time of Collection

- Before start of antibiotics.
- In case patient is already on antibiotics, collect the specimen immediately before the next dose of antibiotic is due.

3. Volume of Blood to be Collected

For adults – 5-10 mL of blood per blood culture bottle.
For pediatric – 1-3 mL of blood per pediatric blood culture bottle.

4. Site from Where Blood is to be Collected

Blood for culture should always be collected in pairs.

- Peripheral (cubital vein)
- Central line (*e.g.* internal juglar vein)

5. Number of Specimens

- At least 2–3 blood culture sets (each set contains one aerobic and another anaerobic blood culture bottle).
- Multiple blood specimens for culture are collected for bacterial endocarditis cases.

6. Technique of Blood Collection

Vene puncture

- All aseptic precautions are to be followed such as washing hands with soap and water, gloves to be worn, use of sterilised/sterile disposable syringes and needles and preparation of site by cleaning with 70% isopropyl alcohol followed by a second antiseptic solution such as povidone-iodine or chlorhexidine (Fig 61.1).
- The antiseptic solution should be applied in circular motion, starting from the center to the periphery.
- Allow the area to air dry before venepuncture.
- Collect the required amount of blood by venipuncture and transfer into blood culture bottle, either a conventional or automated blood culture (Fig 61.2).

7. Transport

- The collected blood is gently mixed with the broth of blood culture bottle. It is then transported immediately to the laboratory.
- If delay in transport is inevitable then incubate blood culture specimen at 37°C.
- **Do not refrigerate** the blood culture specimen. However it can be kept at room temperature.

Step 1 | Step 2 | Step 3 | Step 4 | Step 5

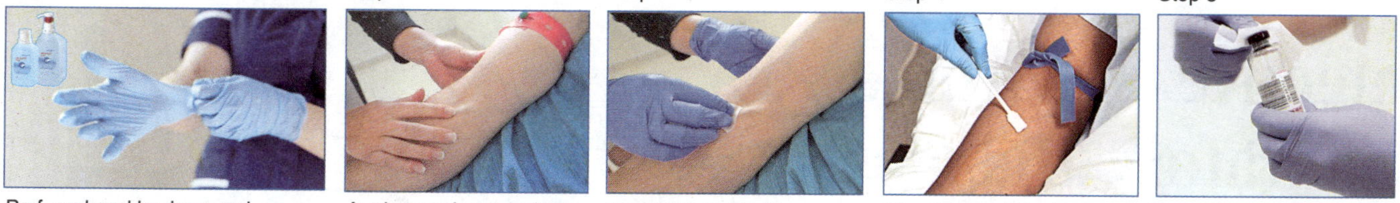

- Step 1: Perform hand hygiene and use sterile gloves
- Step 2: Apply tourniquet, palpate the vein
- Step 3: Use 70% alcohol to disinfect the site upside down and wait for 30 seconds (allow the skin to dry)
- Step 4: Use chlorhexidine/ providone iodine to disinfect the site, concentric from inside out and wait for 1 minute (allow the skin to dry)
- Step 5: Clean the cap of blood culture bottle with alcohol. Collect blood specimen aseptically and inject into blood culture bottle without changing the needle.

Fig. 61.1 Collection of blood for culture

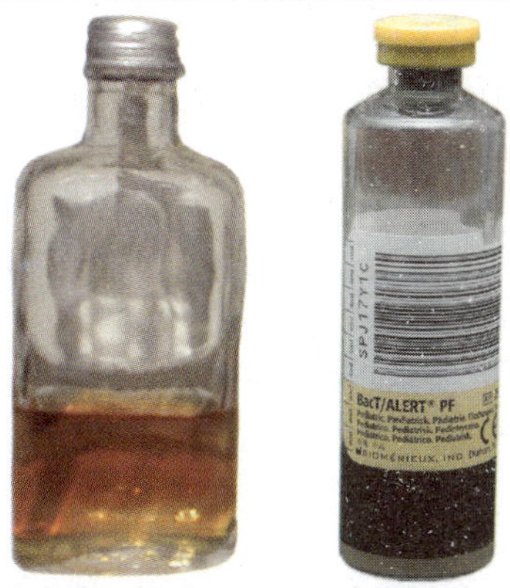

Conventional Automated

Fig. 61.2 Conventional and automated blood culture bottles

VII. FEVER OF UNKNOWN ORIGIN (FUO)

Fever of Unknown Origin (FUO) is commonly used term for any fever without any initial obvious etiology. The term FUO is reserved only for febrile illnesses of prolonged duration in which no etiology could be detected despite intensive evaluation and performing diagnostic tests.

Definition of FUO

The definition of FUO is as follows:

1. Fever of ≥ 38.3°C (≥ 101°F) on several occasions (at least two occasions).
2. For a duration of ≥ 3 weeks.
3. No known immunocompromised state.
4. The diagnosis could not be made after comprehensive history taking, repeated physical examination and a set of laboratory investigations.

Causes of FUO

The causes of FUO include:

- **Infections:** It accounts for one third cases of FUO (majority cases of FUO).
- **Neoplasms** e.g. Hodgkin's lymphoma, leukaemia
- **Non-infectious inflammatory disorders** e.g. systemic lupus erythematosus (SLE)
- Miscellaneous causes such as granulomatous diseases.

All groups of microbial infections can cause FUO such as enteric fever, malaria etc.

KEY POINTS

1. Blood stream infections (BSI) are infections caused by microorganisms present in the blood.
2. It is a serious condition as microorganisms can travel to any organ in the body and produce disease there. It may also lead to multiorgan failure. Hence, timely detection and identification of the causative agent is very important for proper management.

STUDY QUESTION

1. Write short notes on:
   (i) Laboratory diagnosis of blood stream infections caused by bacteria
   (ii) Fever of unknown origin (FUO)

MULTIPLE CHOICE QUESTION (MCQ)

1. Majority of blood stream infections (BSIs) are caused by:
   (a) Bacteria
   (b) Virus
   (c) Fungi
   (d) Parasite

ANSWER (MCQ)

1. (a)

Infective Syndromes: Laboratory Diagnosis

62

I. SORE THROAT

Sore throat is essentially an acute tonsillitis and/or pharyngitis. It is characterised by redness and oedema of mucosa, exudation of tonsils, pseudomembrane formation, oedema of uvula and enlargement of cervical lymph nodes. Viruses are more common cause of sore throat. About two-third cases are of viral origin.

A. Causative Agents

1. Bacteria

Streptococcus pyogenes—This is the most common bacterial cause.

Streptococcus groups C and G
Corynebacterium diphtheriae
Haemophilus influenzae
Bordetella pertussis
Treponema vincentii
Leptotrichia buccalis

2. Fungus

Candida albicans

3. Viruses

Epstein-Barr virus
Adenoviruses
Coxsackievirus A

B. Laboratory Diagnosis

For laboratory diagnosis, refer to the respective chapters.

II. URINARY TRACT INFECTIONS

Urinary tract infection (UTI) is defined as a disease caused by microbial invasion of the genitourinary tract that extends from the renal cortex of the kidney to the urethral meatus.

Normally, kidneys, ureters, urinary bladder and proximal urethra are sterile, but bacteria may be present in distal urethra as transient flora, most of which are derived from the faecal flora.

A. Causative Organisms

1. Gram Negative Bacilli

Gram negative bacilli are by far the most common infecting agents.

1. *Escherichia coli* is the commonest cause of UTI. It is responsible for about 70–80% of acute infections in general population.
2. *Klebsiella* spp.
3. *Proteus* spp., especially *P. mirabilis*
4. *Pseudomonas aeruginosa*

2. Gram Positive Cocci

1. *Enterococci* e.g. *E. faecalis*
2. *Staph. saprophyticus*
3. *Staph. aureus*
4. *Staph. epidermidis*—It is found in urine as a contaminant but may occur as pathogen in immuno-compromised individuals.

3. Miscellaneous

1. *M. tuberculosis*
2. Citrobacter
3. Salmonellae

4. Fungus

Candida albicans may cause UTI in diabetes and immunocompromised patients.

B. Laboratory Diagnosis

Refer to Chapter 24 for laboratory diagnosis of UTI.

III. DIARRHOEAL DISEASES

Diarrhoea is defined as an increase in the frequency, fluidity or volume of bowel movements, relative to the usual habits of an individual. Passage of three or more motions a day can be taken as diarrhoea.

A. Causative Agents

1. Bacteria

1. Vibrios
   (i) *Vibrio cholerae*
   (ii) *V. parahaemolyticus*
   (iii) Other *halophilic vibrios*
2. *Esch. coli* (ETEC, EPEC)
3. *Salmonellae*
   (i) *Salmonella* Enteritidis
   (ii) *S.* Typhimurium
   (iii) Other Salmonella spp.

4. *Shigella* spp.
5. *Campylobacter jejuni*
6. *Yersinia enterocolitica*
7. *Clostridium perfringens*
8. *C. difficile*
9. *Staph. aureus*
10. *Bacillus cereus*

2. Viruses

1. *Rotavirus*
2. *Norwalk virus*

3. Protozoa

1. *Entamoeba histolytica*
2. *Giardia lamblia*

4. Fungus

1. *Candida albicans*

B. Laboratory Diagnosis

For laboratory diagnosis, refer to the respective chapters.

IV. DYSENTERY

Dysentery means passage of *blood* and mucous with motion, often associated with tenesmus.

A. Causative Agents

1. Bacteria

1. *Shigella spp.* (*Sh. dysentriae, Sh. flexneri, Sh. boydii* and *Sh. sonnei*)
2. *Esch. coli* (EIEC, EPEC and EHEC)

2. Protozoa

1. *Entamoeba histolytica*
2. *Balantidium coli*

B. Laboratory Diagnosis

Refer to Chapter 24 for laboratory diagnosis of bacillary dysentery.

V. FOOD POISONING

The term *food poisoning* means an illness acquired through consumption of food or drink contaminated either with microorganisms, their toxins or chemical poisons. But traditionally, it is restricted to acute gastroenteritis caused by microbial contamination of food.

Infective type: Infective doses of microorganisms are ingested with food. Multiplication of bacteria occurs in-vivo. The typical example is food poisoning by salmonellae.

Toxic type: Preformed bacterial toxin is ingested with food, as in staphylococcal food poisoning.

Intermediate type: Bacteria ingested with food release the toxin in the gut. The typical example is *Cl. perfringens* food poisoning.

A. Causative Agents

Infective Type

Salmonella spp. (*S.* Typhimurium, *S.* Enteritidis)
Vibrio parahaemolytius
Campylobacter jejuni

Toxic Type

Staphylococcus aureus
Bacillus cereus
Clostridium botulinum

Intermediate Type

Clostridium perfringens

B. Laboratory Diagnosis

For laboratory diagnosis, refer to the corresponding chapters.

VI. MENINGITIS

Meningitis is an inflammation of the membranes surrounding the brain and spinal cord. It may be caused by viruses, bacteria, fungi or protozoa. Meningitis of bacterial origin may be caused by pyogenic organisms (acute pyogenic meningitis) or by *M. tuberculosis* (tuberculous meningitis). Aseptic meningitis is a term used for meningitis caused by viruses and a few cases caused by bacteria (other than those responsible for acute pyogenic meningitis), fungi and protozoa. Tuberculous meningitis is also included as a part of aseptic meningitis.

ACUTE PYOGENIC MENINGITIS

Diagnosis of acute pyogenic meningitis depends on direct examination of cerebrospinal fluid (CSF) and its bacteriological examination (Table 62.1).

A. Causative Organisms

In children and adults

Streptococcus pneumoniae (pneumococcus)
Neisseria meningitidis (meningococcus)
Haemophilus influenzae
Listeria monocytogenes

In neonates and infants

Esch. coli } important causes in first
Group B streptococci } few months.
Klebsiella spp.
Listeria monocytogenes
H. influenzae
Streptococcus pneumoniae

Meningococcal and pneumococcal meningitis can occur at any age. *H. influenzae* is common in meningitis cases in children from 3 months to 5 years. *Listeria monocytogenes* is very important causative agent in immunocompromised hosts.

Table 62.1: Cerebrospinal Fluid (CSF) in Normal Individuals and in Different Types of Meningitis.

Characteristic	Normal CSF	CSF in		
		Acute pyogenic meningitis	Tuberculous meningitis	Viral meningitis
I. Direct examination				
A. Cell count				
1. Total cell (per cu.mm)	1-3	1,000-20,000	50-500	10-500
2. Predominant cell	Lymphocytes	Neutrophils (90-95%)	Lymphocytes (90%)	Lymphocytes
B. Biochemical analysis				
1. Total proteins (mg%)	30-45	100-600 (Highly increased)	80-120 (moderately increased)	60-80 (Slightly increased)
2. Sugars (mg%)	40-80	Diminished or absent (10-20)	Diminished (30-50)	Normal
II. Bacteriological examination				
A. Microscopy				
1. Gram staining	Nil	Gram negative cocci, Gram positive cocci, Gram negative bacilli or Gram positive bacilli may be found depending upon the causative agent responsible.	—	—
2. Ziehl Neelsen staining	Nil	Nil	Acid-fast bacilli (AFB) may be found	—
B. Culture	Nil	According to the causative agent, specific organism may grow on appropriate media.	*M. tuberculosis* may grow on LJ media.	Viruses may be grown on cell cultures.

B. Laboratory Diagnosis

1. Specimen

CSF is obtained by lumbar puncture under strict aseptic conditions. It is collected in three sterile containers, one each for cell count, biochemical analysis and bacteriological examination. The fluid should be examined immediately after collection or placed in the incubater at 37°C (never refrigerate the CSF as *H. influenzae* may die). Biochemical analysis and cell count give an indication of the type of meningitis (Table 62.1).

2. Bacteriological Examination

The CSF is divided into three portions. One portion is centrifuged and microscopy is performed from the deposit. The supernatant may be used for antigen detection. The second portion of the CSF is inoculated on culture media. The third portion is incubated overnight at 37°C, either as such or after adding an equal volume of glucose broth.

For detail identification of different organisms, refer to the respective chapters.

VII. FEVER OF UNKNOWN ORIGIN (FUO)

Fever of unknown origin (FUO) may be defined as any febrile illness (temperature greater than 38°C) lasting 3 weeks or longer, without any obvious cause and failure to reach a diagnosis despite having a set of investigations.

A. Causes of FUO

Infections account for about one third cases of FUO.

1. Bacterial Infections

- Enteric fever
- Urinary tract infection
- Lung abscess and other deep abscesses
- Septicaemia associated with pneumonia, infective endocarditis etc.
- Tuberculosis
- Brucellosis

2. Parasitic Infections

- Malaria
- Hepatic amoebiasis or liver abscess
- Visceral leishmaniasis (Kala-azar)
- Filariasis
- Toxoplasmosis

3. Viral Infections

- Infectious mononucleosis
- Cytomegalovirus infection
- Hepatitis A virus infection
- Hepatitis B virus infection
- Rubella and other infectious fevers without typical rash
- HIV infection

B. Laboratory Diagnosis

For laboratory diagnosis, refer to the corresponding chapters.

KEY POINTS >>>

1. *Sore throat* is essentially an acute tonsilitis and/or pharyngitis. *Viruses* are more common cause of sore throat. About two-third cases are of viral origin. *Streptococcus pyogenes* is the *most common bacterial* cause. Laboratory diagnosis of sore throat caused by bacteria depends on *direct microscopy* and *culture*.
2. *Escherichia coli* is the *commonest cause* of *Urinary tract infection* (*UTI*). *Midstream urine specimen* (*MSU*) is collected for laboratory diagnosis of UTI. Count *more than* 105 *bacteria* of single species per ml is called *significant bacteriuria*. It indicates active UTI.
3. *Vibrio cholerae, Esch. coli, Salmonellae* are some important bacterial causes of diarrhoeal diseases. Rotavirus is the most important viral etiology of diarrhoea.
4. *Shigella spp.* and *Entamoeba histolytica* cause *bacillary dysentery* and *amoebic dysentery* respectively.
5. *Salmonella typhimurium* and *Vibrio parahaemolyticus* cause infective type of food poisoning while *Staphylococcus aureus* is an example of toxic type of food poisoning.
6. Laboratory diagnosis of diarrhoea, dysentery and food poisoning depends on *isolation of organism* from the relevant specimen.
7. Meningitis of bacterial origin may be caused by pyogenic organisms (*acute pyogenic meningitis*) or by *M. tuberculosis* (*tuberculous meningitis*). *Streptococcus pneumoniae*, *Neisseria meningitidis*, *Haemophilus influenzae* are important bacteria responsible for acute pyogenic meningitis. *Direct microscopy*, *antigen detection* and *culture* are key methods in laboratory diagnosis of acute pyogenic meningitis. These tests are done on a CSF specimen.
8. The causes of FUO include *bacterial, parasitic* amd *viral infections*. *Enteric fever* is the most common bacterial infection as cause of FUO. Culture of different specimens may be performed for isolating the causative organism. *Blood culture* is the most important investigation.

STUDY QUESTIONS

1. Name various organisms causing sore throat. How will you diagnose it in the laboratory?
2. Name various organisms causing urinary tract infection. Discuss the laboratory diagnosis of this condition.
3. Enumerate the different causes of diarrhoea. How will you diagnose it in the laboratory?
4. Discuss in detail the laboratory diagnosis of dysentery.
5. Name various organisms causing meningitis. Discuss the laboratory diagnosis of acute pyogenic meningitis.
6. Define and enumerate the causes of fever of unknown origin (FUO). Discuss the laboratory diagnosis of FUO.

MULTIPLE CHOICE QUESTIONS (MCQs)

1. Which is the most common bacterial cause of sore throat?
   (a) *Streptococcus pyogenes*
   (b) Streptococcus group C
   (c) Streptococcus group G
   (d) Streptococcus group D
2. What is the commonest cause of urinary tract infection?
   (a) *Escherichia coli*
   (b) *Proteus mirabilis*
   (c) *Pseudomonas aeruginosa*
   (d) *Serratia* species
3. Which of the following bacteria can cause diarrhoea?
   (a) *Vibrio cholerae*
   (b) *Escherichia coli*
   (c) *Yersinia enterocolitica*
   (d) All of the above
4. Which of the following organisms can cause dysentery?
   (a) *Shigella dysenteriae*
   (b) *Enteroinvasive Escherichia coli*
   (c) *Entamoeba histolytica*
   (d) All of the above
5. Infective type of food poisoning is caused by:
   (a) *Salmonella* Typhimurium
   (b) *Salmonella* Enteritidis
   (c) *Campylobacter jejuni*
   (d) All of the above
6. Toxic type of food poisoning is caused by:
   (a) *Staphylococcus aureus*
   (b) *Bacillus cereus*
   (c) *Clostridium botulinum*
   (d) All of the above

7. Which of the following bacteria can cause acute pyogenic meningitis?
   (a) *Neisseria meningitidis*
   (b) *Streptococcus pneumoniae*
   (c) *Haemophilus influenzae*
   (d) All of the above

8. Which of the following bacterial infections can result in fever of unkown origin?
   (a) Enteric fever
   (b) Brucellosis
   (c) Urinary tract infection
   (d) All of the above

ANSWERS (MCQs) ...✓

1. (a) 2. (a) 3. (d) 4. (d) 5. (d) 6. (d) 7. (d) 8. (d)

Specimen Collection and Transport

63

I. INTRODUCTION

Proper diagnosis of infectious diseases in Microbiology depends upon:

1. The correct procedure of collection of specimen.
2. Collection of specimen at appropriate timing e.g. blood collection during peak of fever in cases of fever of unknown origin.
3. The proper transport of specimens to the laboratory.

There are certain specimens such as blood and cerebrospinal fluid which are normally sterile. Other specimens such as sputum and faeces contain a large number of commensals. For collection of such normally non-sterile specimens the container may not be absolutely sterile; but must be chemically clean.

The following general points, although glaringly obvious are ignored from time to time.

1. No antiseptic or antimicrobial agents should come into contact with the specimen; all specimen containers should be sterile before use.
2. In collection of specimen, care must be taken to avoid contamination of the outside of the container otherwise the person delivering the specimen to the laboratory and the laboratory staff may be infected.
3. Specimen should be transported to the laboratory immediately. In case of unavoidable delay suitable transport medium has to be used.
4. Proper disposal of the specimen, after use, must be ensured.

II. GENERAL INSTRUCTIONS

These general instructions for collection of any specimen must be taken care of.

1. Specimen should be of adequate quantity.
2. Optimal time of collection of specimen.
3. Specimen should be collected before the administration of antimicrobial agents.
4. Specimen must be collected from actual site of infection with minimum contamination from normal flora of human body.
5. Appropriate container should be choosen for collection of a particular specimen.
6. Proper labelling of specimen container must be done.
7. Specimen handling should not be risky to health care workers.

III. SPECIMENS

The following specimens are commonly collected for microbiological investigations.

1. Blood
2. Respiratory tract specimens
3. Cerebrospinal fluid (CSF)
4. Pus and wound swabs
5. Urine
6. Stool

IV. TRANSPORT

The objectives of proper transport include:

- To maintain the specimen as near to its original state possible.
- To maintain the integrity of specimen even in adverse environmental conditions.

It is recommended that the specimen should reach to the laboratory as soon as possible. If delay is inevitable then this delay should not be more than 2 hours. In case of expected delay, specimen should be stored as per prescribed guidelines and transport media may be used for transportation of specimens to the laboratory.

V. REJECTION CRITERIA FOR SPECIMEN

- Specimen is not labelled.
  Proper labelling of specimen include:
  - Name, age, sex of patient
  - Registration number
  - OPD/IPD status e.g. medicine OPD, medicine ward number
  - Specimen type e.g. sputum, urine etc.
  - Diagnostic test to be performed
- Specimen is not properly transported.
- Time of collection is not known.
- Improper, non-sterile, leaky container is used for collection of specimen.
- Culture swabs which are dry.
- Contaminated, haemolysed or lipaemic specimen of blood has been sent.

- Specimen is not appropriate for requested diagnostic test.

Note: Once the specimen is rejected, it should immediately be communicated to concerned clinician for further action.

VI. COLLECTION OF INDIVIDUAL SPECIMENS

A. Blood Specimen

Blood specimen is collected for diagnosis of following suspected diseases.

- Fever of unknown origin (FUO)
- Infective endocarditis
- Bacteraemia
- Septicaemia
- For detection of antigen and antibody against various disease causing organisms.

1. Types of Blood Specimens

- Whole blood
- Plasma
- Serum: It is plasma without clotting factor.

Whole blood is collected for blood culture or for preparation of peripheral blood smear for identification of parasites. **Serum** is used for antigen and antibody detection for diagnosis of certain diseases. **Plasma** may also be used for detection of antibody in certain conditions.

2. Blood Collection for Culture

(i) Time of collection

- Before start of antibiotics
- During febrile period (mostly at spikes of fever)
- In case patient is already on antibiotics, collect the specimen immediately before the next dose of antibiotic is due.

(ii) Volume of blood to be collected

For infants: 0.5–2 mL
For children: 2–5 mL
For adults: 5–10 mL

(iii) Site from where blood to be collected

Peripheral (cubital vein)
Central line (e.g. Internal juglar vein)

3. Technique of Blood Collection

(i) Vene puncture

Steps

1. Wash hands with soap and water.
2. Wear sterile/sterile desposable gloves.
3. Palpate the vein, clean the site for venepuncture with 70% alcohol for at least 30 seconds. After that clean the site with iodine (tincture iodine) in concentric circles away from puncture site covering an area of 6 cm in diameter.
4. Collect required amount of blood by venepuncture with a sterile needle and syringe.
5. Transfer the blood into blood culture bottle without opening the cap. Blood is transferred into blood culture bottles by inserting the needle of syringe through cap of the bottle which is having hole in it.
6. Shake the blood culture bottles gently to prevent clotting.

Transport

- If delay in transport is inevitable then incubate blood culture specimens at 37°C.

(ii) Blood for serological tests

1. 5 mL of blood is collected by venepuncture.
2. Remove the needle before transferring the blood into a sterile plain vial or test tube.
3. Let the blood clot for 30 minutes at room temperature. Do not shake the container.
4. The container can also be placed in a refrigerator at 4°C for 1–2 hours for clot formation or centrifuge it at 2200-2500 rpm for 15 minutes.
5. Separate serum from clot by a pipette in another container.
6. Serum can be stored at 2°–4°C in a refrigerator for 10 days. Store it at –20°C/–70°C in deep freezer if storage is required for a long duration.

(iii) Preparation of peripheral blood smear

(a) Thin Blood Smear

- The pulp of a finger or lobe of an ear is wiped with spirit and allowed to dry.
- It is pricked with a sterile cutting needle under all aseptic conditions.
- A drop of blood, about the size of pin head, is taken on a grease-free clean glass slide at one end.
- The drop of blood is then touched with the edge of another slide.
- It is held at an angle of 30 degrees and pushed gently to other end, till the blood is exhausted. The smear is formed with 'tails'.
- It is allowed to dry.
- The thin smear should ideally be one cell thick.

(b) Thick Blood Smear

- A thick blood smear may be prepared by taking 4 small drops of blood and joining the corners of the drops with a needle.

- It may also be prepared by taking a thick drop of blood on a slide and spreading with a needle or with the corner of another slide to form a thick smear in about 1 cm square area.
- The smear is allowed to air-dry.
- The thickness of the smear should be such as to allow a newsprint to be read through the preparation.
- Thick blood smear is many cells thick as compared to thin blood smear which is one cell thick.

Peripheral blood smear is generally prepared for diagnosis of parasitic infections such as malaria, filariasis.

B. Respiratory Tract Specimens

Specimens may be collected for upper respiratory tract infections and lower respiratory tract infections.

1. Collection of Upper Respiratory Tract Specimens

(i) Throat swab

- Ask the patient to open mouth wide.
- Hold the tongue down with the help of tongue depressor.
- The sterile swab is guided towards posterior pharynx under proper light and without touching the mouth parts.
- Swab is first rubbed firmly over both the tonsils and then rolled over the posterior pharynx.
- Take out the swab without touching mouth parts.
- If diphtheria is suspected, then collect the specimen from pseudomembrane also.
- Two swabs are collected, one for microscopy and other for culture.
- After collection, the swab is placed immediately into a sterile test tube/container for transport.
- If delay is suspected then refrigerate the specimen.

(ii) Nasopharyngeal swab

- Tilt the patient's head backwards.
- Insert a flexible fine nasopharyngeal swab into one of the nares under proper light.
- Guide the swab backwards and upwards along the nasal septum until it reaches the posterior pharynx.
- Leave the swab in place for few seconds and then gently remove.

(iii) Specimen collection in COVID-19

Specimens to be collected are as follows:

- Oropharyngeal swab
- Nasopharyngeal swab
- Nasal swab

  Specimens for viruses (Influenza, H1N1, SARS-CoV-2 etc.) should be transported in viral transport media (VTM) and immediately placed on ice or cold packs. Specimens can be kept at 2-8°C for no longer than 72 hours. If delay is expected in testing then store the specimen at –70°C or below.

2. Collection of Lower Respiratory Tract Specimens

(i) Sputum

- Ask the patient to rinse the mouth with water.
- Instruct patient to take a deep breath.
- Ask the patient to cough up sputum directly into a wide mouth sterile container.
- In case of delay, refrigerate the specimen.

(ii) Induced sputum

The patient is asked to inhale nebulised hypertonic solution which liquefies airways secretion and promotes coughing.

C. Cerebrospinal Fluid (CSF)

- CSF is obtained from the patient by lumber puncture technique under all aseptic precautions.
- 3–5 mL of specimen is collected in a labelled sterile container by a trained physician.
- CSF should be processed as early as possible after collection but in case of delay the specimen should not be refrigerated but kept at room temperature as refrigeration tends to kill *Haemophilus influenzae*.

D. Pus Specimen

Pus or exudate may be collected from wound. Frank pus or exudate is better than pus swab. Pus/exudate, can be collected by following methods:

- Frank pus/exudate collection in a sterile container from abscess.
- Swabbing of pus/exudate.

  Wound swabbing is the most widely used method.

Collection of Specimen

(i) Pus

- Oozing pus should be directly collected in a sterile test tube/container.

(ii) Swab

- Pus swab should be collected by rotating the tip of swab over 1 cm area of open wound for 5 seconds.

(iii) Specimens if anaerobic organisms suspected

- Pus specimens from deeper area of wound should be collected and placed in **cooked meat broth (CMB)**. Specimens from area in contact with air should not be collected. Swabs are generally not preferred.
- Transport the specimen to laboratory within 30 minutes.

E. Urine Specimen

- The normal urinary tract is devoid of bacteria except for the urethral mucosa which may contain indigenous microbial flora.
- Urine contamination may occur from microflora of urethra, perineum or vaginal canal.

Collection of Urine

(i) Midstream Clean Catch Urine Specimen

- Collection of urine is done by '*clean catch technique*'.
- It is collected preferably prior to administration of antibiotics.
- Specimen is collected in a sterile container.
- Before collecting a sample, genitalia should be cleaned with soap and water and men are instructed to retract the foreskin of glans penis whereas women should keep the labia apart.
- The first portion of urine is allowed to pass, then without interrupting the urine flow, mid-portion of the stream is collected.
- The first portion of urine adequately flushes out the normal urethral flora.

(ii) Urine Collection from Catheter

- A sampling port can be found on the tubing of the catheter drainage bag. Urine should only be collected from this point.
- Clamp the catheter below the port and collect the urine above it.
- Clean the sampling port with an alcohol impregnated swab to reduce the risk of contamination of the specimen.
- Insert the syringe tip into the sampling port and collect the urine.
- Place the specimen in a sterile container and transport to laboratory.

Transport

- Urine specimen should be immediately transported as urine is a good culture medium and bacteria can multiply in it, which may give false results.
- If there is delay of >2 hours in transport then specimen should be refrigerated.
- Preservatives can be used if specimen is not refrigerated. Boric acid (1.8%) is the most commonly used preservative.

F. Stool/Rectal Swab Specimen

1. Stool

- Faecal specimen is collected in a clean, screw capped, wide mouthed container.
- Ask the patient to pass faeces directly into the container.
- Screw the cap on the container and place in a sealed plastic bag.
- Transport the specimen to laboratory as early as possible.
- Stool specimen is preferred over rectal swab.
- Rectal swabs are used for debilitated patients and children.

2. Rectal Swab

- Moisten a cotton swab with sterile saline.
- Insert the swab inside anal sphincter and go 2 to 4 cm inside rectum.
- Gently rotate the swab 90 degree.
- Take out the swab and keep it in transport medium.
- Transport the swab in transport medium to the laboratory.
- The commonly used transport media include Cary-Blair transport medium and alkaline peptone water (APW).

KEY POINTS

1. Proper diagnosis of infectious diseases in microbiology depends upon the correct procedure of collection of specimen and the proper transport of specimens.
2. Rejection criteria for specimen should be known before processing of the specimen.

STUDY QUESTIONS

1. Describe the methods of blood collection for performing blood culture.
2. Describe the method of collection of CSF in case of meningitis.
3. Describe briefly the collection of throat swab in patients suffering from sore throat.
4. Describe the different methods of urine collection in a case of urinary tract infection.

Prophylactic Immunisation

64

Immunisation against infectious diseases has been an important contribution of microbiology to medicine. Aim of immunisation is to produce a degree of resistance sufficient to prevent a clinical attack of the natural infection. It may be active or passive immunisation.

I. ACTIVE IMMUNISATION

Active immunisation is done by use of vaccines. It works through two key elements of adaptive immunity i.e. specificity and memory.

Specificity: Vaccine induces production of specific antibody.

Memory: Due to presence of memory cells, the secondary response is prompt, powerful and prolonged with production of higher level of antibodies than that in primary response.

Vaccines may be ***live attenuated, killed*** or in the form of ***toxoids*** (Table 64.1).

A new type of vaccine, ***subunit vaccine***, prepared by purifying the fragments of major immunogenic components of microorganisms has also been developed. Another new type of vaccine is **recombinant vaccine**.

Table 64.1: Vaccines and Toxoids

Live attenuated vaccines	Killed vaccines	Toxoids
• BCG vaccine • OPV • Measles vaccine • Mumps vaccine • Rubella vaccine • Oral typhoid fever vaccine • Varicella vaccine • Yellow fever vaccine	• Pertussis vaccine • Typhoid fever vaccine • Cholera vaccine • Rabies vaccine • Japanese encephalitis vaccine • Killed polio vaccine • Influenza vaccine • Hepatitis B vaccine • Plague vaccine • Pneumococcal vaccine • Meningococcal vaccine	• Diphtheria toxoid • Tetanus toxoid

A. Live Attenuated Vaccines

A single dose of live vaccine is sufficient for immunisation. The ***attenuated organism*** can multiply in the body to provide a continuous antigenic stimulus and thus serves both as primary and booster dose. The attenuated organisms are the suspensions of living organisms with reduced virulence. These mimic natural infection with antibody production but without symptoms. Examples of some live vaccines are: oral polio vaccine (OPV); mumps, measles and rubella (MMR) and yellow fever.

Sometimes related organisms with shared antigens are used for preparation of live vaccine e.g. a bovine tubercle bacillus for BCG vaccine and vaccinia virus for small pox vaccine.

Live vaccines should not be administered in immunocompromised hosts (leukaemia, malignancy, AIDS etc.) in whom there is an increased incidence of severe complications.

B. Killed (inactivated) Vaccines

These vaccines possess antigens common to the original pathogen but do not replicate. With killed vaccine, usually three doses of vaccines are required to have effective immune response. Booster doses are necessary. Killed vaccines include typhoid, cholera, rabies, hepatitis B, influenza, pertussis and pneumococcal vaccines.

C. Toxoids

Toxoids are modified toxins which have lost toxigenicity but retained the antigenicity. These are usually prepared by treating the toxins with formalin (formol toxoids). Toxoids are used for prophylaxis against those infections in which pathogenesis is attributable to a toxin.

Antigenicity of toxoids is enhanced by adsorption on to a mineral carrier such as aluminium hydroxide or aluminium phosphate. Such adsorbed toxoids remain longer in a depot after injection and serves as a better antigen. In DPT (diphtheria, pertussis, tetanus) vaccine, tetanus toxoid and diphtheria toxoid are mixed with a pertussis vaccine. Pertussis vaccine acts as an **adjuvant**. Tetanus toxoid (TT) and diphtheria toxoid (DT) are two widely used toxoids for immunisation.

D. Special Types of Vaccines

For certain viruses such as hepatitis B virus, only a particular subunit of the virus (hepatitis B surface antigen, HBsAg) is required to initiate the immunity.

Hepatitis B vaccine is produced by inserting the gene coding for surface antigen (HBsAg) into Baker's yeast by recombinant DNA technology.

E. Immunisation Schedule

The national immunisation schedule is shown in Table 64.2.

II. PASSIVE IMMUNISATION

Passive immunisation is used when it is considered necessary to give immediate protection to an anticipated infection. Immunity produced is short-lasting. Human sera and animal sera are used for passive immunisation.

Table 64.2: National Immunisation Schedule

Age	Vaccine	Dose	Route of administration	Site
Infants At birth	BCG (At birth or as early as possible till one year of age)	0.05 mL (0.1 mL for more than one month of age)	Intradermal	Left upper arm
	OPV-zero dose (At birth or as early as possible within first 15 days)	Two drops	Oral	Oral
	Hepatitis B vaccine (At birth or as early as possible within 24 hours)	0.5 mL	Intramuscular	Anteriolateral side of mid thigh
6 weeks	Pentavalent-1•	0.5 mL	Intramuscular	–Do–
	OPV-1•	Two drops	Oral	Oral
	f IPV	0.1 mL (Fractional dose)	Intradermal	Right upper arm
	Rotavirus vaccine••	5 drops	Oral	Oral
	PCV•••	0.5 mL	Intramuscular	Anteriolateral side of mid thigh
10 Weeks	Pentavalent-2•	0.5 mL	Intramuscular	Anteriolateral side of mid thigh
	OPV-2*	Two drops	Oral	Oral
	Rotavirus vaccine••	5 drops	Oral	Oral
14 weeks	Pentavalent-3•	0.5 mL	Intramuscular	Anteriolateral side of mid thigh
	OPV-3*	Two drops	Oral	Oral
	f IPV	0.1 mL (Fractional dose)	Intradermal	Right upper arm
	Rotavirus vaccine••	5 drops	Oral	Oral
	PCV•••	0.5 mL	Intramuscular	Anteriolateral side of mid thigh
9-12 months	MR vaccine (1st dose) (Can be given till 5 years of age)	0.5 mL	Subcutaneous	Right upper arm
	JE-1••••	0.5 mL	Subcutaneous	Left upper arm
	PCV Booster	0.5 mL	Intramuscular	Anteriolateral side of mid thigh
	Vitamin A (1st dose) at 9 months	1 mL (One lakh IU)	Oral	Oral
16 to 24 months	DPT** Booster-1	0.5 mL	Intramuscular	Anteriolateral side of mid thigh
	OPV*** Booster	Two drops	Oral	Oral
	MR••••• (2nd dose)	0.5 mL	Subcutaneous	Right upper arm
	JE-2••••	0.5 mL	Subcutaneous	Left upper arm
	Vitamin A•••••• (2nd to 9th dose)	2 mL (Two lakh IU)	Oral	Oral
5-6 years	DPT** Booster-2	0.5 mL	Intramuscular	Upper arm
10 years	Td	0.5 mL	Intramuscular	Upper arm
16 years	Td	0.5 mL	Intramuscular	Upper arm
For pregnant women As early as possible during pregnancy (first contact)	Td•••••••	0.5 mL	Intramuscular	Upper arm

Antibiotic Resistance and Antimicrobial Sensitivity Testing

65

Pathogenic bacteria exhibit great strain variations in susceptibility to antibiotics. It is, therefore, essential to determine the susceptibility of isolates to antibiotics that are likely to be used in the treatment.

I. ANTIBIOTIC RESISTANCE

The emergence of antibiotic resistance is a major problem in antimicrobial therapy. At first, there is an emergence of a small number of resistant bacteria which soon multiply selectively in the presence of antibiotic at the cost of sensitive bacteria. The resistance may be of two types as follows:

1. Chromosomal Resistance

This occurs as a result of spontaneous mutation. In clinical practice, mutational resistance is of great importance in tuberculosis. The antimicrobial drugs selectively suppress susceptible organisms but resistant mutants will multiply unchecked. If two or more antituberculous drugs are used for treatment, resistant mutant does not occur, as a mutant resistant to one drug will be destroyed by the other drug. This is the rationale behind multiple drug therapy used in tuberculosis.

2. Extrachromosomal Resistance

This occurs by transfer of plasmids and genetic material. Transferable drug resistance mediated by the R factor is the most important. R factors are plasmids that contain genes that code for drug resistance against one and often several antimicrobial drugs. Inactivation of drugs occur by plasmid coded enzymes e.g. β-lactamases destroy the β-lactam ring which is responsible for the antibacterial action of β-lactam antibiotics (penicillins and cephalosporins). The plasmid mediated drug resistance can be transmitted from one bacterium to another either by transduction or conjugation.

(a) Transduction

Acquisition of resistance by transduction is common in staphylococci. Plasmid (carrying gene for β-lactamase production) enclosed in a bacteriophage is transferred from a penicillin-resistant staphylococcus to a susceptible staphylococcus.

(b) Conjugation

R factors carrying genes for drug resistance are transferred by conjugation. This is the most common method of spread of multiple drug resistance among different genera of Gram negative bacteria.

II. MULTIDRUG RESISTANT ORGANISMS (MDROs)

Definition

A multidrug resistant organism (MDRO) is an organism which is resistant to one or more classes of antimicrobial agents.

MDROs are difficult to treat since many antibiotics will not be effective against these organisms. Examples of MDROs include methicillin resistant *Staphylococcus aureus* (MRSA), vancomycin resistant enterococci (VRE), vancomyccin resistant *Staphylococcus aureus* (VRSA). MDROs can cause urinary tract infections (UTIs), pneumonia, blood infections, wound infections etc. Most MDRO infections spread by direct contact with an infected persons body fluids such as blood, sputum, urine, stool. They may also spread by contact with equipment or surfaces, which may have contaminated with these organisms. They often affect persons who are older or very ill.

To prevent MDROs infections, the following measures will be helpful.

1. Enhanced standard precautions
   - Hand hygiene
   - Respiratory hygiene and cough etiquette.
   - Personal protective equipment (PPE)
   - Safe injection practices
   - Care of environment
2. Use of contact precautions until patients become culture negative for MDRO.
3. Active surveillance cultures
4. Enhanced environmental cleaning
5. Education

MRSA

Staph. aureus which are tested in laboratory as oxacillin resistant, or positive by molecular testing for mecA genes and PBP_{2a}. MRSA are resistant to many antibiotics.

III. ANTIMICROBIAL SENSITIVITY TESTS

Antimicrobial sensitivity tests are of two types:

A. Diffusion tests
- Stokes disc diffusion method
- Kirby-Bauer disc diffusion method

B. Dilution tests
- Broth dilution method
- Agar dilution method

A. Diffusion Tests

The 'disc diffusion' method uses filter paper discs charged with appropriate concentration of the drugs. The test bacterium is inoculated on the medium and antibiotic discs are applied. Sensitivity to the drug is determined from the inhibition of bacterial growth around the disc.

Medium

Mueller-Hinton agar may be used for testing aerobes and facultative anaerobes. Nutrient agar is another alternative medium used.

Antibiotic Discs

Antibiotic discs may be prepared in the laboratory or purchased commercially. Filter paper discs of 6 mm in diameter are used.

1. Stokes Disc Diffusion Method

The test bacterium is inoculated on the central one third and control on upper and lower thirds of the plate. However, in modified Stokes disc diffusion method, the test bacterium is inoculated over the upper and lower thirds of the plate and control on central one third. Antibiotic discs are applied between the standard and test inocula (Fig. 65.1). The plates are then incubated at 37°C for 16-18 hours.

Reporting

The reporting of results is done by comparing the zones of inhibition of control and test bacterium. Measure the zone size i.e. the distance in mm from edge of the disc to the zone edge. It is interpreted as follows:

Sensitive

- The zone of test bacterium is equal to, or larger than that of control strain.
- If zone size of test bacterium is smaller than that of control, the difference between the two should not be more than 3 mm.

Intermediate sensitive

The zone size of the test bacterium should be at least 2 mm and the difference between the zone of test and control strain should be at least 3 mm.

Resistant

The zone size of the test bacterium is smaller than 2 mm.

2. Kirby-Bauer Disc Diffusion Method

Inoculate the Mueller-Hinton agar plate by streaking the swab over the entire agar surface. Allow 3-5 minutes for surface of agar to dry before applying the antibiotic discs. The plates are then incubated at 37°C for 16-18 hours. The zones of complete growth inhibition around each of the discs are measured (Fig. 65.2). The interpretation of zone size into sensitive, intermediate or resistant is based on interpretation chart. Control strains should be tested each time when a new batch of discs or agar is used.

3. Epsilometer or E-Test

Epsilometer or E-test is antimicrobial sensitivity test to detect minimum inhibitory concentration (MIC) of antibiotic (Fig. 65.3). It is a recent modification of the agar diffusion sensitivity test. It uses an absorbent strip with a known gradient of antibiotic concentration along its length. When the strip is placed on the agar plate inoculated with the test organism, the antibiotic diffuses into the medium. The minimum inhibitory concentration (MIC) is recorded as the lowest concentration of the gradient which inhibits the growth of the organism.

B. Dilution Tests

1. Broth Dilution Method

Serial dilutions of the drug in Mueller-Hinton broth are

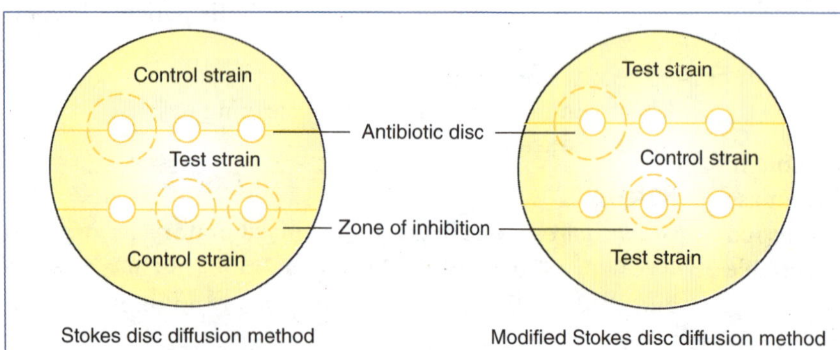

Fig. 65.1 Stokes disc diffusion method and modified Stokes disc diffusion method

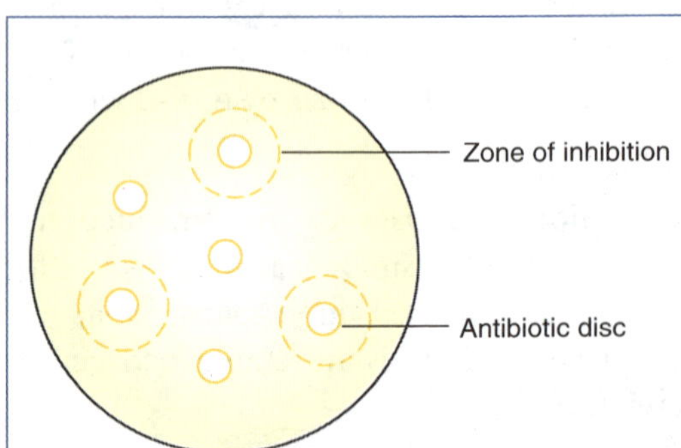

Fig. 65.2 Kirby-Bauer disc diffusion method

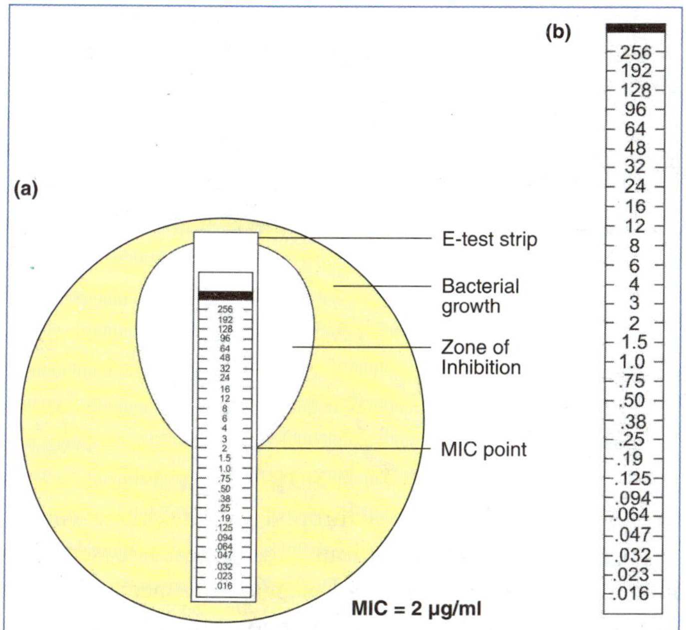

Fig. 65.3 (a) Epsilometer or E-test on the agar plate (b) Details of E-test strip

taken in tubes and a standardised suspension of the test bacterium inoculated. An organism of known sensitivity should also be titrated. Incubate at 37°C for 16-18 hours. The minimum inhibitory concentration (MIC) is read by noting the lowest concentration of the drug at which there is no visible growth. The minimum bactericidal concentration (MBC) is determined by subculturing from each tube showing no growth on to a nutrient agar plate without any antimicrobial agent. Incubate the plates and examine them for growth, if any. The tube containing the lowest concentration of the drug that fails to show growth, on subculture, is the MBC of the drug for that test strain. MIC inhibits the bacterial growth while MBC kills the bacterium.

2. Agar Dilution Method

Serial dilutions of the drug are prepared in agar and poured into plates. Many strains can be inoculated on each plate containing an antibiotic dilution. This method is more convenient when several strains are to be tested at the same time.

KEY POINTS

1. Antimicrobial sensitivity tests are of two types: *diffusion tests* and *dilution tests*.
2. *Stokes* disc diffusion method and *Kirby-Bauer* disc diffusion method are examples of diffusion tests.
3. *Epsilometer* or *E-test* is a modification of the agar diffusion sensitivity test. It uses an absorbent strip with a known gradient of antibiotic concentration along its length.
4. The *minimum inhibitory concentration* (*MIC*) *inhibits* the bacterial growth while the *minimum bactericidal concentration* (*MBC*) *kills* the bacterium.

STUDY QUESTION

1. Write short notes on:
   (i) Antibiotic resistance (ii) Strokes disc diffusion method (iii) Kirby-Bauer disc diffusion method.

MULTIPLE CHOICE QUESTIONS (MCQs)

1. How does *Staphylococcus aureus* acquire drug resistance?
   (a) Transformation
   (b) Transduction
   (c) Mutation
   (d) Conjugation
2. Which medium is the most ideal for antibiotic sensitivity testing of bacterial isolates?
   (a) Mueller-Hinton agar
   (b) Nutrient agar
   (c) Blood agar
   (d) MacConkey agar
3. In Stokes disc diffusion method, if the size of zone of inhibition of test bacterium is equal to, larger than or not more than 3 mm smaller than the control strain zone, bacterial strain is considered as:
   (a) Sensitive
   (b) Intermediate sensitive
   (c) Resistant
   (d) None of the above
4. In Stokes disc diffusion method, if the zone size of inhibition of test bacterium is smaller than 2 mm, bacterial strain is considered as:
   (a) Sensitive
   (b) Intermediate sensitive
   (c) Resistant
   (d) None of the above
5. In which method, an absorbent strip with a known gradient of antibiotic concentration along its length is used for antibiotic sensitivity testing?
   (a) Kirby-Bauer disc diffusion method
   (b) Epsilometer test
   (c) Primary disc diffusion test
   (d) Agar dilution method

ANSWERS (MCQs)

1. (b) 2. (a) 3. (a) 4. (c) 5. (b)

66 Vehicles and Vectors

Infectious agent may be transmitted from the reservoir or source of infection to a susceptible individual in many different ways. Vehicles and vectors are two important ways of transporting an infectious agent to a susceptible individual.

I. VEHICLES

Various vehicles for transmission of the infectious agent include:

- water
- food (including raw vegetables, fruits, milk and milk products)
- ice
- blood
- serum
- plasma
- Other biological products e.g. tissues and organs.

Water and food are the most frequent vehicles of transmission, because they are used by everyone.

A. Diseases Transmitted by Water and Food

Acute diarrhoeas
Cholera
Typhoid fever
Poliomyelitis
Hepatitis A virus infection
Food poisoning
Intestinal parasitic infestations

B. Diseases Transmitted by Blood

Diseases caused by the following infectious agents may be transmitted by blood.

1. Viruses

Hepatitis B and other hepatitis viruses
Human immunodeficiency viruses
Human T cell lymphotropic viruses
Cytomegaloviruses

2. Bacteria

Treponema pallidum

3. Parasites

Plasmodia
Trypanosoma cruzi

II. VECTORS

Vector is defined as an arthropod or any living carrier that transports an infectious agent to a susceptible individual. Vector transmission may be mechanical or biological. In biological transmission, the disease agent has a developmental cycle or multiplication in the vector.

A. Mechanical Transmission

The infectious agent is only mechanically transported and there is no development or multiplication of the agent on or within the vector.

B. Biological Transmission

The infectious agent undergoes replication or development or both in vector and requires an incubation period before its transmission. Biological transmission is of three types:

Propagative

The agent only multiplies in the vector, but there is no change in its form e.g. plague bacilli in rat fleas.

Cyclopropagative

The agent changes its form and number e.g. malarial parasites in mosquito.

Cyclodevelopment

The agent undergoes only development but no multiplication, e.g. microfilaria in mosquito.

Vertical transmission of the infectious agent from the infected female to her progeny in the vector is known as *transovarial transmission*.

MEDICAL ENTOMOLOGY

A study of the arthropods of medical importance is known as medical entomology. Arthropods act as vectors or carriers of diseases (Table 66.1).

Table 66.1: Diseases Transmitted by Arthropods as Vectors	
Mosquito	Malaria, filaria, Japanese encephalitis, dengue, West-Nile, yellow fever, dengue haemorrhagic fever
Sandfly	Kala-azar, oriental sore, sandfly fever, oroya fever, Chandipura
Rat flea	Bubonic plague, endemic typhus, chiggerosis, *Hymenolepis diminuta*
Hard tick	Tick typhus, Kyasanur forest disease (KFD), tularaemia, human babesiosis
Soft tick	Q fever, endemic relapsing fever
Trombiculid mite	Scrub typhus, Rickettsial-pox
Cyclops	Guinea-worm disease, fish tapeworm
Louse	Epidemic typhus, epidemic relapsing fever, trench fever
Reduviid bug	Chagas disease
Tsetse fly	Sleeping sickness
House fly	Typhoid and paratyphoid fevers, diarrhoea, cholera, dysentery, gastroenteritis.

KEY POINTS

1. *Vehicles* and *vectors* are two important ways of transporting an infectious agent to a susceptible individual.
2. *Water*, *food*, *blood*, *sera* and other biological products are various vehicles for transmission of the infectious agent.
3. *Acute diarrhoeas*, *cholera*, *typhoid fever* are the diseases transmitted by water and food.
4. Hepatitis B, human immunodeficiency viruses are the viruses transmitted by *blood* and *blood products*.
5. *Vector* is defined as an *arthropod* or *any living carrier* that transports an infectious agent to a susceptible individual.
6. Malaria, filaria, dengue, kala-azar are some diseases transmitted by arthropods as vectors.
7. A study of the arthropods of medical importance is known as *medical entomology*.

STUDY QUESTIONS

1. Discuss the role of vehicles and vectors in transmission of infectious agents.
2. Write short notes on:
   (i) Water-borne diseases
   (ii) Diseases transmitted by blood and blood products
   (iii) Diseases transmitted by arthropods as vectors

Unit IX

MICROBIOLOGY AT A GLANCE

Essentials of Microbiology at Glance

67

I. SYSTEMIC BACTERIOLOGY

Disease producing bacteria may be gram positive or Gram negative. These may be cocci or bacilli. Some bacteria are acid-fast on Ziehl-Neelsen staining. Characteristic features of different bacteria are shown in Table 67.1.

1. **Gram positive cocci**
   (i) *Staphylococcus* (present in clusters)
   (ii) *Streptococcus* (present in chains)
   (iii) Pneumococcus (present in pairs)
2. **Gram negative cocci**
   (i) *Neisseria* (present in pairs)
3. **Gram positive bacilli**
   (i) *Corynebacteria* (can be stained with Albert's staining)
   (ii) *Clostridium* (Anaerobic)
4. **Gram negative bacilli**
   (i) Members of Enterobacteriaceae (oxidase negative)
   (ii) *Vibrio* (curved bacilli and oxidase positive)
   (iii) *Pseudomonas* (oxidase positive)
5. **Acid-fast bacilli**
   (i) *Mycobacteria*
6. **Helical bacteria**
   (i) *Spirochaetes*

Table 67.1: Characteristics of Different Bacteria

S. No.	Group	General features	Bacteria	Morphology	Culture	Diseases	Diagnosis
1.	Staphylococcus	• Gram positive cocci • Non-motile • Arranged in grape-like clusters	*Staphylococcus aureus*	• Gram positive cocci • Non-motile • 1μm in diameter • Arranged in grape like clusters	On blood agar, colonies are 2-4 mm (pin head size) in diameter, circular, smooth, convex, opaque, with beta haemolysis.	• Boils • Carbuncles • Abscesses • Wound infections • Osteomyelitis • Food poisoning • Nosocomial infections	• Direct microscopy to demonstrate Gram positive cocci • Isolation of bacteria by culture on blood agar
2.	Streptococcus	• Gram positive cocci • Non-motile • Arranged in chains	*Streptococcus pyogenes*	• Gram positive cocci • Non-motile • 0.5μm in diameter • Arranged in chains	On blood agar, colonies are small (0.5-1.0 mm, pinpoint), circular, semitransparent, low convex with a wide zone of beta haemolysis around them.	• Sore throat (acute tonsillitis and/or pharyngitis) • Impetigo • Cellulitis • Scarlet fever • Acute rheumatic fever • Acute glomerulonephritis	• Smear examination of specimen to demonstrate Gram positive cocci in chains • Isolation of bacteria by culture on blood agar • Anti streptolysin 'O' (ASO) test for diagnosis of acute rheumatic fever
3.	Pneumococcus	• Gram positive cocci • Non-motile • Arranged in pairs	*Strcptococcus pneumoniae*	• Gram positive cocci • Non-motile • 1μm in diameter • Arranged in pairs	On blood agar, colonies are small (0.5-1 mm), dome shaped, with alpha haemolysis.	• Pneumonia • Meningitis	• Gram staining of smear reveals Gram positive diplococci • Isolation of bacteria by culture on blood agar

Contd.

Table 67.1 (Contd.)

Table 67.1: Characteristics of Different Bacteria

S. No.	Group	General features	Bacteria	Morphology	Culture	Diseases	Diagnosis
4.	Neisseria	• Gram negative cocci • Non-motile • Arranged in pairs • Oxidase positive	*Neisseria meningitidis*	• Gram negative cocci • Non-motile • 0.6μm-0.8μm in diameter • Arranged in pairs (diplococci) with adjacent sides flattened	On blood agar/ chocolate agar, colonies are small (1 mm in diameter), round, convex, translucent	• Meningitis • Meningococcal septicaemia	• Gram staining of CSF smear shows Gram negative diplococci present mainly inside polymorphs (intracellular) • Antigen detection in CSF • Isolation of bacteria by culture on blood agar on chocolate agar
			Neisseria gonorrhoeae	• Gram negative cocci • Non-motile • Arranged in pairs (diplococci) with adjacent sides concave (pear or bean shaped)	On chocolate agar, colonies are small, round, grey, translucent, convex	• Gonorrhoea • Ophthalmia neonatorum	• Gram staining of urethral discharge shows Gram negative intracellular diplococci • Isolation of bacteria by culture on chocolate agar
5.	Corynebacteria	• Gram positive bacilli • Non-motile	*Corynebacterium diphtheriae*	• Gram positive bacilli • The bacilli look green and metachromatic granules appear bluish black when Albert stain is used. • Arranged in chinese letter pattern • 3-6 μm × 0.6-0.8 μm	On Tellurite blood agar, colonies are grey or black in colour	• Diphtheria	• Direct microscopy for demonstration of bacilli • Isolation of bacteria by culture on tellurite blood agar
6.	Clostridium	• Gram positive bacilli • Spore forming • Anaerobic	*Clostridium perfringens*	• Gram positive bacilli with subterminal spore • 4-6μm × 1μm • Non-motile • Capsulated	• It can be grown in Robertson cooked meat broth (RCM) and blood agar	• Gas gangrene	• Direct microscopy to demonstrate Gram positive bacilli • Isolation of bacteria by culture on RCM and blood agar
			Clostridium tetani	• Gram positive bacilli with spherical, terminal spores (*drumstick* appearance) • 4-8μm × 0.5μm • Non-capsulated	• It can be grown in Robertson cooked meat broth (RCM) and blood agar	• Tetanus	• Direct microscopy may show Gram positive bacilli with drumstick appearance • Isolation of bacteria by culture on RCM and blood agar
7.	Enterobacteriaceae	• Gram negative bacilli • Non-motile or motile • Oxidase negative • Non capsulated • Non sporing	*Escherichia coli*	• Gram negative bacilli • Motile • 1-3μm × 0.4-0.7μm	• Can grow on blood agar • On MacConkey's agar, colonies are circular, non-mucoid, pink due to lactose fermentation (Lactose fermenter colonies–LF)	• Urinary tract infection (UTI) • Diarrhoea • Septicaemia	• Isolation of bacteria by culture

Contd.

Table 67.1 (Contd.)

Table 67.1: Characteristics of Different Bacteria

S. No.	Group	General features	Bacteria	Morphology	Culture	Diseases	Diagnosis
			Shigella sp.	• Gram negative bacilli • Non-Motile • 1-3μm × 0.5μm	• Can grow on ordinary media • On MacConkey's agar, colonies are circular, convex, colourless (non-lactose fermenting-NLF)	• Bacillary dysentery	• Isolation of bacteria by culture
			Salmonella sp.	• Gram negative bacilli • Motile • 1-3μm × 0.5μm	• Can grow on ordinary media. • On MacConkey's agar, colonies are circular, colourless due to non-lactose fermentation-NLF).	• Enteric fever • Gastroenteritis • Septicaemia	• Isolation of bacteria by culture • Demonstration of antibody in serum
8.	Vibrio	• Gram negative • Curved or comma shaped bacilli • Motile • Oxidase positive	*Vibrio cholerae*	• Gram negative • Curved or comma shaped bacilli • 1.5 μm × 0.2-0.4 μm • Actively motile (darting motility)	• Selective media such as bile salt agar (BSA) is used for isolation of *V. cholerae* from faeces.	• Cholera	• Isolation of bacteria from faeces by culture on selective media
9.	Pseudomonas	• Gram negative bacilli • Motile • Oxidase positive	*Pseudomonas aeruginosa*	• Gram negative bacilli • Motile • 1.5-3 μm × 0.5 μm	• Can grow on ordinary media ie. nutrient agar. • On MacConkey's agar, colonies are pale or colourless (non-lactose fermenters, NLF).	• Nosocomial infections • Urinary tract infection • Wound and burns infections	• Isolation of bacteria by culture
10.	Haemophilus	• Gram negative bacilli • Non-motile • Non-sporing	*Haemophilus influenzae*	• Gram negative bacilli • 1.5 μm × 0.3 μm • Non-motile • Non-sporing • Plemorphic	• On blood agar or chocolate agar, small opaque colonies appear	• Meningitis • Acute epiglottitis • Pneumonia • Bronchitis	• Direct microscopy to demonstrate Gram negative coccobacilli • Antigen detection in specimen by latex agglutination, coagglutination or CIEP • Isolation of bacteria by culture
11.	Mycobacteria	• Slender bacilli • Acid fast bacilli (AFB) • Non-motile • Non-capsulated • Non-sporing	*Mycobacterium tuberculosis*	On Ziehl-Neelsen (ZN) staining • These are seen as slender straight or slightly curved bacilli. • Acid-fast • Non-motile • 3 μm × 0.3 μm	• The bacilli grow slowly (in weeks). • Lowenstein Jensen (LJ) medium is used for growing it. • Colonies on this medium are dry, rough, tough, buff coloured. It has a luxuriant growth (eugonic growth)	• Tuberculosis – Pulmonary – Extrapulmonary	• Direct microscopy of specimen to demonstrate AFB by ZN staining • Isolation of bacteria by culture on LJ medium

Contd.

Table 67.1 (Contd.)

Table 67.1: Characteristics of Different Bacteria

S. No.	Group	General features	Bacteria	Morphology	Culture	Diseases	Diagnosis
			Mycobacterium leprae	On ZN staining • Slender straight or slightly curved bacilli, arranged in clumps • Acid-fast but less so than *M.tuberculosis* • 1-8 μm × 0.2-0.5 μm	• *M. leprae* has not yet been grown on artificial culture media or tissue culture.	• Leprosy – Tuberculoid – Lepromatous	• Ziehl-Neelsen (ZN) staining of slit skin smears to demonstrate the bacilli. • Skin and nerve biopsy. • Lepromin test to differentiate tuberculoid leprosy and lepromatous leprosy.
12.	Spirochaetes	• Large helical bacteria • Motile	*Treponema pallidum*	• Thin, delicate spirochaete with tapering ends, having about ten spirals • 10 μm × 0.1-0.2 μm • Motile • Does not take ordinary bacterial stains. • Cannot be seen by light microscope. • It can be seen by dark ground microscopy.	• Cannot be grown in artificial culture media.	• Syphilis	• Demonstration of treponemes by dark ground microscopy. • Serological tests to demonstrate antibody in serum. • Venereal Disease Research Laboratory (VDRL) test is the commonly used serological test. • Other serological tests include Treponema pallidum haemagglutination assay (TPHA) and Fluorescent treponema antibody absorption (FTA-ABS) test.
13.	Chlamydia	• Small obligate intracellular parasite • Non-motile • Gram negative	*Chlamydia trachomatis*	• Exist in two forms, the elementary body (EB) and reticulate (Initial) body (RB)	Isolation by • Animal inoculation • Yolk sac inoculation • Tissue culture	• Trachoma • Inclusion conjunctivitis • Non-gonococcal urethritis • Lymphogranuloma venereum (LGV)	• Direct detection of antigens by light microscopy, immuno-fluorescence, ELISA • Isolation as under heading 'culture' • Serology for antibody detection by CFT, Microimmuno-fluorescence, ELISA

II. VIROLOGY

Viruses are the smallest obligate intracellular infective agents. They have no metabolic activity outside the living cells.

A. General Properties

1. Viruses contain only one type of nucleic acid (DNA or RNA) as their genome.
2. They lack the enzymes necessary for protein and nucleic acid synthesis.
3. They are dependent on synthetic machinery of host.
4. They multiply by a complex process and not by binary fission.
5. They do not grow in inanimate media.
6. They are unaffected by antibiotics.

B. Morphology of Viruses

1. Size

(i) The size of viruses range from 20 to 300 nm in diameter.

(ii) The largest virus is the smallpox virus (300 nm) and the smallest is the parvovirus (20 nm).

2. Shape

The overall shape of virus particles varies in different groups.

(i) Pox virus is brick shaped.

(ii) Rabies virus is bullet shaped.

3. Structure (Fig. 67.1)

(i) Virus consists of a nucleic acid core (DNA or RNA) surrounded by a protein coat called **capsid**.

(ii) The capsid is composed of protein subunits known as **capsomers**.

(iii) Certain viruses also contain envelope that surrounds the nucleic acid.

(iv) Protein subunits on the surface of the envelope, are called peplomers.

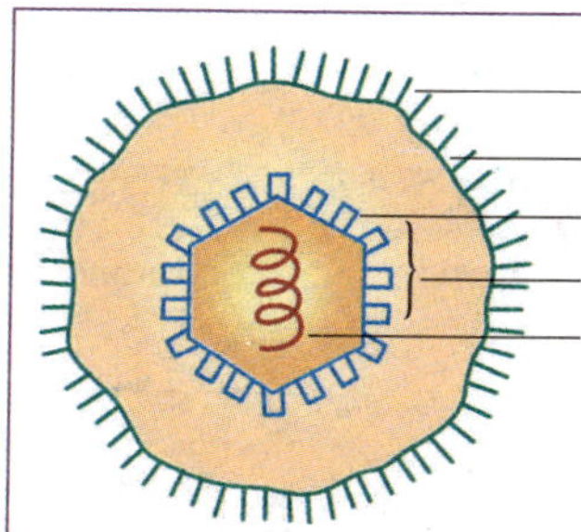

Fig. 67.1 Virus particle

C. Cultivation of Virus

As viruses multiply only in living cells, they cannot be grown on any of the inanimate culture medium. Three methods are employed for the cultivation of viruses:

1. **Animal inoculation:** Infant mice are used in the isolation of arboviruses.
2. **Embryonated egg inoculation:** Embryonated hen's eggs are inoculated with the specimen using syringe. The eggs are incubated and observed for the growth of organisms.
   Different routes of inoculation are used for different viruses.
3. **Cell Culture:** Cell culture is routinely employed for diagnostic virology. Tissues are dissociated into the component cells. These cells are washed and suspended in a growth medium. The cell suspension is distributed in glass or plastic bottles. These cell cultures are inoculated by the specimen. Growth of viruses is observed.

D. Classification of Viruses

Viruses are broadly classified into DNA and RNA viruses. Some of these viruses are given below:

1. DNA Viruses (Table 67.2)

(i) Poxvirus
(ii) Herpesvirus
(iii) Adenovirus
(iv) Papovavirus

2. RNA Viruses (Table 67.3)

(i) Orthomyxovirus
(ii) Paramyxovirus
(iii) Picornavirus
(iv) Rhabdovirus
(v) Togavirus
(vi) Flavivirus
(vii) Retrovirus
(viii) Coronavirus

Table 67.2: DNA Viruses

S. No.	Group	Morphology	Viruses	Disease	Route of infection	Diagnosis
1.	Poxviruses	• Brick shaped • Can be seen by light microscope • DNA genome	• Variola • Molluscum contagiosum	• Small pox • Benign wart	• Respiratory tract • Sexually transmitted	• Grows in chorioallantoic membrane (CAM) of chick embryo and tissue culture
2.	Herpesviruses	• Enveloped • Double stranded DNA genome • 100-200 nm in diameter	• Herpes simplex virus (HSV)	• Acute gingivostomatitis • Herpes labialis • Keratoconjunctivitis • Eczema herpeticum • Genital herpes • Neonatal herpes • Aseptic meningitis	• Respiratory tract • Skin lesions • Sexually transmitted • Birth canal	• Direct examination to observe inclusion bodies • Tissue culture • Polymerase chain reaction (PCR)

Contd.

Table 67.2 (Contd.)

Table 67.2: DNA Viruses						
S. No.	Group	Morphology	Viruses	Disease	Route of infection	Diagnosis
			• Varicella zoster	• Chickenpox	• Respiratory tract	• Direct examination to observe inclusion bodies • Tissue culture • Polymerase chain reaction (PCR)
			• Cytomegalovirus	• Congenital infection	• Sexually transmitted • Blood transfusion • Organ transplantation	• Cytomegalic cells demonstration • Tissue culture • Antigen detection • PCR • Serology
			• Epstein-Barr virus (EBV)	• Infectious mononucleosus • Burkitt's lymphoma • Nasopharyngeal carcinoma	• Oral contact (kissing)	• Atypical lymphocytes demonstration in blood • Paul-Bunnell test • Antigen detection • PCR
3.	Adenoviruses	• Non-enveloped • Double stranded DNA genome • 70-75 nm in diameter	• Adenovirus	• Respiratory infections • Eye infections • Urinary tract infections	• Through conjunctiva • Through nasal mucosa • Faeco-oral route	• Virus particles seen by electron microscope • Viral antigens demonstration by immunofluorescence • Tissue culture
4.	Hepatitis viruses		• Hepatitis B	Described under Hepatitis Viruses in Table 67.4		

Table 67.3: RNA Viruses						
S. No.	Group	Morphology	Viruses	Disease	Route of infection	Diagnosis
1.	Picornaviruses	• Non-enveloped • Single stranded RNA genome • 27-30 nm in diameter	• Poliovirus	• Poliomyelitis	• By Ingestion • By Respiratory secretions	• Direct demonstration of virus in faeces by electron microscopy • Tissue culture
			• Hepatitis A virus	Described under Table 67.4 Hepatitis viruses		
2.	Orthomyxoviruses	• Enveloped • Single stranded RNA genome • 80-120 nm in diameter	• Influenza virus	• Influenza	• Through respiratory tract	• Demonstration of viral antigens in nasopharyngeal secretions by immunofluorescence • Isolation of virus in chick embryo • Serology
3.	Rhabdoviruses	• Bullet shaped • Single stranded RNA genome • 75 × 180 nm	• Rabies virus	• Rabies	• By bite of rabid dog or other animals	• Demonstration of viral antigen in corneal smear by immunofluorescene • Demonstration of Negri bodies in brain • Isolation of virus by intracerebral inoculation in mice
4.	Arboviruses	• Enveloped • Single stranded RNA genome • 40-50 nm in diameter	• Dengue virus	• Dengue fever	• By bite of infected *Aedes aegypti* mosquito	• Demonstration of IgM antibody in serum by ELISA • Demonstration of NS1 antigen in serum
			• Hepatitis C virus	Described under Table 67.4 Hepatitis Viruses		

Contd.

Table 67.3 (Contd.)

Table 67.3: RNA Viruses

S. No.	Group	Morphology	Viruses	Disease	Route of infection	Diagnosis
		• Enveloped • Single stranded RNA genome • 50-70 nm in diameter	• Rubella virus	• Rubella (German measles) • Congenital rubella	• By inhalation • Through placenta	• Isolation of virus • Serology (ELISA for antibody detection)
5.	Reovirus	• Non-enveloped • Double stranded RNA genome (segmented) • 55-75 nm in diameter	• Rotavirus	• Diarrhoea in children	Faeco-oral	• Demonstration of virus in the faeces by ELISA • Detection of antibody in blood by ELISA.
6.	Retroviruses	• Enveloped • Single stranded RNA genome • 90-120 nm in diameter • Contains reverse transcriptase enzyme	• Human immunodeficiency virus (HIV)	• Acquired immunodeficiency syndrome (AIDS)	• Sexual contact • Blood transfusion • Needle stick injury • Mother to new born either transplacentally or perinatally • Faeco-oral	• Detection of antibody in serum by ELISA

Table 67.4: Hepatitis Viruses

Group	Morphology	Viruses	Disease	Route of infection	Diagnosis
Hepatitis viruses	• Non-enveloped • Single stranded RNA genome • 27 nm in diameter	• Hepatitis A Virus (HAV)	• Acute viral hepatitis	• Oro-faecal route	• Demonstration of HAV by ELISA • Antibody detection (IgM, IgG)
	• Double shelled • Double stranded DNA genome • 42 nm in diameter	• Hepatitis B Virus (HBV)	• Acute viral hepatitis • Chronic hepatitis	• Blood transfusion • Needle stick injury • Sexual contact • Mother to newborn during birth	• Detection of HBsAg in serum by ELISA
	• Enveloped • Single stranded RNA genome • 50-60 nm in diameter	• Hepatitis C Virus (HCV)	• Acute viral hepatitis	• Blood transfusion • Needle stick injury • Sexual contact • Mother to newborn during birth	• Detection of anti HCV antibody in serum by ELISA
	• Single stranded RNA virus • Only infective with the help of hepatitis B virus	• Hepatitis D Virus (HDV)	• Acute viral hepatitis • Simultaneous infection with both HDV and HBV (coinfection) is required	• Blood transfusion • Needle stick injury • Sexual contact • Mother to newborn during birth	• Detection of IgM anti-delta antibody in serum by ELISA
	• Non-enveloped • Single stranded RNA genome • 27-38 nm in diameter	• Hepatitis E Virus (HEV)	• Hepatitis similar to that of hepatitis A virus	• Faeco-oral route	• Detection of IgM and IgG antibody in serum by ELISA • PCR

III. MYCOLOGY

Fungi are eukaryotic organisms. They are obligate or facultative aerobe. They exist as saprophytes, parasites or commensals.

A. General Properties

1. Fungi possess rigid cell walls.
2. The cytoplasmic membrane contains sterols.
3. The cytoplasm contains true nuclei with nuclear membrane, mitochondria and endoplasmic reticulum.
4. Fungi may be unicellular or multicellular.
5. They divide asexually, sexually or by both processes.

Characteristic features of fungi under superficial mycoses, subcutaneous mycoses, systemic mycoses and opportunistic mycoses are shown in Tables 67.5 to 67.8.

B. Laboratory Diagnosis

Laboratory diagnosis of mycoses consists of following:

1. **Direct Microscopy**
   (i) **KOH preparation:** Specimen is placed in a drop of 10% KOH for detecting fungal elements. This preparation is examined under microscope. It is used in specimens such as skin, hair, nails and tissue.
   (ii) **Gram staining:** It is done to observe Gram positive yeasts as in case of Candida species.
   (iii) **India Ink Preparation:** India ink preparation may be used for detection of capsulated yeast.
2. **Culture**
   Culture is used for growing fungi. The culture media used for fungi include:
   (i) Sabouraud's dextrose agar (SDA)
   (ii) SDA with antibiotics
   (iii) Brain heart infusion agar (BHI)

Table 67.5: Superficial mycoses

S. No.	Disease	Name of the fungus	Clinical features	Specimens	Diagnosis
1.	Dermatophytosis Infections of skin, hair and nail.	• *Trichophyton sp.* • *Microsporum sp.* • *Epidermophyton sp.*	• Infection of skin hair and nail	• Skin, Hair, Nail	• KOH preparation shows. branched septate hyphae. • Spores surrounding the hair. • Culture on SDA.

Table 67.6: Subcutaneous Mycoses

S. No.	Disease	Name of the fungus	Clinical features	Specimens	Diagnosis
1.	Mycetoma	• A number of fungi are involved.	• Foot is the most commonly affected. • Multiple sinuses with deep abscesses are present.	• Pus	• Granules are examined for their characteristic appearance.
2.	Rhinosporidiosis	• *Rhinosporidium seebri*	• Friable polyps in the submucosa confined to nose, eye or mouth.	• Polyp biopsy	• Tissue section stained with H & E stain shows characteristic large number of endospores within the sporangia.

Table 67.7: Systemic Mycoses

S. No.	Disease	Name of the fungus	Clinical features	Specimens	Diagnosis
1.	Histoplasmosis	• *Histoplasma capsulatum*, a dimorphic fungus	• Asymptomatic (in most persons) • Pulmonary disease resembling tuberculosis • Disseminated disease • Lymphadenopathy, hepatosplenomegaly, fever, anaemia • Ulcerative lesions on skin or mucosa	• Lung biopsy • Skin scrapings	• Culture on Sabouraud's dextrose agar reveals hyphae at 25°C and yeasts at 37°C.
2.	Blastomycosis	• *Blastomyces dermatitidis*, a dimorphic fungus	• Asymptomatic • Mild pulmonary disease • Disseminated lesions • Cutaneous blastomycosis	• Sputum • Pus • Biopsy of affected tissue	• Culture on Sabouraud's dextrose agar reveals hyphae at 25°C and yeasts at 37°C.
3.	Paracoccidiodomycosis	• *Paracoccidioides brasiliensis*, a dimorphic fungus	• Primary pulmonary infection • May spread to mouth, nose, lymph nodes and adjacent skin.	• Sputum • Pus • Biopsy of affected tissue	• Culture on Sabouraud's dextrose agar reveals hyphae at 25°C and yeast at 37°C.

Contd.

Table 67.7 (Contd.)

Table 67.7: Systemic Mycoses					
S. No.	**Disease**	**Name of the fungus**	**Clinical features**	**Specimens**	**Diagnosis**
4.	Coccidioidomycosis	• *Coccidioides immitis*, a dimorphic fungus	• Asymptomatic • Primary pulmonary disease • Disseminated disease	• Sputum • Tissue biopsy	• Culture on Sabouraud's dextrose agar reveals hyphae at 25°C and yeasts at 37°C.

Table 67.8: Opportunistic Mycoses					
S. No.	**Disease**	**Name of the fungus**	**Clinical features**	**Specimens**	**Diagnosis**
1.	Aspergillosis	• *Aspergillus fumigatus* • *A. niger* • *A. flavus*	• Respiratory disease • Aspergillus asthma • Aspergilloma • Invasive aspergilloma • Mycotic keratitis • Otomycosis	• Sputum • Lung Biopsy	• KOH preparation shows septate hyphae. • Culture on SDA.
2.	Candidiasis	• *Candida albicans*	• Oral thrush (white patches on the tongue) • Vulvovaginitis • Keratitis • Napkin dermatitis–skin infection • Urinary tract infection • Intestinal candidiasis • Pulmonary candidiasis • Septicaemia	• Swab • Scrapings from skin • Sputum • Urine	• KOH preparation shows budding yeast cells. • Culture on SDA.
3.	Cryptococcosis	• *Cryptococcus neoformans*	• Asymptomatic • Mild pneumonitis • Meningitis (Headache, fever, vomiting etc.)	• Sputum • CSF	• India ink stain of CSF shows encapsulated yeast. • Gram staining shows Gram positive yeast. • Antigen detection in CSF. • Culture on SDA.
4.	Pneumonia in immuno-compromised patients	• *Pneumocystis jiroveci*	• Dyspnoea • Fever • Non-productive cough • Chest discomfort • Weight loss	• Bronchoalveolar lavage • Induced sputum • Lung biopsy	• Demonstration of trophozoites and cysts by Giemsa, toludine blue, methenamine silver and calcofluor white stains • Serological tests • PCR

Unit X

PRACTICAL MICROBIOLOGY

68 Practical Microbiology

Practical in Microbiology includes the folowing exercises for undergraduate students.

1. Special staining

Smear is provided for special staining.

2. Identification of bacterial culture

Bacterial growth is provided for identification on a culture plate as well as in liquid medium.

3. Stool/Faeces examination

Faeces specimen is given for isolation and identification of pathogenic findings *i.e.* ova and/or cysts.

4. Spots

Spots in the form of specimens, slides, glassware, media etc. are kept for identification.

In this chapter, staining methods, preparation of hanging drop and stool/faeces examination will be discussed followed by identification of bacterial culture.

I. STAINING METHODS

For practical purposes, staining methods can be conveniently divided into *special staining* and *Gram staining*.

A. Special Staining

1. Albert's Staining

Staining of Corynebacteria (*Corynebacterium diphtheriae* and other corynebacteria) is done by this technique.

METHOD

1. The smear is heated gently by flaming the slide from underneath. It will fix the smear. Do not overheat.
2. Cover the smear with Albert I (Albert's stain) for 5 minutes.
3. Drain off the whole stain without washing.
4. Pour Albert II (iodine solution) over the smear so as to cover it completely, leave it for 2 minutes.
5. Drain off the Albert II solution without washing.
6. Blot dry the smear with the help of filter paper.
7. Examine this preparation under oil immersion (X100) objective.

{**Important Note:** Washing with water is ***not*** done in this staining, only blot dry the smear.}

REAGENTS

A. Albert I or Albert stain

1.	Toludine blue	..	0.15 gm
2.	Malachite green	..	0.20 gm
3.	Glacial acetic acid	..	1 ml
4.	Alcohol (95 per cent ethanol)	..	2 ml
5.	Distilled water to make	..	100 ml

B. Albert II or Albert's iodine solution

1.	Iodine	..	2 gm
2.	Potassium iodide	..	3 gm
3.	Distilled water to make	..	300 ml

OBSERVATIONS

In case of *Corynebacterium diphtheriae*, green coloured bacilli with bluish black metachromatic granules are observed. Bacilli are arranged in *Chinese letter* or *cuneiform arrangement* (Fig. 68.1).

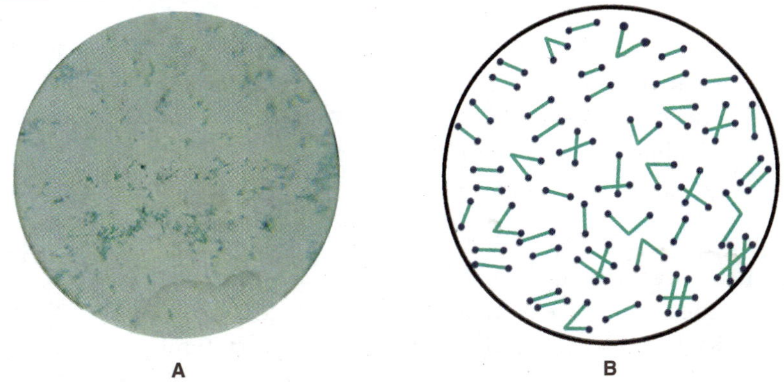

Fig. 68.1 *Corynebacterium diphtheriae* on Albert's staining: Green bacilli with metachromatic granules (A) as seen under X100 magnification (B) diagrammatic representation

2. Ziehl-Neelsen (ZN) Staining or Acid-Fast Staining

Staining of Mycobacteria (usually tubercle and lepra bacilli) is done by this technique.

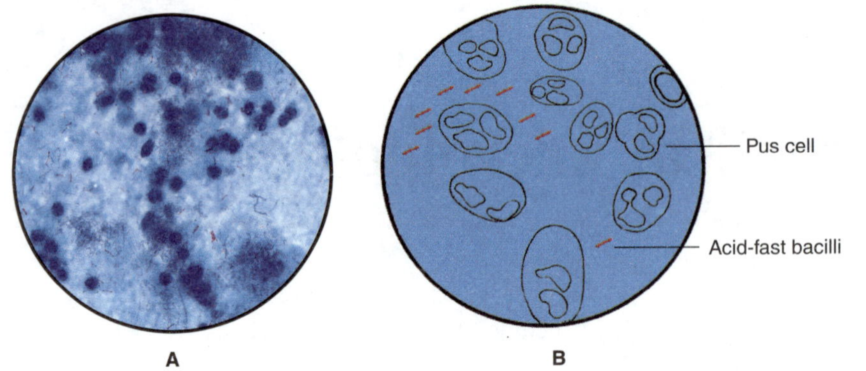

Fig. 68.2 *Mycobacterium tuberculosis* on Ziehl-Neelsen (ZN) staining: Acid-fast bacilli (AFB) (A) as seen under X100 magnification (B) diagrammatic representation

Method

1. The smear is heated gently by flaming the slide from underneath. This will fix the smear.
2. The carbol fuchsin stain is poured on a slide so as to cover the fixed smear.
3. Gentle heat is applied to the underside of the slide, by means of a spirit flame, until the stain just commences to steam.
4. The carbol fuchsin is left on the slide for 5-10 minutes with intermittent heating during that period. Care must be taken to ensure that the stain *does not dry out;* to counteract drying more solution of stain is added to the slide and the slide reheated. Heating of the stain is required for penetration of the dye into the cell wall.
5. Wash with tap water.
6. The stained smear is decolourised with 20% sulphuric acid and washed with water. This step should be repeated till the pink/red colour stops coming out.
   {**Note**: In case of lepra bacilli 5% sulphuric acid is used as *M. leprae* is less acid-fast. Alternative method for decolourisation is acid-alcohol (3 ml HCl and 97 ml ethanol).}
7. The smear is counterstained with methylene blue for 1-2 minutes. Malachite green can also be used as counterstain instead of methylene blue.
8. Wash with water and air dry.
9. Examine under oil immersion (X100) objective.

Reagents

A. Zeihl-Neelsen's Carbol fuchsin

1. Basic fuchsin .. 1 gm
2. Phenol (crystalline) .. 5 gm
3. Alcohol (95 per cent or absolute) .. 10 ml
4. Distilled water to make .. 100 ml

B. Methylene blue

1. Saturated solution of methylene blue in alcohol .. 30 ml
2. KOH, 0.01 per cent in water .. 100 ml

Observations

In case of *Mycobacterium tuberculosis,* bacilli are seen as bright red (acid-fast) while the tissue cells are stained blue (Fig. 68.2). These bright red bacilli are called *acid-fast bacilli (AFB).*

B. Gram Staining

Gram staining is done for identification of bacterial culture provided to you. The smear is prepared from culture plate provided to you, it is first fixed and then stained.

Preparation of the Smear

1. Take a drop of water on a glass slide with the help of wire loop.
2. With a straight wire or loop, touch the bacterial colony and emulsify in drop of water to make a smooth suspension. It is called *smear.*
3. Let the smear be air dried. Don't heat the smear for drying purposes.
4. Dried smear is heated gently by flaming the slide from underneath. This is done to fix the smear.

Method

1. Fixed smear is fully covered with crystal violet solution (*primary stain*) for one minute. (Other dyes such as gentian violet or methyl violet may also be used as primary stain.)
2. Pour Gram's iodine over the smear for one minute.
3. Wash the smear with water.
4. Decolourise the smear with acetone for 10–30 seconds taking care *not* to overdecolourise. (Alcohol can be substituted for acetone.)
5. Immediately wash with water to remove the decolouriser.
6. Cover the smear with a dye safranin (*counterstain*) for 1-2 minutes. (Dilute carbol fuchsin or neutral red may also be used as counterstain.)
7. Wash the smear with water.
8. The smear is then blot dried.
9. Examine under oil immersion (X100) objective.

Reagents

A. Crystal violet solution

1. Crystal violet .. 0.5 gm
2. Distilled water to make .. 100 ml

B. Gram's iodine

1. Iodine	..	1 gm
2. Potassium iodide	..	2 gm
3. Distilled water to make	..	100 ml

C. Acetone

D. Safranin

1. Safranin	..	0.5 gm
2. Distilled water to make	..	100 ml

II. HANGING DROP PREPARATION

Hanging drop is used to observe the *motility* of bacteria. It is prepared from the bacterial growth provided in liquid culture medium in a test tube.

Method (Fig. 68.3)

1. Make a ring of plasticin provided to you and place it in the centre of a clean glass slide (*Step 1*).
2. Take a loopful of liquid bacterial culture and put it in the centre of a clean coverslip (*Step 2*).
3. Invert the glass slide containing the plasticin ring (*Step 1*) and place it on the coverslip (*Step 2*) in such a manner so that the coverslip sticks with the plasticin and the drop remaining in the centre of the plasticin ring (*Step 3*).
4. Bring back the glass slide along with coverslip into the original position (*Step 4*).
5. The drop now hangs beneath the coverslip, that is why it is called *hanging drop.*
6. Examine the preparation under the microscope (Refer below).

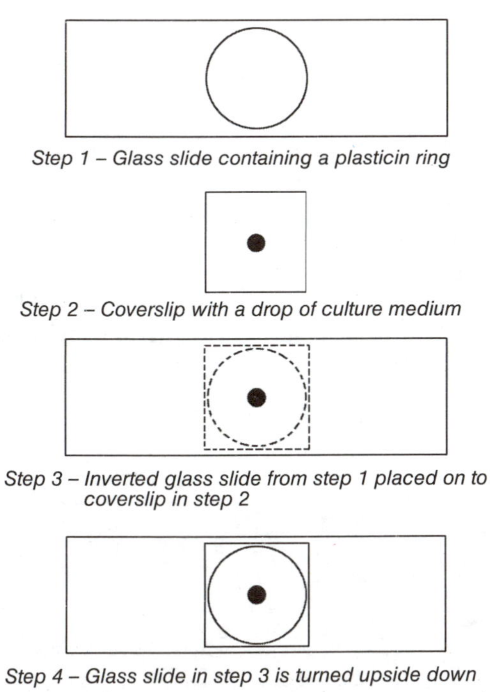

Fig. 68.3 Hanging drop preparation

Precautions

(i) Do not make the plasticin ring very thick or very thin. It should be of appropriate thickness.

(ii) There is difficulty in focussing the hanging drop preparation when thick plasticin ring is used. It might result in breakage of coverslip while objective lens is being lowered for focussing.

(iii) In case of thin plasticine ring, the hanging drop preparation touches the glass slide and examination of drop becomes difficult.

Examination (Fig. 68.4)

1. Always first focus the edge of a hanging drop preparation under low power objective (X10) of microscope.
2. Turn the focus to high power objective (X40) and observe for the motility of bacteria. Make sure that the edge of the hanging drop should also be visible under high power.

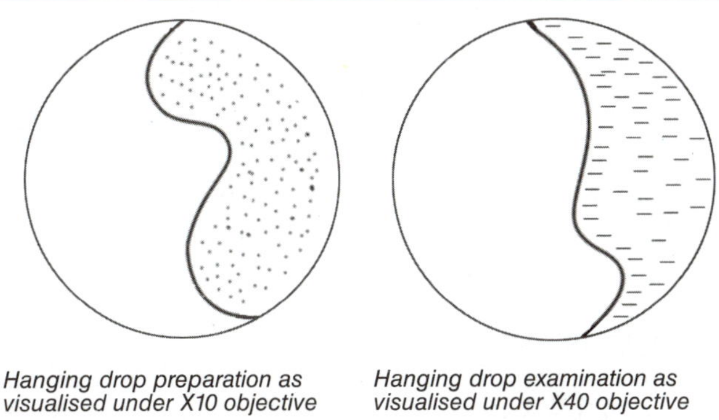

Fig. 68.4 Examination of hanging drop under the microscope

Precautions

(i) Never use oil immersion objective (X100) for hanging drop examination.

(ii) Always look for the motility of bacteria under the high power objective (X40) and *not* under the low power objective (X10).

(iii) *Never* examine the hanging drop preparation if it has dried up. Dry preparation may show false results, *i.e.,* motile bacteria may be seen as non-motile. Therefore, it is always better to repeat the hanging drop preparation for proper interpretation.

III. STOOL/FAECES EXAMINATION

Stool examination is done to find out *ova and cysts* of different parasites.

Method (Fig. 68.5)

Wet preparations of stool specimen are prepared as follows:

1. Saline preparation as well as iodine preparation of stool are made on the same glass slide.

2. A drop of normal saline (0.9 per cent) is put at one end of a clean glass slide while on the other end of the same slide, a drop of iodine solution is put.
3. A minute portion of faeces is added in both the drops with the help of a small wooden stick to make a uniform suspension.
4. A coverslip is gently placed over each suspension (saline and iodine) separately, taking care that no air bubble forms.
5. Examine the preparation under low power objective lens of microscope (see below).

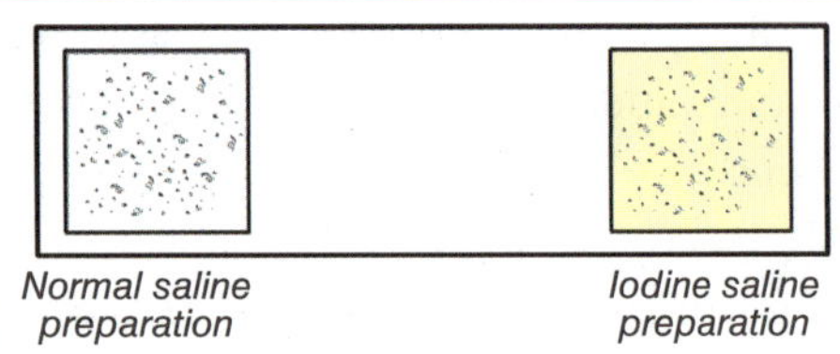

Fig. 68.5 Stool preparation

Precautions

(i) Before adding faeces either to saline or iodine drops, faeces in container should be mixed properly with wooden stick. Sometimes ova or cysts may settle down in the container, mixing ensures the uniform distribution of these within the faeces.

(ii) If preparation has dried up, prepare another slide for examination purposes.

Examination

1. Examine both the preparations (saline and iodine) under low power objective (X10) starting from one end to another in a particular given direction (Refer Fig. 68.6).

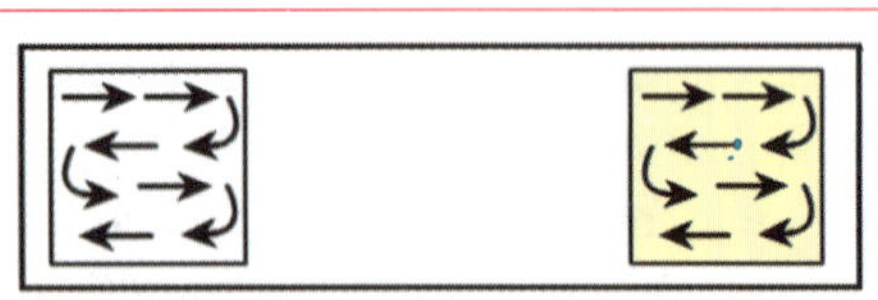

Fig. 68.6 Stool examination: It should be done in the direction of arrows starting from one end

2. Any suspicious object, if found, should be studied under high power objective (X40) for identification/confirmation of the ova, trophozoites or cysts.
3. Always show your findings to the examiner under high power objective (X40).

Precautions

(i) Never show your findings to the examiner under low power (X10) or oil immersion lens (X100).

(ii) Do not report normal non-pathogenic findings, *i.e.*, cyst of *Entamoeba coli.*

Identification Features of Eggs and Cysts

1. Eggs

Roundworm

Scientific name for roundworm is *Ascaris lumbricoides.* Eggs are of two types; fertilized eggs and unfertilized eggs.

Fertilized egg (Fig. 68.7)

(i) It is round or oval in shape measuring 60–75 µm in length and 40–50 µm in breadth.

(ii) It is bile stained and thus brownish in colour.

(iii) It is surrounded by a thick, translucent shell with an outer albuminous coat in the form of rugosities. This outer coat is sometimes lost (decorticated egg).

(iv) It contains a large unsegmented ovum with a clear crescentric area at each pole.

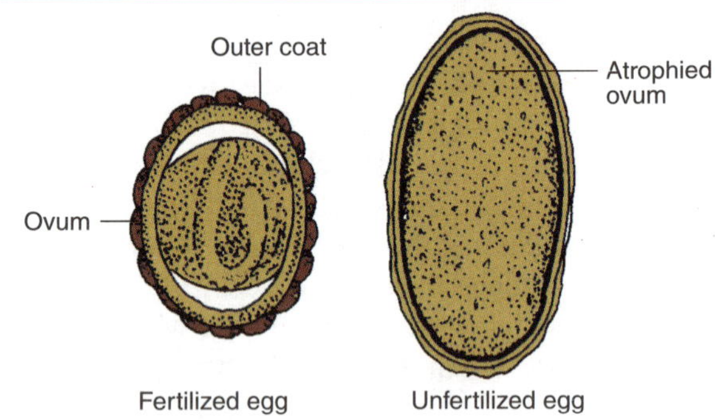

Fig. 68.7 Eggs of Ascaris lumbricoides

Unfertilized egg (Fig. 68.7)

(i) It is narrower and longer measuring 80 µm in length and 55 µm in breadth.

(ii) It is bile stained and brownish in colour.

(iii) It has a thinner shell with an irregular coating of albumin.

(iv) It contains a small atrophied ovum.

Hookworm (Fig. 68.8)

(i) The egg is oval measuring 65 µm in length and 40 µm in breadth.

(ii) Colourless, *i.e.*, not bile-stained.

(iii) It is surrounded by a thin transparent hyaline shell membrane.

(iv) It contains a segmented ovum with four blastomeres.

(v) There is a clear space between the egg shell and the segmented ovum.

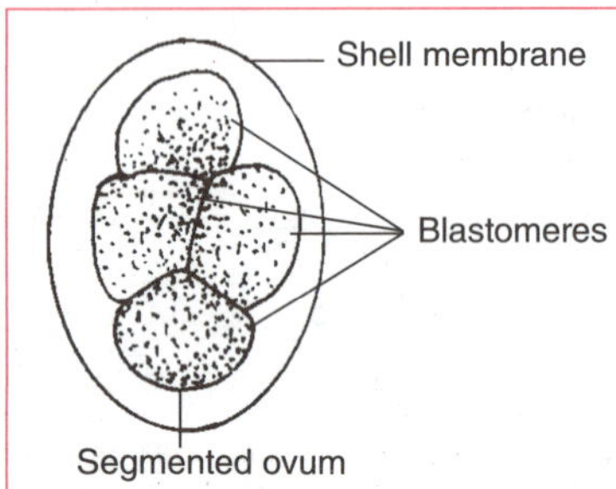

Fig. 68.8 Egg of hookworm

ENTEROBIUS VERMICULARIS (Fig. 68.9)

(i) Colourless, *i.e.,* not bile-stained.
(ii) Planoconvex in shape, *i.e.,* flattened on the ventral side and convex on the dorsal side.
(iii) Dimensions: 50 to 60 μm × 30 μm (length × breadth).
(iv) Contains a tadpole-like larva.
(v) Surrounded by a transparent shell.

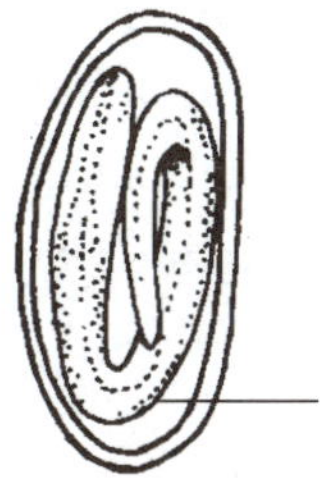

Fig. 68.9 Egg of Enterobius vermicularis

TRICHURIS TRICHIURA (Fig. 68.10)

(i) 50 μm in length and 25 μm in breadth.
(ii) Brown-coloured (bile-stained).
(iii) Barrel-shaped with a mucous plug at each pole.
(iv) Contains an unsegmented ovum.

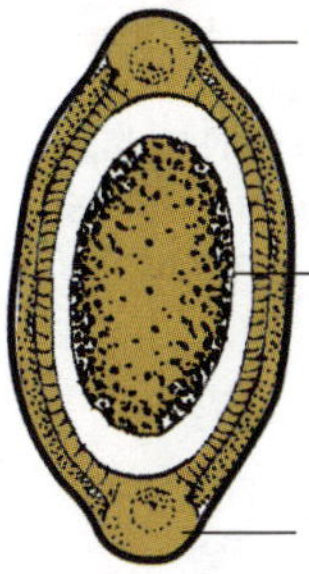

Fig. 68.10 Egg of Trichuris trichiura

HYMENOLEPIS NANA (Fig. 68.11)

(i) Spherical or oval in shape.
(ii) 30 to 45 μm in diameter.
(iii) The outer membrane is thin and colourless.
(iv) It contains an oncosphere with three pairs of hooklets.

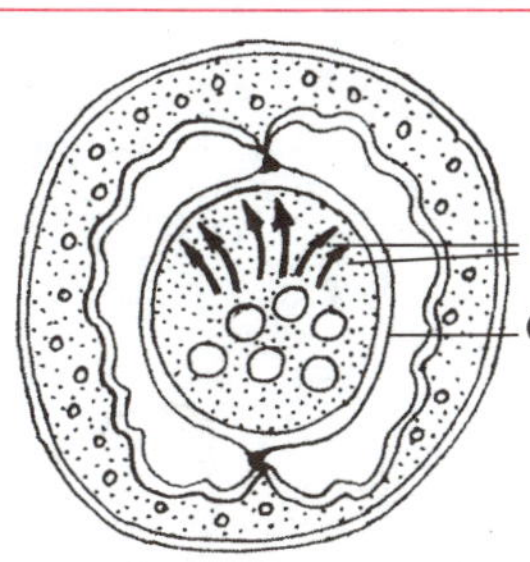

Fig. 68.11 Egg of Hymenolepis nana

TAENIA SP. (Fig. 68.12)

(i) Spherical and bile-stained.
(ii) 31 to 43 μm in diameter.
(iii) The inner embryophore is thick-walled, radially striated and brown in colour.
(iv) It contains an oncosphere (measuring 14 to 20 μm in diameter) containing 3 pairs of hooklets.

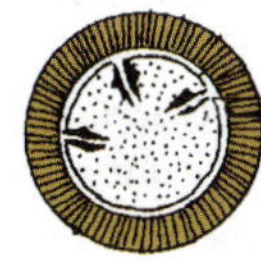

Fig. 68.12 Egg of Taenia sp.

2. *Cysts*

ENTAMOEBA HISTOLYTICA (Fig. 68.13)

(i) It is round 10–15 μm in diameter and is surrounded by a highly refractile membrane, called the *cyst wall.*
(ii) It contains four nuclei (***quadrinucleate***) and central karyosome is present in the nucleus.

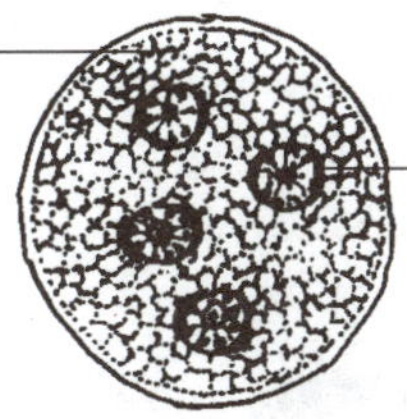

Fig. 68.13 Cyst of Entamoeba histolytica

GIARDIA LAMBLIA (Fig. 68.14)

(i) The cyst is oval in shape and it is 12 μm long and 7 μm broad.
(ii) It contains four nuclei.
(iii) The axostyles lie diagonally, forming a dividing line within the cyst-wall.

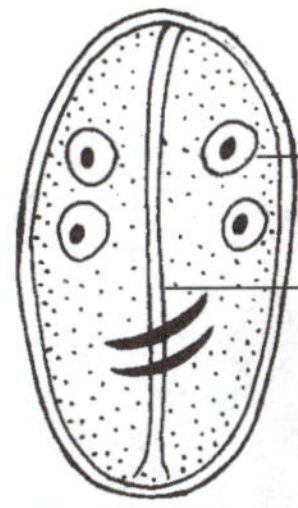

Fig. 68.14 Cyst of Giardia lamblia

IV. IDENTIFICATION OF BACTERIAL CULTURE

One of the following media with bacterial growth may be provided for identification:

	Medium	Probable organism
1.	Nutrient agar	– *Pseudomonas aeruginosa*
2.	Blood agar	– *Staphylococcus aureus* – *Streptococcus pyogenes* – *Proteus species*
3.	MacConkey's agar	A. Lactose fermenter – *Esch. coli* – *Klebsiella sp.* B. Non-lactose fermenter – *Salmonella sp.* – *Shigella sp.*

You will be provided with the bacterial growth on one of the solid media mentioned above and as well as in the liquid medium such as peptone water or glucose broth.

Morphology of colony on solid medium and characteristics of liquid medium gives a presumptive diagnosis. Gram staining from solid medium and hanging drop preparation from liquid medium helps in further identification. Biochemical reactions and slide agglutination test are done to confirm the diagnosis of individual bacteria.

Some coloured photographs of bacterial colonies on different media and Gram staining morphology are shown in Fig. 68.15 to Fig. 68.24.

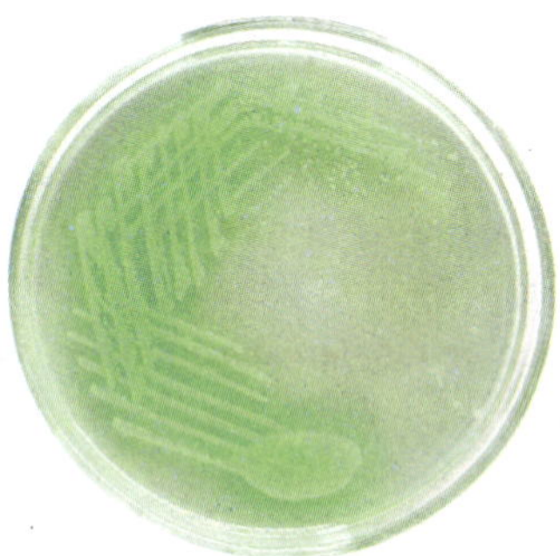

Fig. 68.15 Green pigmented growth of *Pseudomonas aeruginosa* on the nutrient agar

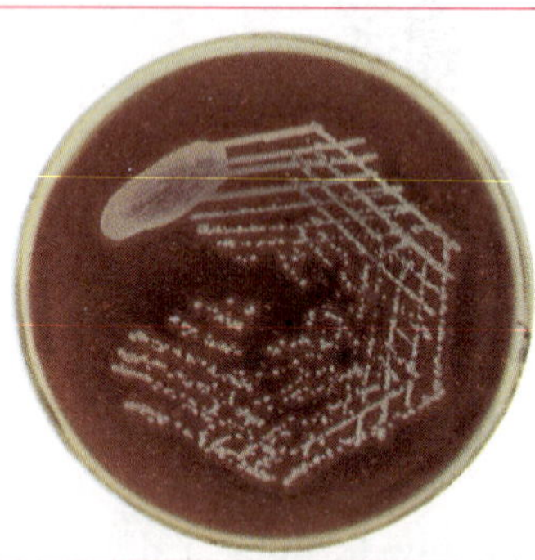

Fig. 68.16 Growth of *Staphylococcus aureus* showing beta haemolysis and golden pigment on blood agar

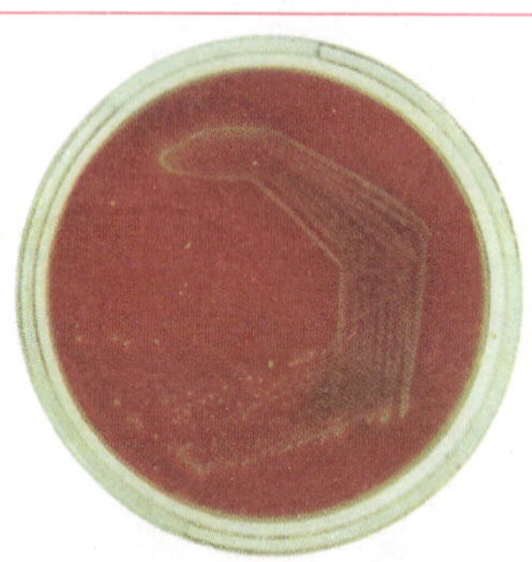

Fig. 68.17 Growth of *Streptococcus pyogenes* showing beta haemolysis on blood agar

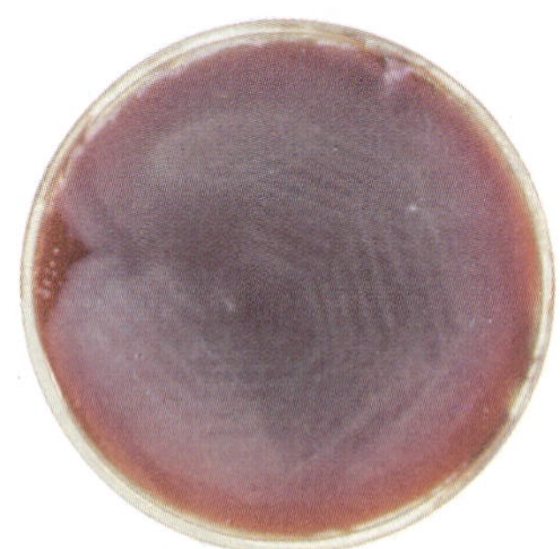

Fig. 68.18 Growth of *Proteus sp.* showing swarming on blood agar

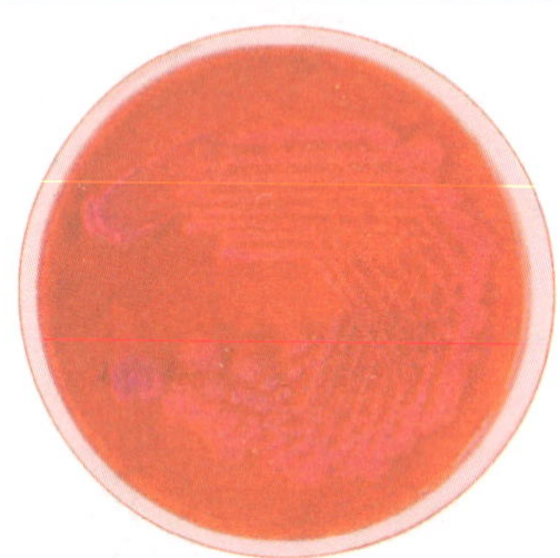

Fig. 68.19 Lactose fermenter colonies (non-mucoid) of ***Esch. coli*** on MacConkey's agar

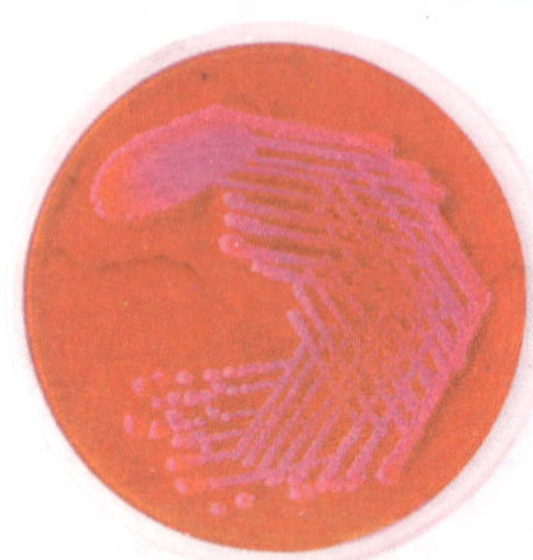

Fig. 68.20 Lactose fermenter colonies (mucoid) of *Klebsiella sp.* on MacConkey's agar

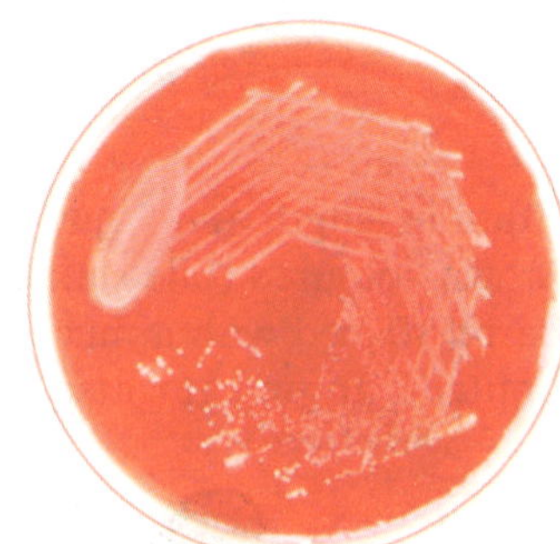

Fig. 68.21 Non-lactose fermenter colonies of *Salmonella sp.* on MacConkey's agar

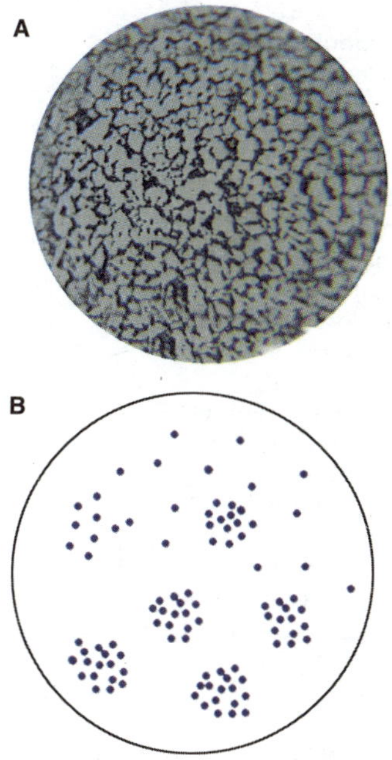

Fig. 68.22 Gram positive cocci in clusters (*Staphylococcus aureus*): (A) as seen under X100 magnification (B) diagrammatic representation

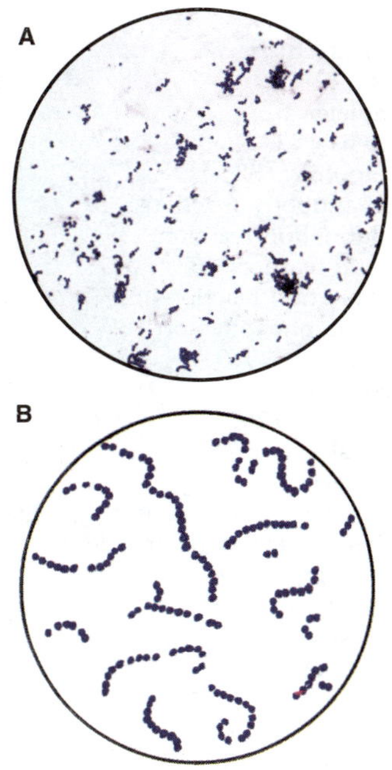

Fig. 68.23 Gram positive cocci in chains (*Streptococcus pyogenes*): (A) as seen under X100 magnification (B) diagrammatic representation

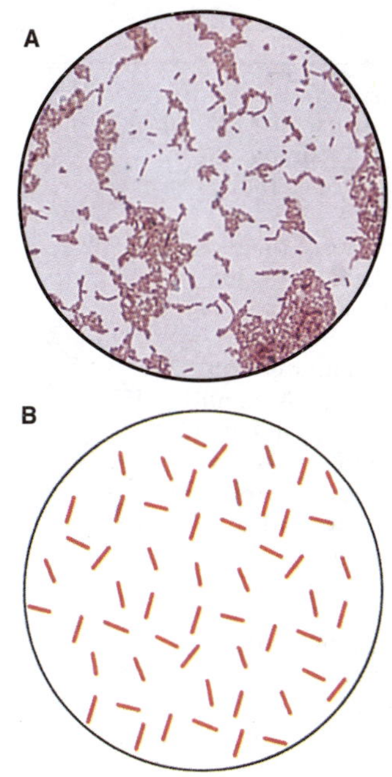

Fig. 68.24 Gram negative bacilli on Gram staining: (A) as seen under X100, (B) diagrammatic representation

Index

C

D

E

I

J

K

L

M